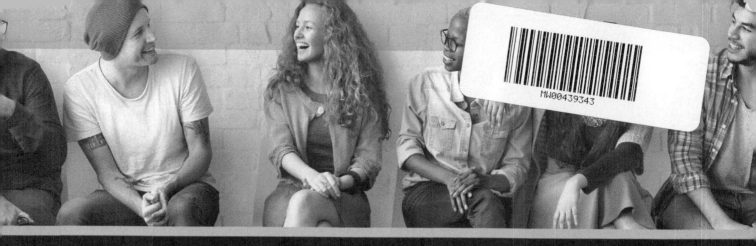

Communication
DISORDERS

Foundations and Clinical Applications for Emerging Clinicians

Rachel Glade | Kimberly Frazier

University of Arkansas—Fayetteville

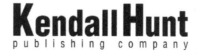

Kendall Hunt
publishing company

Cover image: © Shutterstock.com

Kendall Hunt
publishing company

www.kendallhunt.com
Send all inquiries to:
4050 Westmark Drive
Dubuque, IA 52004-1840
Preliminary Edition (c) 2019 by Kendall Hunt Publishing Company

Preliminary Edition ISBN 978-1-5249-4704-0
First Edition text with KHQ: 978-1-5249-8928-6
Text ISBN 978-1-5249-9343-6

Published in the United States of America

Contents

Preface

The American Speech Language Hearing Association (ASHA) reported that 90% school (and preschool) speech language pathologists (SLPs) spend their time treating individuals with autism spectrum disorder, language disorders, or speech sound disorders. (*ASHA, Schools Survey Report: SLP Caseload Characteristics Trends 2000–2018*). Data analyzed from 2009–2017 indicated SLPs in medical settings spent over half their time providing treatment for individuals with swallowing disorders and 43% of their treatment time treating aphasia, traumatic brain injury (TBI) or a related cognitive communication disorder (*ASHA, SLP Health Care Survey Report: Caseload Characteristics and Trends 2005–2017*). This book is written for early clinicians and educators in the field of communication disorders. Given these statistics and considering the target audience of this book, chapters were carefully chosen to reflect undergraduate training in communication disorders. The purpose of each chapter is to provide a brief review of a relevant content area in speech-language pathology and then provide application-based questions related to the content area reviewed. This book is not meant to be a comprehensive review of each content area. References and resources are provided throughout each chapter for additional discussion in each targeted content area. This innovative text format combines foundational knowledge with early clinical application skills.

At the end of each chapter there are either study questions or application-based scenarios. Case scenarios are designed to be at an introductory level of professional development to assist young clinicians with developing goal and objective writing skills as well as to develop critical thinking skills for intervention. Sample goals and objectives are provided throughout the book; however, educators and students are encouraged to have candid discussions to develop developmentally appropriate and individualistic goals and objectives based on the scenarios provided.

Students and clinicians early in their career are encouraged to view **Appendix B**, *Tips for Emerging Clinicians*. This is a list of helpful tips for planning and conducting intervention across the lifespan.

Acknowledgments

This book would not have been possible without support from the following volunteer undergraduate researcher assistants:

Alex andra Little

Alexia Allen

Rachel Holland

Ellie Coffee

Erin Smith

Bailey Pearson

Emily Richter

Additionally, support from family and colleagues throughout the writing and editing process was invaluable. A special thank you to Mrs. Frances Frazier, Mrs. Alex Clark, M.S., CCC-SLP, and Mrs. Krista Scruggs, M.S., CCC-SLP for taking time to complete reviews and provide candid feedback on chapter content.

Dr. Glade would like to especially thank her husband Andrew and her sons Maddux and Mason for being incredibly gracious with their support and also sharing their "mommy time" to allow time for writing and brainstorming this project.

Contributors

Andrea Hanson, M.S., CCC-SLP, has over 10 years of experience working in university, elementary, and pediatric practice settings. She has experience working with children who have Autism, Down syndrome, dyslexia, Cerebral Palsy, Verbal Apraxia, Selective Mutism and speech and language impairments. She has also completed the following trainings: Picture Exchange Communication System (PECS), Seeing STARS, TEACCH and Take Flight. Recently she completed the requirements to become an academic language therapist and she enjoys providing professional development on the topics of language and literacy development for school-age children.

Julie C. Hill, Ph.D, NCC, is an assistant professor of rehabilitation counseling at Auburn University in the department of Special Education, Rehabilitation, and Counseling. She has conducted several national presentations and authored or co-authored book chapters and articles in peer-reviewed rehabilitation journals on topics related to disability and chronic illness. She completed her PhD in Counselor Education and Supervision with an emphasis in Rehabilitation at the University of Arkansas. Her research interests include psychosocial adaptation to chronic illness and disability and career implications of chronic illness.

Christine Holyfield, Ph.D., CCC-SLP, is an Assistant Professor in Communication Disorders at the University of Arkansas. Her research focuses on the development and evaluation of technology and instruction to benefit individuals who have limited or no functional speech and require augmentative and alternative communication (AAC) as the result of an intellectual and developmental disability. She teaches courses on AAC, early language learning for individuals with multiple disabilities, and language disorders in children. Her past clinical experiences include AAC and language assessment and intervention for children in public schools.

Elizabeth Rosenzweig, M.S., CCC-SLP, LSLS Cert. AVT, is an Auditory Verbal Therapist in private practice. She serves families around the world via teletherapy and mentors aspiring LSLS professionals. Elizabeth is a member of the National Leadership Consortium in Sensory Disabilities and a PhD candidate at Teachers College, Columbia University. You can find her online at www.AuditoryVerbalTherapy.net.

Elaine Smolen, MAT, LSLS Cert. AVEd, is a PhD candidate and National Leadership Consortium in Sensory Disabilities scholar at Teachers College, Columbia University. She serves as an adjunct faculty member at Teachers College and at The College of New Jersey. An experienced teacher of the deaf and certified Listening and Spoken Language Specialist, she provides consulting and professional mentoring services in the New York area. Prior to beginning her doctoral studies, Smolen served young children with hearing loss and their families as a head classroom teacher and in an itinerant role. Her research interests include family engagement, public policy, and language and literacy development. Smolen received her master's degree in education of the deaf and hard of hearing from The College of New Jersey. She holds teaching certification in the areas of deaf education, elementary education, and English.

Ashlen Thomason, Ph.D., CCC-SLP, is a member of the outpatient speech pathology team at Arkansas Children's Hospital. She is a graduate of the Arkansas Consortium for the Ph.D. in Communication Sciences and Disorders with a major research emphasis in pediatric stuttering and minor in cleft palate and craniofacial anomalies. Ashlen is an adjunct instructor for the University of Arkansas for Medical Sciences/University of Arkansas at Little Rock Department of Audiology and Speech Pathology graduate program teaching courses in Fluency Disorders and Craniofacial Anomalies. She is the director of the Arkansas Stuttering Network, a nonprofit organization, service-learning initiative, and clinical research platform designed to elevate the level of holistic care available to Arkansans who stutter. Ashlen is also part of the Arkansas Children's Hospital Cleft Lip and Palate Team and the 2018 President of the Arkansas Speech-Language Hearing Association.

CONTRIBUTORS

CHAPTER 1

Professionalism in Writing

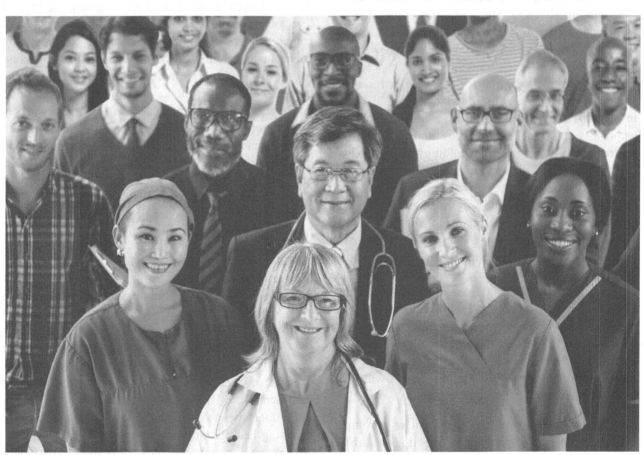

Rawpixel.com / Shutterstock.com

"Since you cannot always carry and display your diploma, kindly act like you have one. Professionalism. Include that to your dictionary."

—Joshua De Vera Bautista

PROFESSIONALISM

Professionalism is what separates you, the aspiring speech–language pathologist (SLP) or audiologist, from someone with a computer and access to Google. Professionalism is what defines our profession and the way we serve our clients. You will be judged on your clinical writing. Your reports and treatment plans are a lasting document of your work with your client. Assuring the highest quality in writing is the hallmark of professionalism.

PROFESSIONAL WRITING IN COMMUNICATION DISORDERS

SLPs prevent, diagnose, and treat communication disorders involving the following areas: articulation, phonology, language, voice, fluency, and swallowing. Difficulty producing certain speech sounds, producing speech fluently, or speaking with appropriate voice or resonance are considered speech disorders. Language disorders involve difficulty expressing ideas, feelings, or thoughts (expressive language), or difficulty understanding others (receptive language). SLP treat individuals who have these issues across the lifespan and work in a variety of settings from public schools to health care settings. Each setting will have a unique way in which professional communication is handled, but the guidelines presented in this chapter are universal and applicable whether you are working with preschool children in a daycare setting, or assisting a family in coping with the communication challenges dementia brings in a home health setting. SLPs also work collaboratively with a variety of other professionals. From audiologists, teachers, physicians, to social workers, SLPs are valuable members of an interdisciplinary team and professional behavior is of paramount importance when working in concert with other team members for the benefit of our clients.

Prevention, assessment, and treatment of communication disorders are the primary functions that SLPs perform. This chapter will cover writing basics for the practice of speech–language pathology.

PROFESSIONAL CONDUCT

Professionally appropriate and career advancing interactions in the workplace are closely akin to walking a tightrope at the County Fair. It all looks easy, and it all looks like fun, but one slip and you can come crashing down never to recover. Throughout your work experience, you will have countless opportunities to present yourself as a person of integrity, empathy, and skill, and your profession will, in part, be judged by you. The ASHA Code of Ethics is to be adhered to by all speech-language pathologists, and those violating this code may lose ASHA certification or membership or both.

ASHA's Code of Ethics is a guide of minimally accepted behaviors and is composed of the following Four Principles of Ethics: (1). Individuals shall honor their responsibility to hold paramount the welfare of persons they serve professionally or participants in research and scholarly activities and shall treat animals involved in research in a humane manner; (2) Individuals shall honor their responsibility to achieve and maintain the highest level of professional competence; (3) Individuals shall honor their responsibility to the public by promoting public understanding of the professions, by supporting the development of services designed to fulfill the unmet needs of the public, and by providing accurate information in all communications involving any aspect of the professions including dissemination of research findings and scholarly activities; (4) Individuals shall honor their responsibilities to the professions and their relationships with colleagues, students, and members of allied professions. Individuals shall uphold the dignity and autonomy of the professions, maintain harmonious interprofessional relationships, and accept the professions' self-imposed standards (ASHA Code of Ethics).

Maintaining our client's right to privacy confidentiality, and welfare are addressed at length in the ASHA Code of Ethics. Legal protection of a client's right privacy is also guaranteed by federal and state laws. Additionally, HIPAA is the Health Insurance Portability and Accountability Act of 1996 provides specific procedures regarding the protection of client confidentiality. HIPAA was originally drafted so that individuals who switched jobs would not be at risk of losing health insurance coverage. All practitioners who receive government payments must do so electronically which necessitates compliance to HIPAA. HIPAA may be seen as a framework for managing billing practices for clinicians while assuring clients that their data are secure. Most graduate programs in communication disorders will provide HIPAA compliance training for their students.

In addition to maintaining HIPAA compliance, all clinical documentation is subject to potential subpoena in a court case. This includes diagnostic reports, POCs, and SOAP notes. Also, funding sources may request all of these documents as part of routine chart audits.

PROFESSIONAL DRESS

A first impression will forever be "A First Impression," and that impression should say loud and clear, especially in the work arena, "I know who I am, I know why I'm here, and I know what I'm doing; now how may I help you?" There are several "do's and don'ts" which contribute to a favorable initial evaluation. Progression up the career ladder can certainly be influenced by the way one presents oneself in the work environment, and that is to a large degree determined by colleagues' and supervisors' views of employees in their daily interactions.

In order to be perceived as a professional in your chosen vocation, consider the following: clothes that are clean, pressed, and always in good repair. Jackets and blazers which give one an air of professionalism are a wise choice. Hairstyles also must be considered. In general, short hair for men and short hair for women or hair worn up are wise choices. Immaculate nails worn short for men and women while women may opt to add subdued polish, and subtle makeup. When deciding on shoes, it's a good idea to choose comfort over flash and leave athletic shoes to the athletes and sandals to the social scene.

Our college graduates are stylish, competent, caring, hardworking, and ethical. Our goal is to assist you in presenting yourselves in such a way that prospective employers will recognize how valuable you will be to their program and clients will trust your expertise.

ASSESSMENT =evaluation

A valid assessment of your client's abilities is the foundation on which all future clinical activities are based—it is the starting point. Assessment involves the gathering of valid and reliable data and integrating and interpreting the data in order to reach diagnoses and conclusions about behaviors of interest. In order to make a diagnosis, the SLP will consider information from the case history, test results, and observations to determine if a problem exists, the nature of the problem and its severity. The terms assessment and evaluation can be used synonymously. A good assessment will be comprehensive and will require skill to administer. The SLP must have knowledge of development milestones and effective techniques for eliciting behaviors. It is imperative that the SLP have good observation skills and is able to relate to clients both empathetically and effectively.

The assessment provides the opportunity to scrutinize all behavioral aspects of communication. In order to distinguish a client's problem, it is necessary to know how he/she performs to a variety of tasks presented in a variety of conditions. For the SLP, assessment provides information that can lead to not only diagnoses and conclusions, but also the need for treatment, the focus of treatment, as well as the frequency of treatment and the degree to which caregivers should be involved in the therapy process. Assessment may also reveal the need to refer to other professionals (e.g., audiologists, dentists, and physicians) (Shipley & McAfee, 2016). According to ASHA guidelines (ASHA Scope of Practice in Speech–Language Pathology, 1970) for preferred assessment practices, a thorough assessment should include the following elements.

Case history

The case history provides invaluable information that is relevant to the speech–language assessment and crucial in determining speech and language related diagnoses.

Reason for the referral—Who made the referral and why? Provide a description of the presenting behaviors and concerns in other areas related to the suspected issue.

Medical status—List all relevant medical information both current was well as previous. List any health issues and existing conditions (e.g., diagnosis of cerebral palsy) that might impact learning (i.e., frequent ear infections, vision, seizures, cleft palate, oral motor issues, physical limitations, etc.).

Education history—Include the student's name, age, classroom grade level and level of academic support, and the school attended. List history of schools attended and the duration, client's academic and social strengths and concerns, teacher comments, attendance and discipline history, and any relevant information documented in school records. List previous assessments, diagnoses, and therapy the child may have received from outside agencies or from previous assessments. Document general education interventions (e.g., Response to Intervention) and the outcomes of the interventions.

Developmental milestones/developmental history—List any language related developmental milestones, including family history of speech or language issues.

Family information—With whom does the client live? List any history of household changes, including changes in family members in the household. What is the home language? Describe family relationships and any indicators that the home may impede educational performance.

Information from related service providers—List other suspected disabilities, along with any confirmed diagnoses.

Patient/client/student and family interview

The interview provides a mechanism to clarify information obtained in the case history or gather missing information. The interview is the opportunity to ask the client or family to describe their concerns and gives them the opportunity to articulate the reason for the evaluation.

Review of auditory, visual, motor, and cognitive status

It is important to consider the results of previous assessments. Screen the client's hearing and refer for a vision screening if a current one doesn't exist.

ASSESSMENT OF SKILLS

Select measures to sample and evaluate the client's speech in the areas of articulation, voice, and fluency; also measure the client's receptive and expressive language abilities. List standardized, nonstandardized, and criterion-referenced measures for speech, language, cognitive-communication, and/or swallowing assessment used during the evaluation. Include all types of measures such as oral-motor examination, oral mechanism exam, speech sample analysis, and phonetic inventory. Administer assessments that will provide information in the area of suspected disability and if need be investigate other areas of disability that may arise. Include a statement detailing that selected tests and assessment materials and procedures used for the purposes of assessment were selected and administered so as not to be racially, culturally, linguistically,

or sexually discriminatory. Also, verify that the client's dominant language was considered in selecting assessment instruments and that tests were validated for the specific areas of educational need. List how the structural and functional integrity of the oral-facial mechanism was evaluated.

INTEGRATE AND INTERPRET ASSESSMENT INFORMATION

This is one of the most vital aspects of the assessment procedure and includes the evaluation of all data collected. Careful analysis and evaluation will determine clinical impressions, diagnosis and conclusions, prognosis, and recommendations.

ASSESSMENT MECHANICS

Psychometrics is a field of study devoted to the measurement of human traits, abilities, skills, behaviors, and processes. SLPs rely on psychometric principles in order to assess a client's communication. Clinical decisions are based on information derived from the assessment process. Assessment, also known as evaluation, helps us understand the client's communication abilities and needs, and can culminate in a diagnosis, which is a clinical decision as to whether a disorder is present or not. A diagnosis is helpful in determining not only the need for treatment but also, aids in the planning of treatment in terms of length, focus, and structure and whether recommendations for additional services are warranted. Assessment starts with the collection of relevant information which is then analyzed and interpreted to determine if a disorder exists, and if so, to establish its nature, severity, and impact on the daily living skills of the client. In communication disorders, clinicians measure behaviors of interest using a variety of instruments and tools. Becoming familiar with psychometric terminology is important for the student of communication disorders.

NORM-REFERENCED TESTS, CRITERION-REFERENCED TESTS, AND AUTHENTIC ASSESSMENT

There are many different types of measures that have been designed to assess, diagnose, and aid in treatment planning. There are several different paths to evaluation, and oftentimes, clinicians use a combination of methods to gain a complete picture of their client's abilities. **Norm-referenced** tests are widely used because of their objective nature, efficiency of administration, and are broadly recognized. Another reason for their popularity is that they are preferred by insurance companies and third parties for payment of services. Additionally, public school favor them for qualification for services. Norm-referenced instruments allow for comparison of an individual client to a larger group, called the normative group. Norm-referenced instruments are also always standardized which means that there is a set method of test administration and scoring. While all norm-referenced instruments are standardized, not all standardized instruments are norm referenced. Norm-referenced instruments are helpful when determining how an individual client is performing compared to a group of similar individuals. The normative group used during the standardization of the test comprises individuals who have already taken the test and are similar in parameters such as age or grade level. Most often the normative group is drawn from national peers and yields a normal distribution which is most often represented as a bell-shaped curve. From the standardization procedures, a variety of scores can be obtained to describe the performance of the client. These scores will be discussed later in this chapter.

Criterion-referenced tests do not compare a client's performance to a larger group as norm-referenced instruments do; instead, these measures give an indication of what a client can and cannot do in relation to a predetermined criterion. Criterion-referenced instruments will not yield standard scores and percentile ranks like norm-referenced measures; instead, these instruments will yield a cut-score with and place the client's performance in categories such as "basic," "proficient," and "advanced." Criterion-referenced tests are used most often in the field of communication disorders to assess abilities of children under the age of three, individuals with voice and/or fluency issues, or individuals with neurogenic disorders. Unlike norm-referenced tests, criterion-referenced ones may or may not be standardized.

Authentic Assessment is very similar to criterion-referenced assessments in that they identify what a client can or cannot do. The difference is that authentic assessment focuses on contextualized evaluation stimuli in the most realistic environment. For example, it is difficult to measure a client's social-pragmatic language using norm-referenced and criterion-referenced instruments due to the context-specific nature of social performance. An authentic assessment would allow a clinician to measure requisite social skills in a realistic situation such as the client's interaction with peers during recess. The important thing to remember is that use of these approaches is not mutually exclusive. It is acceptable and even preferred to use a combination of approaches to gain the most realistic picture of a client's true communication abilities.

SCORES

Regardless of the type of testing that you perform, test results will be displayed by a number of different scores. Some of the most common scores for the field of communication disorders include raw scores, scaled scores, standard scores, and percentile ranking. A norm-referenced assessment will result in a **standard score** which will compare your client's performance to that of a normative group. A standard score, sometimes called a scaled score, is calculated by taking the **raw score** (the number of items that the client answered correctly) and transforming it to a common scale. A standard score is centered on a normal distribution and has mean and a standard deviation. The same information may be expressed by Z-scores, T-scores, or scaled scores, but do so based on a different numerical system with different means and standard deviation units. **Percentile ranks** are derived from the standard score and are another commonly used comparison of a client's standing in comparison to the normal distribution. The percentile rank tells the percentage of individuals scoring at or below a given score. **Age-equivalent scores** are used to compare a client's performance to age groups whose average scores are in the same range. Age-equivalent scores should be used with caution because the information they provide is limited and can be somewhat misleading, particularly for clients who score within the average range of performance.

RELIABILITY AND VALIDITY

It is imperative that the tools and instruments used to draw clinical conclusions are both reliable and valid. **Validity** means that the test measures what it claims to measure. There are metrics used to determine the validity of standardized instruments. This is usually accomplished by comparing the instrument to other well-established instruments which measure the same skills. **Reliability**, on the other hand, refers to the test's ability

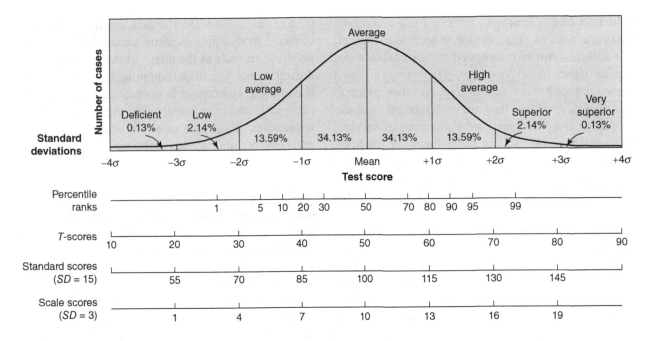

to yield consistent results. If the test yields stable or similar results on repeated administrations or with different examiners, the test would be considered reliable. There are different types of test validity and reliability that you will be introduced to in a clinical assessment course.

INTERVENTION PLANNING

Once the assessment has been completed, intervention planning begins with the development of a Plan of Care (POC). Assessment data should drive the intervention plan for the client. The behaviors that will be targeted during the course of therapy are called **long-term goals**. These are broad in nature, and once these goals have been accomplished, therapy may be discontinued. For example, an assessment revealed that five-year-old Ellie has a severe phonological processes disorder characterized by final consonant deletion, stridency deletion, cluster reduction, stopping, gliding, and vowelization. Long-term goals for Ellie could include the following:

- Ellie will increase her speech intelligibility by producing targeted speech patterns correctly.
- Ellie will increase speech intelligibility to communicate wants and needs.
- Ellie will reduce the occurrence of deviant phonological processes by producing targeted phonemes at the word level.

After long-term goals have been established, the clinician must determine the best way to reach these goals.

Short-term objectives or behavioral objectives are the steps recommended to achieve long-term goals. There are three components of a behavioral objective: a *do* statement, a *condition*, and a *criterion*.

The *do* statement is the action that the client will perform. This statement should contain action verbs that can be observed as measured. Appropriate *do* statements for Ellie might include:

- Ellie will produce final consonants in CVC words
- Ellie will raise her hand

The *condition* specifies the situation in which the target behavior is to be performed. It is the *when*, *where*, and *with whom* the behavior will occur and with what materials or cues will it happen. Examples of possible conditions for Ellie might include:

- In response to pictures
- Following a clinician's model
- While playing games with a peer

Lastly, the *criterion* stipulates how well the target must be performed for the objective to be met. Examples of possible criteria for Ellie might be:

- With 80% accuracy across three sessions.
- With 90% accuracy, 4/5 data collections.
- Do so consistently over a 10-minute period.

Please refer to the sample Plan of Care in Appendix D.

REPORT WRITING

Once an assessment has been completed, it is imperative that the findings and recommendations are shared. The diagnostic report is the mechanism that SLPs and audiologists use to convey information to families and other professionals. It is the result of the complex procedure of assessing, defining and interpreting your clients' communication skills and necessitates the integration of a variety of information collected during the evaluation. Because the report provides a lasting record of what occurred during the diagnostic session, it serves as a link to the session for the client, the family of the client, and other stakeholders, and as such "must be all things to all people." The diagnostic report will become a part of the Client's permanent file and is a legal document. It is an important document that is permanent and can be referred to and that communicates impressions from the assessment session. Depending on the type of facility in which you are employed report writing will vary.

The following are some tips for writing a thorough diagnostic report that will be meaningful to not only the client and family, but to other service providers as well.

A good diagnostic report starts with good clinical observations. The resulting report will only be as strong as your skills as a diagnostician. It is imperative that you write down everything during the evaluation that might be significant. Also, it's important to obtain a thorough and complete case history. The case history information will be invaluable for crafting the introduction and background sections of the report. The client or parent interview is another essential element to the diagnostic report. It's a good idea to review the case history with the client/parent during the interview to obtain missing information or clarify information. For my reports, I like to include a quote from the client describing the reason the evaluation was requested. When writing the report be sure to use past tense consistently throughout. When using phonetic symbols always enclose them in either virgules or brackets. Brackets are typically used when notating what the client actually said, while virgules indicate that the symbols used are IPA (International Phonetic Alphabet) symbols. It is acceptable to use numbers when listing dates and test scores, however, all other numbers must be spelled out. For example, "Ellie's score on the PLS-5 was XXX." "Samantha is a four-year, three-month-old female." "Maddie could count from one to ten." Vary your word usage, including how the client is referred. It

can become cumbersome to read the same phrases and terms repeatedly. Determine how the report sounds by reading it to assess wording, clarity, and smoothness. The first time you reference a particular test, write out the name and use capitalization and include the abbreviation so that subsequent mentioning of the test can use abbreviation only. For example, Preschool Language Scale-5 (PLS-5). Be sure to give a brief explanation of the tests in terms of the specific skills they measure. In order to gain relevant information both from functional and developmental standpoints, use a variety of assessment tools and strategies. It is also important to select materials that may be administered in the client's native language or mode of communication, if possible. Racially, culturally, or sexually discriminatory materials and procedures must be avoided.

ASSESSMENT TEAMS

There are different types of assessment teams. For a multidisciplinary team, each professional evaluates clients individually and submits their findings in a report which may be later shared with members of the team for review and recommendation of services. Transdisciplinary assessment teams gather similar data only in a different manner. A transdisciplinary team will assess the client together with each member being assigned a role during the assessment process. Transdisciplinary teams are often used in health care; clinician from various professions work together and share ideas to develop a total assessment or treatment plan that covers all necessary diagnoses and interventions for a patient.

Refer to Appendixes H, I, and J for ASHA's Scope of Practice and Clinical Competence Guidelines.

TREATMENT PLANS AND THE WRITING OF GOALS AND OBJECTIVES

Writing treatment goals and objectives can be very challenging for students. The first step for developing a treatment plan is to identify the areas of concern. Diagnostic reports, developmental checklists, speech and language developmental milestones, common core curriculum benchmarks/standards, or any other skills assessments will drive the client's treatment plan and serve as a reference when developing treatment, including goals and objectives. The clinician should also keep in mind the needs of the client and the client's family and include them in the process of determining goals. It is important to keep in mind what you want the end result of therapy to be when writing goals. In other words, "keep your eye on the prize." What is it that you ultimately want your client to be able to do, and what will the impact on communication be? Also keep in mind that setting too many goals can hinder your treatment plan. When prioritizing goals, think about what limitations are the most challenging for the client in day-to-day life. A well-written and thoughtful treatment plan will provide a task analysis and hierarchical plan that will facilitate treatment. The acronym *SMART* is helpful for new clinicians as they take on the challenge of goal writing. *SMART: specific, measureable, attainable, relevant, and timely.* Let's start! **Goal: Ellie will learn the names of primary colors.** This is not a *SMART* goal. Let's discover how this goal is lacking and how it can be improved. We can improve the goal by making sure it is:

Specific—All goals should specifically state what the client will do, in what setting the client will do it, to what accuracy it will be done, and what supports will be required. Questions to ask yourself: What are the client's communicative strengths and weaknesses? What skills should be targeted first and why? What supports will be needed when targeting the skill?

Measurable—All goals should specifically state how the skill will be measured. This includes how data will be collected and exactly what percentage/accuracy will be attained. Questions to ask yourself: How will you measure progress? When will you consider the goal accomplished?

Attainable—All proposed goals should be accomplished by the client in a given time frame. This can be very hard to determine, particularly if you have limited familiarity with the client and do not know how quickly the client will progress. Keep in mind, that the treatment plan can be adjusted if the client is making faster or slower progress than expected. Questions to ask yourself: Do you think the client can actually accomplish the skill in your given timeframe? If not, ask yourself what can reasonably be accomplished.

Relevant—All goals should be relevant and customized to meet each client's individual needs. Questions to ask yourself: Will the attainment of the goal serve an important communicative function for the client? Will it serve a purpose in the client's life considering the limits and ramifications of the diagnosis and cultural and social needs?

Time-Bound—All goals should explicitly state the time frame in which the goal will be achieved (e.g., by the end of the IEP cycle, by a certain date, or specified timeframe). Questions to ask yourself: Does the goal contain a timeframe and can it be accomplished given the timeframe?

Let's practice recognizing *SMART* components for goal writing:

- By _____ (T*ime-Bound*: when the client will master the goal)
- Client will _____ (*Specific, Attainable, and Relevant*)
- In _____ setting/context (*Specific*: where will the skill be measured? In the classroom? In the therapy room? In conversational speech? At the sentence level? During peer interactions?)
- As measured by _____ (*Measurable*: how will progress be measured? With data collection? By teacher or parent report? A language sample? A checklist? A tally sheet?)
- With _____ accuracy (*Measurable*: how accurate must the client be? Examples: 80% accuracy, in 4 of 5 trials, on 3 of 4 observed opportunities, on 5 consecutive data collection days)
- With _____ supports (*Specific*: can the client have any supports and still be considered to have met the goal? Examples: Independently, with reminders, with verbal prompts, with physical prompts, with partial physical assistance, with visual cues)

Here is an example of a goal that includes all *SMART* components: *By the end of the Spring semester, Maddie will correctly produce the pronouns "he" and "she" when retelling a story that has just been read aloud by the clinician as measured by data collection with at least 80% accuracy across 3 therapy sessions with no more than 2 reminders as needed.*

Several chapters in the text provide practice in the development of *SMART* goals.

BENCHMARK OR SHORT-TERM OBJECTIVES

Benchmarks and short-term objectives should follow the same criteria outlined above for goal writing. These goals list the steps that lead up to a bigger goal. Think of these as the skills that the client will need to learn before a larger goal can be accomplished. Benchmarks follow a logical progression of skills that the client will need for mastery of larger goals. Benchmarks also help in determining if clients are on track to meeting long-term goals.

DOCUMENTATION

Documentation provides crucial information for third-party reimbursers (e.g., Medicaid, insurance companies) and is critical for making sound decision regarding client care. Documentation should clearly outline clinical information about the client's diagnosis, as well as the course and outcome of treatment. Documentation formats vary across institutions. State or federal agencies governing schools, Medicaid reimbursement, or audiology and speech–language pathology regulations may have specific requirements for documentation. Documenting each individual session is how you provide evidence about the quality and efficacy of your treatment plan. Unclear, vague, or incomplete documentation may result not only in reimbursement issues, but can also result in compliance violations and possibly ethical charges. A good rule to keep in mind: "If you didn't document it; it didn't happen."

SOAP NOTES

SOAP is an acronym which stands for subjective, objective, assessment, and plan. The *SOAP* process will assist in documenting your client's performance and information during each therapy session. A unique note is required for each and every therapy session. *SOAP* notes will help organize your client's performance by keeping track of your clinical observations and assessments, and the treatment plan. Therapy techniques and interventions should be clearly justified. *SOAP* notes should be detailed yet as concise as possible. Provide enough information to give a solid overview of what each session involved, how the client is progressing, and what you anticipate working on in the near future.

Following a consistent structure will assist you with reference, organization, and comparisons later on. Length requirements, exact formats, and abbreviations may vary across clinical settings. The best time to complete *SOAP* notes is immediately after a session when everything is fresh in your mind. The further removed you are from a session, the less you will be able to remember important details when it comes time to write the notes. Make prompt writing of *SOAP* notes a habit; you'll be glad you did. Let's take a look at each aspect of the *SOAP* note:

Subjective—This section contains information related by the client, or behaviors that you have observed during the session. Example: "Client related that her teacher said that she can understand her better."

Objective—This section contains only quantifiable, measurable, and observable data. Example: "The client produced the /s/ in the initial position of words with 90% accuracy with minimal cueing."

Assessment—This section is an analysis of the information listed in the *Subjective* and *Objective* portions. Example: "The client's made a 20% improvement in correct tongue placement since last session, which has been noticed by others."

Plan—This section lists the anticipated number of sessions required to meet goals and the activities for the next section. Example: The client continues to improve with /s/ in the initial position of words and should require one more session to reach her goal of 90% accuracy across three therapy sessions. The next session will continue to focus on /s/ in the initial position with minimal cueing.

REFERENCES

ASHA Scope of Practice in Speech-Language Pathology. (1970, January 01). Retrieved from https://www.asha.org/policy/sp2016-00343/

McAfee, J. G. (2016). *Assessment in speech-language pathology: A resource manual.* Australia: Cengage Learning.

CHAPTER 2

Introduction to Auditory Skill Development

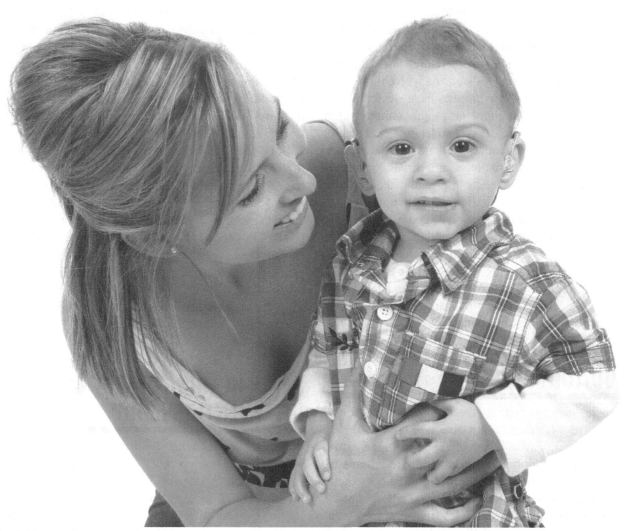

Lopolo / Shutterstock.com

"Kindness is the language which the deaf can hear and the blind can see."

—Mark Twain

OVERVIEW

Hearing loss is affecting all generations of Americans in all facets of society, and its impact is undeniable. "The prevalence of congenital (present at birth) hearing loss is estimated at 3 in 1,000 births, making it the most frequently occurring birth defect." (Flexer & Madell, 2008, p. 13; White, 2003). Hearing loss is not only a concern for the pediatric population. Bainbridge and Wallhagen (2014), as referenced in the National Health and Nutrition Examination Survey (NHANES), note "the prevalence of hearing loss increases dramatically with age . . . . . bilateral hearing loss of at least mild severity doubles for every 10 years of life after the age of 50" (p.141). The impact hearing loss is having on all generations is undeniable.

The purpose of this chapter is to review hearing anatomy and physiology and auditory skill development. Auditory skills are the foundation of speech and spoken language development; therefore, this chapter is most relevant for clinicians working with children who have hearing loss whose families have elected to pursue either spoken language or a total communication approach (sign language + spoken language). It is often the role of the interventionist to provide parents and caregivers with information about various communication approaches as well as informational counseling regarding hearing loss, basic information about hearing technologies, and educational supports. Regarding the communication approach or language the family chooses for their child, all can have successful outcomes. It is best practice for clinicians to educate families about communication options and defer to the family to decide what communication methodology or language works best for the family.

AUDITORY ACCESS

Hearing involves getting the *brain* access to sound. The sense of hearing occurs when a sound wave enters the outer ear, travels down the ear canal, and causes the tympanic membrane (i.e., eardrum) to vibrate. On the opposite side of the eardrum from the ear canal is the middle ear space that houses the smallest bones in the body knows as the ossicles (malleus, incus, and stapes). The vibration of the eardrum starts a chain reaction of events. The original acoustic signal changes to a mechanical signal in the middle ear travels down the chain of ossicles (i.e., the ossicular chain) where sound is amplified or volume is increased. The last bone in the ossicular chain, the stapes, has a footplate that sits in the oval window of the inner ear. As the sound continues to move toward to brain from the vibration of the eardrum down the ossicular chain, the stapes vibrates the oval window causing the fluid in the inner ear (composed of the cochlea and vestibular system) to be set into motion, thus converting the mechanical signal to a hydraulic signal. Three fluid-filled channels of the cochlea are set in motion by the movement of the oval window. The channels are separated by a thin membrane so that movement from one channel impacts the movement of another channel. The middle channel of the cochlea (also called the organ of Corti) is lined with small hair cells that have nerve fibers which help to send the signal (transmitted from the movement of the fluid to the hair cells) to the auditory nerve. The signal is then transmitted to the auditory cortex in the brain. As fluid moves in the cochlea, the hydraulic signal is converted into an electrical signal at the level of the auditory nerve as the hair cells in the organ of Corti create nerve impulses. This pathway allows for sound to be transmitted to the auditory cortex of the brain located in the temporal lobes on both the right and left sides of the brain (Fucci & Lass, 1999; Seikel, King, & Drumwright, 2000). A breakdown in any part of this process, from the initial acoustic signal to the outer ear to the electrical pulse created in the inner ear that travels to the brain, can cause hearing loss. The National Institute on Deafness and Other Communication Disorders (NIDCD) produced an animated video to depict this process. See the link for *The Journey of Sound:* https://www.youtube.com/watch?v=inAHoYuTS7U. See Table 2.1, Hearing Related Websites, for a list of websites recommended to learn more about hearing, hearing loss, and related technologies.

EARLY HEARING DETECTION AND INTERVENTION (EHDI)

In 1993, the National Institutes of Health (NIH) Consensus Development Conference on Early Identification of Hearing Loss recommended that all infants should be screened for hearing loss prior to leaving their birthing hospital. At the time, only 11 hospitals were screening over 90% of infants born in their centers. Currently, all 50 states in the Unites States have Early Hearing Detection and Intervention (EHDI) laws in place or universal newborn hearing screening (UNHS) programs. For additional information about

Table 2.1 Hearing Related Websites

Website	Website
www.audiology.org	www.successforkidswithhearingloss.com
www.audiologist.org	www.medel.com
www.asha.org	www.cochlear.com
www.entnet.org	www.advancedbionics.com
www.babysfirsttest.org	www.jtc.org
www.babyhearing.org	www.hearingjourney.com
www.jcih.org	www.hearingloss.org
www.infanthearing.com	www.hearingfirst.org
www.boardofaudiology.org	www.heartolearn.org
www.agbell.org	www.handsandvoices.org
www.audiologyonline.com	www.nidcd.nih.gov (click on Hearing)

UNHS programs, readers are encouraged to visit *www.infanthearing.org*.

HEARING SCREENING

A hearing screening is a quick test to determine how well someone is hearing. It is within the scope of practice for a speech-language pathologist, speech-language pathology assistant to provide a hearing screening. In fact, no license or certification is required to administer a hearing screening. An individual administering a hearing screening is allowed only to determine a "pass" or "fail" status of the hearing screening. Only an audiologist may complete a full hearing evaluation and determine a diagnosis of hearing loss. It is recommended that a hearing screening be an initial step in all evaluations for speech and language across the lifespan. If a child or adult fails their hearing screening, it is recommended that the evaluation be discontinued and that he or she be referred to their managing primary care physician or audiologist for a follow-up screening. After the diagnosis of hearing loss is ruled out (or determined and treated as may be the case with a diagnosis of hearing loss), the evaluation for speech and language is continued. For details regarding recommendations for administering hearing screenings (including videos and informative handouts), readers are encouraged to visit *www.infanthearing.org/earlychildhood/index.html* and *https://www.asha.org/PRPSpecificTopic.aspx?folderid=8589935406&section=Key_Issues*.

AUDIOGRAMS

To plot or map hearing loss, an audiogram is used; see Figure 2.1, Audiogram explained, below. Loudness or hearing level (HL) is measured in decibels (dB) from very quiet sounds at the top of the chart to very loud louds at the bottom of the chart. The pitch of frequency of sound is measured in cycles per second (Hertz (Hz)) and is represented as very low sounds to the far left of the chart to very high pitched sounds to the far right of the chart.

In 2015, Tye-Murray stated "Hearing loss may be categorized along four dimensions: degree, onset, causation, and time course." (p. 12) Degree of hearing loss is discussed first. The range of normal hearing for a child is 15 dB HL across all speech frequencies. The range of normal hearing for an adult is 25 dB HL across all speech frequencies. Hearing loss that falls between 26 dB HL (or 15 dB HL for children) and 40 dB HL is classified as a mild hearing loss. Hearing loss that falls between 41 and 55 dB HL is referred to as a moderate hearing loss; while, hearing loss that falls between 56 and 70 dB HL is referred to as moderate-to-severe hearing loss. Severe hearing loss is that which falls between 71 and 90 dB HL and hearing loss beyond 90 dB HL is classified as profound hearing loss (Clark, 1981, p. 497).

"A child with a 35- to 40-dB hearing loss without hearing technology can miss up to 50% of class discussions" (Cole & Flexer, 2016, p. 45). Children with moderate

Normal ≤ 25 dB HL

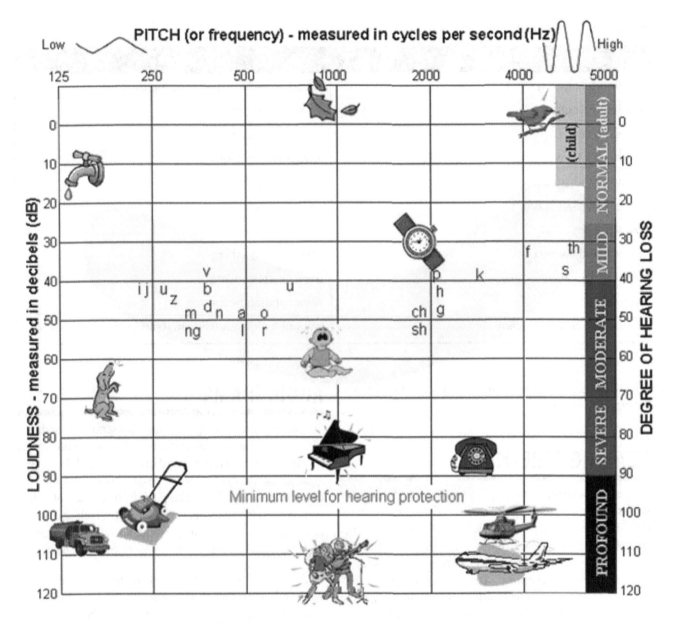

Figure 2.1 Audiogram explained.

Reprinted by permission of A.G. Bell. (www.agbell.org)

hearing losses may miss 50–75% of speech information (Killion & Mueller, 2010). A child with a moderately severe hearing loss (a hearing loss greater than 55 dB across speech frequencies) can miss *one hundred percent* of the information shared in the classroom if the hearing loss remains untreated (Killion & Mueller, 2010). These same performances can apply to adults.

Hearing loss is also classified based on when it was identified or is believed to have occurred. It can be classified as congenital, pre-lingual (occurring prior to learning speech and language), post-lingual (occurring after learning speech and language), peri-lingual (occurring when the child has developed some language, but not all language has been acquired), or acquired (occurs post-lingually as a person ages).

Hearing loss is also classified based on the believed causation of the hearing loss. Hearing loss that is caused by a breakdown in the acoustic signal in the outer or middle ear is referred to as a conductive hearing loss. For example, an obstruction in the ear canal or even something as simple as an ear infection could cause a conductive hearing loss. If the sound signal passes through the outer and middle ear with no problem, but has a breakdown at the level of the inner ear (and/or the auditory nerve or auditory cortex in the brain), it is termed a sensorineural hearing loss. A mixed hearing loss is a combination of both a conductive hearing loss and a sensorineural hearing loss. In addition, hearing loss may be categorized as a progressive hearing loss (gets worse over time) or sudden onset (happened unexpectedly) (Tye-Murray, 2015, pp. 14–16).

HEARING TECHNOLOGY

Hearing loss causes what Cole and Flexer (2016) term a "doorway problem," in which sound cannot properly travel from the ears (the "doorway") to the brain. Because the development of the auditory brain depends on meaningful auditory input through the ears to the brain, the consistent use of appropriate *hearing technology* is critical for children with hearing loss who are learning to listen and talk. Hearing technology is also a key component in successful auditory therapy for adults who have experienced hearing loss later in life.

You are probably familiar with *hearing aids*, which are perhaps the most widely known form of technology used by individuals who are deaf or hard of hearing. Programmed by an audiologist according to the patient's audiogram, digital hearing aids amplify (or make louder) the sound waves they receive. These amplified sound waves then travel to the inner ear, where they are converted to neural signals that the brain perceives as speech or other sounds (National Institute on Deafness and Other Communication Disorders [NIDCD], 2017). Children usually use behind-the-ear (BTE) hearing aids, which transmit sound through an ear mold worn in the outer ear.Because hearing aids transmit sound through the outer and middle ears, they are most effective for individuals with sensorineural hearing loss, who have typical middle-ear functioning (National Institute on Deafness and Other Communication Disorders [NIDCD], 2017). Children and adults with

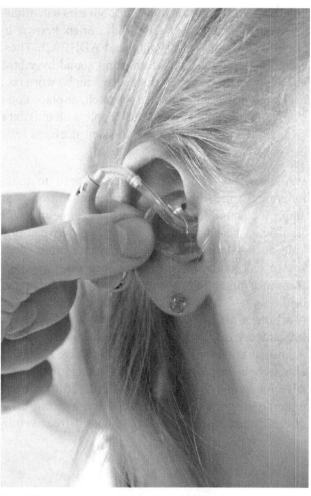

Traditional, behind-the-ear (BTE) hearing aid.

Life in View/Science Source

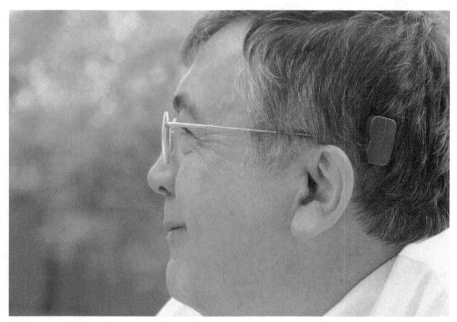

Bone conduction hearing aid.

Life in View/Science Source

conductive hearing loss in one or both ears sometimes use bone-conduction hearing aids, often known by brand names like Baha, Ponto, and ADHEAR. These special hearing aids, which transmit sound by vibrating the mastoid bone behind the ear, can be worn on a headband, used with an adhesive patch, or placed on a surgically implanted post. Some people with unilateral profound hearing loss, or single-sided deafness, also use bone-conduction hearing aids.

While hearing aids provide great benefit to many individuals, they are limited in the amount of clear, amplified sound that they can provide to people with significant hearing loss. *Cochlear implants* can provide access to sound for children and adults with severe to profound hearing loss who do not benefit from hearing aids, as well as those with single-sided deafness and hearing loss in the high frequencies (Carlson et al., 2018). In the United States, cochlear implants are officially approved by the Food and Drug Administration for infants 12 months of age and older, although an increasing number of younger babies are now receiving the devices (Gifford, 2016).Patients undergo surgery to implant a device with an array of electrodes in their inner ear. Sound is received by

an external speech processor, usually worn behind the ear, and then transmitted as electrical impulses through magnets on top of and under the skin to the electrode array. The array receives the electrical impulses and transmits them to the auditory nerve, where they are perceived as sound (NIDCD, 2016).

Before beginning to work with a child who has hearing loss, it is important to gather all the background information the professional typically would for any pediatric client (e.g., social history, diagnosed or suspected conditions, intervention/educational history). When working with a child who has hearing loss, the clinician will also need to ask for details about the child's hearing loss, such as the type and degree, as well as the hearing technology he or she uses. Information about the child's hearing history should also be gathered in order to develop a treatment plan based on the child's *listening age*.

LISTENING AGE

Chapter 4 introduced the concept of developmental age, or a child's level of functioning based on

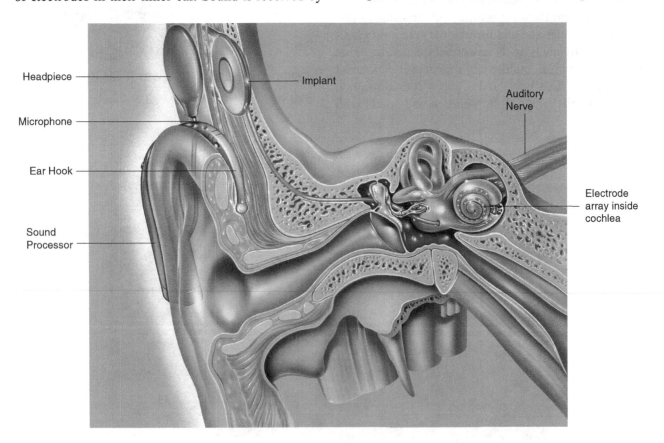

Figure 2.2

John Bavosi/Science Source. Adapted by Kendall Hunt Publishing Company.

his or her achievement of developmental or language milestones.For children who are deaf or hard of hearing, it is also important to consider *listening age*. *Listening age* refers to the length of time the child has had clear, consistent access to sound through hearing technology, such as hearing aids or cochlear implants. It is calculated by subtracting the age at which the child began using technology consistently from his or her current chronological age. For example, a 24-month-old boy with profound hearing loss, who received cochlear implants at 13 months of age, would have a listening age of 11 months (24 months – 13 months = 11 months). A girl whose hearing loss was identified by newborn hearing screening and who received technology shortly thereafter, may have a listening age and a chronological age which are very close. In contrast, a child whose hearing loss was identified late may have a listening age that is much younger than his or her chronological age.Note that listening age is based on the age at which the child first consistently used appropriate hearing technology. If a baby received hearing aids at 1 month of age, but did not begin to wear them during all waking hours until 9 months of age, the child's listening age would be calculated from 9 months old. So, at 10 months of age (chronologically), the child would have a listening age of 1 month. Similarly, using technology that is not appropriately fit for the child's hearing loss or wearing hearing aids, but receiving little benefit before cochlear implantation, may affect calculation of a child's listening age.

Just as the clinician must select activities that are appropriate for the developmental age of a child with developmental delays, considering listening age is critical for developing long- and short-term goals and treatment plans for a child with hearing loss. Because auditory-based therapy follows a developmental model, auditory goals should be developed based on a child's listening age, or the amount of time the child has had consistent, meaningful access to sound. For example, considering only a 4-year-old's chronological age might lead the clinician to expect the child to follow complex, multi-step directions. However, if that child has only been using appropriately fit hearing aids for 1 year, the clinician should plan goals and activities based on the auditory development of a typical 1-year-old. This may mean that the treatment plan includes following simple, one-step directions with common objects. Of course, if the child is otherwise developing

typically, toys and other materials appropriate for a four-year-old should be incorporated into these listening activities.

LING SIX SOUND CHECK

Knowing about a child's hearing loss, technology, and listening age is important for planning auditory-based intervention. It is equally important to perform a *listening check* at the beginning of each session to be sure the child has optimal access to sound. The best-laid treatment plans quickly become irrelevant if the child cannot access auditory input because of a problem with technology, or because of a temporary or permanent drop in his hearing levels. An effective listening check thus begins with checking the child's hearing aids, cochlear implants, or other hearing technology. The clinician might use a device called a stethoset or listening tube to listen to the child's hearing aids or specialized headphones to check the microphones of the child's cochlear implant processor. Indicator lights on the device might also give information about how well it is functioning. Consult the child's educational or personal audiologist to learn the most effective ways to check specific technology.

After making sure the child's device is functioning properly, the clinician then checks the child's listening with the device using the *Ling Six Sound Check*. Developed by auditory-verbal pioneer Daniel Ling, the Ling Six Sound Check allows a professional or parent to assess the child's hearing across the speech spectrum and, when performed before each session, to track this hearing over time (Ling, 2002). Performing and recording the results of the Ling Six Sound Check every day allow the clinician and family immediately to note changes in a child's hearing or the functioning of the hearing technology. The Ling Six Sound Check is fast and flexible and can be performed in close proximity or at a distance, in quiet or noisy conditions, and with both ears together or separately. The six sounds in the check, roughly ordered from low to high frequency, are:

- /m/,
- /u/ ("oo"),
- /i/ ("ee"),
- /a/ ("ah"),
- /ʃ/ ("sh"),
- /s/,
- and a seventh "sound": silence.

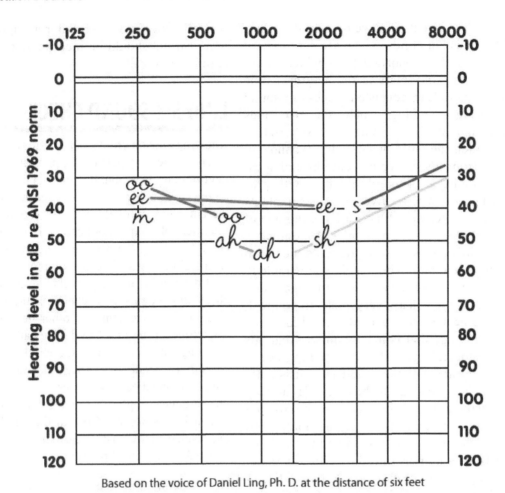

Based on the voice of Daniel Ling, Ph. D. at the distance of six feet

Figure 2.3

© John Tracy Clinic. www.jtc.org. Used with permission.

To perform a basic Ling Six Sound Check, the clinician or parent presents each sound individually, including a few periods of silence to prevent random guessing. The child can indicate when a sound appropriate for auditory functioning is heard. For example, the child might be expected to complete a movement (such as dropping a toy in a bucket), choose a picture card that corresponds to the sound, or repeat the sound(s) heard. (Designing activities that are appropriate for clients on each level of the auditory hierarchy is discussed in detail in the next section.) It is important to document the child's responses to each sound at the beginning of each therapy session. The results can be analyzed quickly to note any patterns or changes in the child's hearing. For instance, a child who did not respond when /m/ or /u/ were presented might not have adequate access to low-frequency sounds, while a child who misses /s/ might have experienced a drop in access to high-frequency sounds. These children should be referred to their audiologists for further assessment.

ERBER'S HIERARCHY

While we may use terms like "listen" and "hear" relatively interchangeably in everyday conversation, auditory perception is actual a complex phenomenon with many precursor steps that must occur before an individual is able to truly "listen" for comprehension of auditory messages. What are the steps to building auditory skills?

In 1982, Norman P. Erber described what is now commonly referred to as "Erber's Hierarchy" consisting of four levels: *detection, discrimination, identification,* and *comprehension.*

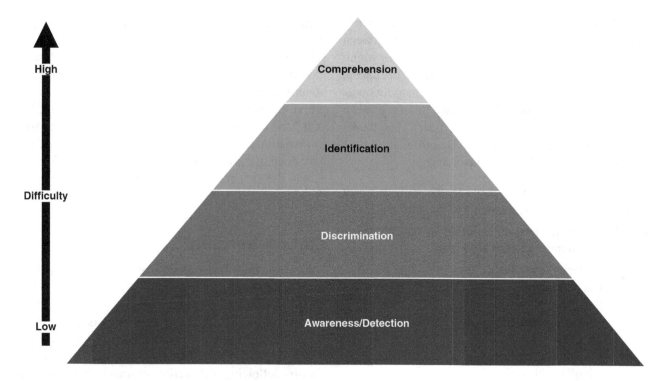

Figure 2.4 Visual Depiction of Erber's Hierarchy

Rachel Glade

Detection

Detection refers to the ability to determine the presence or absence of a sound. The listener need not respond to the sound in a particular way (e.g. hand raising, saying, "I hear it!") nor is he required to determine the sound's source (see *Localization*, below). A patient at the detection level may respond to sound in a variety of ways: by widening the eyes, changing sucking patterns (Siqueland & Delucua, 1969), turning the head, or giving a verbal response, such as, "I heard that."

Localization

Localization refers to the ability to not only detect a sound, but also to identify its source. While there is some localization ability in the left/right horizontal plane present at birth, human infants cannot reliably localize to sounds emitting from their left or right sides until roughly 5–6 months of age (Field, Muir, & Pilon, Sinclair, & Dodwell, 1980; Muir & Field, 1979; Wertheimer, 1961).

It is important to note that development of localization abilities is dependent upon having auditory access from both ears. Interaural (between-ears) timing differences are the cues that alert listeners to the position of the sound (e.g., a sound coming from ones right side will hit the right ear slightly before it hits the left ear. Though this millisecond-long difference is not perceived, the brain does perceive the sound and alerts the individual that the sound has come from the right side). For listeners who do not have access to sound on both sides (for example, a person with unilateral [one-sided] hearing loss), localization ability will be limited (Bess & Tharpe, 1984). Listeners who use hearing technology such as cochlear implants or hearing aids have been shown to exhibit localization ability if they are binaurally aided (have technology for both ears), though this localization ability may be less accurate and less developed than in typically-hearing listeners (Grieco-Calub & Litovsky, 2010).

Discrimination

Given that a listener has established a detection response ("I hear something!"), the next step in the auditory hierarchy is the development of discrimination skills. Auditory discrimination refers to the ability to determine whether sounds are the same or different. At this level, the listener needs to be able to repeat the auditory stimulus (see *Identification*, below), just to indicate, when given choices, whether the sounds presented are the same as, or different from, one another.

For a beginning listener, regardless of age, discrimination begins with the ability to discriminate between pairs of sounds differing in duration. For a baby or young child, this may mean the difference between "up, up, up, up" (a short, repeated sound) and "dooooooooooown" (a long sound). For an older listener, this may mean discrimination by syllable length ("pear" [1 syllable] versus "hamburger" [3 syllables]).Discrimination then moves to more complex tasks involving:

- Words of the same syllable length with different consonant and vowel content (e.g. "dog" vs. "cat")
- Minimal pairs (words differing in one phoneme [speech sound] but otherwise identical)
  - Differing by vowels ("boot" vs. "bat")
  - Consonants differing by manner of articulation ("shoe" vs. "two")
  - Consonants differing by voicing ("fan" vs. "van")
  - Consonants differing by place of articulation ("bat" vs. "back")

Discrimination of minimal pairs is most difficult when the phoneme that differs is in the final position and varies by place of production (e.g., "pat" vs. "pack" is harder than "tap" vs. "cap").

While discrimination tasks may be targeted using minimal pair stimulus cards, it is also possible (and preferable!) to use naturalistic materials and stimuli for discrimination tasks to promote generalization of these skills to everyday conversational contexts. For example, a clinician could target discrimination by duration with a three-year-old child who has just received cochlear implants by playing with farm animals and asking the child to select the cow (moooooo/ long sound) or the dog (woof woof woof/ short sound) from a set of two with prior modeling of the sound associated with each animal toy. A good resource for minimal pair stimulus cards can be found at: https://successforkidswithhearingloss.com/for-professionals/listening-training-resources/ (Click "Compass Test of Auditory Discrimination")

Identification

Once a listener has established detection ("I hear something!") and discrimination ("I can tell what it is and what it's not."), the next task in the auditory hierarchy is the identification of sounds and speech stimuli. Identification is the ability to repeat what is heard, write what is heard, or point to what is heard (if given pictures or a list of words/sentences).

Identification does not require an understanding of the message (see *Comprehension*, below), simply selecting (or repeating) what is heard. The listener's identification ability gives the clinician information about the clarity of the message received. For example, if the clinician says, "hat" and the listener replies "cat," the clinician has received important diagnostic information about the listener's perceptual skills, and may need to move back to the *Discrimination* level to assess the listener's ability to discriminate between the phonemes /h/ and /k/.

Comprehension

Following the development of detection ("I hear something!"), discrimination ("I know what it is and what it's not."), and identification ("I can label it."), the pinnacle of the auditory hierarchy is comprehension—the ability to understand the spoken message without visual cues and demonstrate that comprehension by following a direction or answering questions about the information heard.Unlike previous steps in the auditory hierarchy, comprehension abilities depend on vocabulary and overall linguistic knowledge, rather than auditory perception skills alone.

Auditory Memory

After a listener has established identification skills and is able to select (write, point to, imitate) single words, the clinical focus shifts to the development (or rehabilitation) of auditory memory abilities. Auditory memory is the ability to retain, manipulate, and use information presented through audition (oral presentation) (Stredler-Brown & Johnson, 2004).

Complex Comprehension Tasks

Simple comprehension may be the ability to demonstrate understanding by following a simple one-step direction ("Clap your hands.") presented through audition alone. As linguistic knowledge and comprehension skills grow, a listener will be able to complete more complex comprehension tasks, such as:

- Answering a variety of wh- questions
  - About self
  - About objects
  - About increasingly lengthy passages presented through audition alone (e.g. sentences, paragraphs, books)

Auditory Learning Guide

SOUND AWARENESS (Speech and Environmental Sounds)	PHONEME LEVEL** (Speech Babble)	DISCOURSE LEVEL (Auditory Processing of Connected Speech)	SENTENCE LEVEL	WORD LEVEL
Step 1 - Detect * the presence of any speech syllable.	Step 1 - Imitate physical actions (before speech imitations).	Step 1a - Imitate motions of nursery rhymes/songs with accompanying vocalization.	Step 1 - Identify familiar stereotypic phrases or sentences.	Step 1a - Identify and imitate approximations of "Learning To Listen" sounds varying in suprasegmentals and vowel content, e.g., (a-a-a)/airplane, (u)-(u)/train, (oi) (oi)/pig in isolation, at the end, and in the middle of a sentence.
Step 2 - Detect * vowel variety, [u] [a] [i] and raspberries [b-r-r].	Step 2 - Imitate any phoneme that child produces spontaneously when given hand cue (or other cue).	Step 1b - Identify nursery rhymes or songs.	Step 2 - Recall two critical elements in a message.	Step 1b - Identify one, two, and three syllable words in isolation, e.g., cat vs. chicken vs. kangaroo.
Step 3 - Detect * consonant variety, e.g., [m-m-m], [b^] [b^] [b^] and [wa] [wa].	Step 3 - Imitate varying suprasegmental qualities in phonemes (vary intensity, duration, and pitch) aeeee (long) vs [ae ae] (pulsed); [ae-ae] loud/quiet/whispered; [ae] high/mid/low pitch.	Step 2 - Answer common questions with abundant contextual support, e.g., "What's that?", "Where's mama?", "What is _____ doing?"	Step 3 - Recall three critical elements in a message.	Step 2 - Identify words having the same number of syllables but different vowels/diphthongs and consonants, e.g., horse vs. cow vs. sheep.
Step 4 - Detect * the presence of environmental sounds at loud, medium and soft levels at close range, at a distance of 6-12 ft and at a distance of greater than 12 ft.	Step 4 - Imitate vowel and diphthong variety, e.g., [u], [ae], [au], [i], etc.	Step 3 - Identify a picture that corresponds to a story phrase in a three or four scene-story.	Step 4 - Complete known linguistic messages from a closed set (ex: nursery rhymes, songs, familiar stories).	Step 3a - Identify words in which the *initial* consonants are the same but the vowels and final consonants are different, e.g., ball vs. bike.
Step 5 - Detect * whispered [hae] [hae] and [p] [p] [p].	Step 5 - Imitate alternated vowels and diphthongs, e.g., [a-u] [e-i] [a-i].	Step 4 - Identify an object from several related descriptors (closed set).	Step 5 - Answer common questions about a disclosed and familiar topic: a) without pictorial cues b) over the telephone c) on audio/video.	Step 3b - Identify words in which the *final* consonants are the same but the vowels and initial consonants are different, e.g. food vs. card.
Step 6 - Detect * the sounds of the Six Sounds Test.	Step 6 - Imitate consonants varying in manner (fricatives, nasals, and plosives). Use phonemes previously produced, e.g., /h/ vs. /m-m-m/ vs. /p/.	Step 5 - Follow a conversation with the topic disclosed.	Step 6 - Recall four or more critical elements in a message to follow multiple element directions.	Step 4 - Identify words in which the initial and final consonants are identical but the vowels/diphthongs are different, e.g., book vs. back.
Step 7 - Detect * the sounds of the Six Sounds Test at various distances.	Step 7 - Imitate consonants differing in voiced vs. unvoiced cues, e.g., [b^] [b^] vs. [p] [p] and then with vowel variety, [bobo] [pae-pae].	Step 6a - Answer questions about a story with the topic disclosed.	Step 7 - Complete known linguistic messages (open set).	Step 5a - Identify words in which the vowels and final consonants are identical but the *initial* consonants differ by three features - manner, place of articulation, and voicing, e.g., mouse vs. house.
Step 8 - Locate the direction of sound if amplified bianurally.	Step 8 - Alternate consonants varying in place cues, first with varying vowels, e.g., /ma-ma/ /no-no/; /go-go/ /bi-bi/, etc.	Step 6b - Answer questions about a story with the topic disclosed; story is teacher-recorded.	Step 8 - Follow open set directions and instructions (disclosed).	Step 5b - Identify words in which the vowels and initial consonants are identical but the *final* consonants differ by three features - manner, place of articulation, and voicing, e.g., comb vs. coat.
	Step 9 - Alternate syllables with varying consonants and same vowel, e.g., [bi], [di], [ho], [go].	Step 7 - Recall details of a story (topic disclosed).	Step 9 - Recall specific elements in a sentence by answering questions about an undisclosed but familiar topic.	Step 6 - Identify words in which the vowels and the final/initial consonants are identical but the initial/final consonants differ by two features: a) manner and place (voicing in common), moat vs. goat; b) manner and voicing (place in common), man vs. pan; c) place and voicing (manner in common), boat vs. coat.
		Step 8 - Sequence the events of a story (topic disclosed).	Step 10 - Repeat each word in a sentence exactly. a) predictable sentences "I'm going to the grocery store to buy cereal and milk." b) less predictable sentences "A woman hit me so I told her to calm down."	Step 7a - Identify words in which the vowels and final consonants are identical but the *initial* consonants differ by only one feature - manner of articulation, e.g., ball vs. mall.
		Step 9 - Retell a story with the topic disclosed, recalling all the details in sequence.	Step 11 - Recall specific elements in a sentence by answering questions on an undisclosed topic.	Step 7b - Identify words in which the vowels and the initial consonants are identical but the *final* consonants differ by only one feature - manner of articulation, e.g. cloud vs. clown.
		Step 10 - Make identification based on several related descriptors (open set).		Step 8a - Identify words in which the vowels and final consonants are identical but the *initial* consonants differ by only one feature - voicing, e.g., coat vs. goat.
		Step 11 - Follow a conversation of an undisclosed topic.		Step 8b - Identify words in which the vowels and initial consonants are identical but the *final* consonants differ by only one feature - voicing, e.g., bag vs. back.
		Step 12 - Retell a story about an undisclosed topic, recalling as many details as possible.		Step 9a - Identify words in which the vowels and final consonants are identical but the *initial* consonants differ by only one feature - place of articulation, e.g. bun vs. gun.
		Step 13 - Process information in noise and at various distances.		Step 9b - Identify words in which the vowels and initial consonants are identical but the *final* consonants differ by only one feature - place of articulation, e.g. sheep vs. sheet.
		Step 14 - Process group conversations.		

KEY

The color codes in the chart designate auditory behaviors to be mastered by the end of the specified year, given optimally fitted hearing devices.

Year 1
Year 2
Year 3
Year 4

This guide is intended to aid professionals in the *beginning* stages of learning an auditory-based approach. As professionals acquire more experience in auditory teaching, children should progress more rapidly.

The information on this chart was adapted from Judy Simser's article in the *Volta Review* (1993) (**items), from the Auditory Skills Program, New South Wales Department of School Education, from the Foreworks Auditory Skills Curriculum (1976, North Hollywood, CA), and from teacher input.

Notes:
*A detection response could include turning head, pointing to ear, clapping, dropping a toy in a container, etc.

Reference:
Simser, J.I. (1993). Auditory-verbal intervention: Infants and toddlers. *Volta Review* 95(3): 217-229.

Acknowledgement:
Originally developed for First YEARS, a training program for professionals in listening and spoken language developed in partnership and offered by The University of North Carolina at Chapel Hill and The Alexander Graham Bell Association for the Deaf and Hard of Hearing with funding from the Oberkotter Foundation. ©Beth Walker, 2009

Revised: 09/15/16

Figure 2.5

- Following directions of increasing length with concepts such as temporal (before/after), conditional ("If I touch my nose, get the ball."), ordinal (first, second), locational (behind, beside, etc.)
- Higher-level cognitive functions
  - Opposites
  - Convergent thinking (answering riddles and questions where there is one correct answer, (e.g., "What is an animal that swims in the water and has eight legs?" "An octopus.")
  - Divergent thinking (generating a variety of ideas in response to a prompt, (e.g., "What are different modes of transportation?" "Car, train, boat, bicycle. . .")

The pinnacle of auditory comprehension is conversational discourse skills. All aspects of the auditory hierarchy build to the individual's ability to participate in everyday conversational interactions using spoken language (with a variety of communication partners, on a variety of topics) without the need for visual support.

For an additional reference on the development of auditory skills, see Figure 2.5.

SUMMARY

This chapter presented a brief overview of normal hearing, hearing technology, and the development of auditory skills. Hearing is the foundation for the development of speech and spoken language. A child's speech mirrors what is heard. For adults, especially adults who are post-lingually (after learning speech and language) deafened, hearing loss can impact quality of life and lead to communication breakdowns. Therefore, it is important that professionals who work with individuals who have communication disorders prioritize hearing screenings and subsequent audiological follow up (if needed) during initial assessments and continued dynamic assessment regardless of the age of the individual with whom they are working.

REFERENCES

Bainbridge, K., & Wallhagen, I. (2014). Hearing loss in an aging American population: Extent, impact, and management. *Annual Review Public Health*, 35, 139–152.

Bess, F. H., & Tharpe, A. M.(1984). Unilateral hearing impairment in children. *Pediatrics, 74*(2), 206–216.

Carlson, M. L., Sladen, D. P., Gurgel, R. K., Tombers, N. M., Lohse, C. M., & Driscoll, C. L. (2018). Survey of the American Neurotology Society on Cochlear Implantation: Part 1, candidacy assessment and expanding indications. *Otology & Neurotology, 39*(1), e12–e19.

Clark, John G. (1981). Uses and abuses of hearing loss classification. *American Speech-Language Hearing Association (ASHA), 23*, 493–500.

Clifton, R. K., Gwiazda, J., Bauer, J. A., Clarkson, M. G., & Held, R. M.(1988). Growth in head size during infancy: Implications for sound localization. *Developmental Psychology, 24*(4), 477–483.

Cole, E., & Flexer, C. (2016). *Children with hearing loss: Developing listening and talking birth to six* (3rd ed.). San Diego, CA: Plural Publishing.

Erber, N. P. (1982). *Auditory training.* Washington DC: AG Bell Association for the Deaf.

Field, J., Muir, D., Pilon R., Sinclair, P., & Dodwell, P.(1980). Infants' orientation to lateral sounds from birth to three months. *Child Development, 51*(1), 295–298.

Flexer, C., & Madell, J. (2008). *Pediatric audiology.* New York, NY: Thieme Medical Publishers, Inc.

Fucci, D., & Lass, F. (1999). *Fundamentals of speech science.* Needham Heights, MA: Allyn & Bacon.

Gifford, R. H. (2016). Expansion of pediatric cochlear implant indications. *The Hearing Journal, 69*(12), 8–10.

Grieco-Calub, T. M., & Litovsky, R. Y.(2010). Sound localization skills in children who use bilateral cochlear implants and in children with normal acoustic hearing. *Ear & Hearing, 31*(5), 645–656.

Killion, M. C., & Mueller, H. G. (2010). Twenty years later: A NEW count-the-dots method. *The Hearing Journal, 63*(1), 10–12.

Ling, D. (2002). *Speech and the hearing-impaired child: Theory and practice* (2nd ed.). Washington, DC: Alexander Graham Bell Association for the Deaf and Hard of Hearing.

Muir, D., & Field, J.(1979). Newborn infants orient to sounds. *Child Development, 50*(2), 431–436.

National Institute on Deafness and Other Communication Disorders. (2016). *Cochlear implants.* (NIH Pub. No. 00–4798). Retrieved from https://www.nidcd.nih.gov/health/cochlear-implants.

National Institute on Deafness and Other Communication Disorders. (2017). *Hearing aids.* (NIH Pub. No. 13–4340). Retrieved from https://www.nidcd.nih.gov/health/hearing-aids.

Seikel, J. A., King, D. W., & Drumwright, D. G. (2000). *Anatomy and physiology for speech, language, and hearing* (2nd ed.). San Diego, CA: Singular Publishing Group.

Siqueland, E. R., & Delucua, C. A.(1969). Visual reinforcement of nonnutritive sucking in human infants. *Science, 165*(3898), 1144–1146.

Stredler-Brown, A., & Johnson, C. D. (2004). Functional auditory performance indicators: An integrated approach to auditory skill development. Retrieved from https://www.phonakpro.com/content/dam/phonakpro/gc_hq/en/resources/counseling_tools/documents/child_hearing_assessment_functional_auditory_performance_indicators_fapi_2017.pdf

Tye-Murray, N. (2015). *Foundations of aural rehabilitation: Children, adults, and their family members.* Stamford, CT: Cengage Learning.

Wertheimer, M.(1961). Psychomotor coordination of auditory and visual space at birth. *Science, 134*(3491), 1692.

White, K. (2003). The current status of EHDI programs in the United States. *Mental Retardation and Developmental Disabilities Research Reviews, 9*, 79–88.

Case Scenario 2-1

NAME: _____   DATE: _____

Caroline is a 12-month-old female with profound sensorineural hearing loss bilaterally. She was referred for further testing when her hearing was tested shortly after birth, and her hearing loss was identified at 1 month of age. Caroline began wearing binaural hearing aids loaned to her family by her audiologist when she was two months old. Although Caroline reportedly sometimes turned to loud sounds, such as fire engines, with her hearing aids, her parents reported that she did not visibly react to speech sounds, like someone calling her name. Caroline recently received bilateral cochlear implants. She and her family will soon begin auditory-based speech therapy with you. Results of Caroline's recent comprehensive developmental evaluation revealed delays in receptive and expressive language (*Strengths: participates in visual/gestural routines and fingerplays, uses gestures to request objects, demonstrates consistent eye contact, shakes her head "no." Weaknesses: does not quiet or excite in response to novel sounds, does not respond when her name is called, does not echo duration or pitch, rarely vocalizes to request objects/actions or respond to others*). Her cognitive, adaptive, social-emotional, and fine- and gross-motor skills were all rated within the average range.

1. Calculate the patient's listening age

   _____

2. On what level of Erber's Hierarchy will you begin to work with this patient? Why?

   _____

   _____

3. What is an appropriate LONG-TERM GOAL?

   _____

4. What are three appropriate SHORT-TERM OBJECTIVES? (Hint: Short-term objectives should correlate with the long-term goal listed above.)

   A.

   _____

   _____

   B.

   _____

   _____

C.

_____

_____

5. List the TASK you would use to target the short-term objectives listed above. The task for 3A should pair with the short-term objective listed for 2A. Please list MATERIALS you plan to utilize.

A.

_____

_____

B.

_____

_____

C.

_____

_____

6. How would you introduce and explain the purpose of each short-term objective and task in the therapy session to the parent/caregiver?

A.

_____

_____

B.

_____

_____

C.

_____

_____

Case Scenario 2-2

NAME: _____ **DATE:** _____

Jason is a 4-year-, 2-month-old male with bilateral moderate-to-severe hearing loss. He was referred for further testing when his hearing was tested at birth, but, due to challenging family circumstances, his hearing loss was not confirmed by an audiologist until he was 18 months old. Although Jason was fitted with binaural hearing aids at 20 months of age, he did not begin wearing them consistently until he was 26 months old. Jason has been receiving auditory-based, family-centered speech therapy since that time. He has reportedly been making steady progress in his auditory skill development, though his receptive and expressive language remain delayed. Jason's family reports that he easily detects both environmental and speech sounds, discriminates between minimal pairs of familiar words, and identifies words by repeating or pointing. Jason also demonstrates comprehension of simple sentences by following one- and two-step directions and responding to simple "what" and "where" questions. Jason's family would like to continue to develop his comprehension skills by focusing on more complex tasks. His teachers report no concerns with his vision, cognition, adaptive, social-emotional, or motor skills at this time.

1. Calculate the patient's listening age.

   _____

2. On what level of Erber's Hierarchy will you begin to work with this patient? Why?

   _____

   _____

3. What is an appropriate LONG-TERM GOAL?

   _____

4. What are three appropriate SHORT-TERM OBJECTIVES? (Hint: Short-term objectives should correlate with the long-term goal listed above.)

   A.

   _____

   _____

   B.

   _____

   _____

C.

_____

_____

5. List the TASK you would use to target the short-term objectives listed above. The task for 3A should pair with the short-term objective listed for 2A. Please list MATERIALS you plan to utilize.

A.

_____

_____

B.

_____

_____

C.

_____

_____

6. How would you introduce and explain the purpose of each short-term objective and task in the therapy session to the parent/caregiver?

A.

_____

_____

B.

_____

_____

C.

_____

_____

Case Scenario 2-3

NAME: _____   DATE: _____

Ms. Snyder is a 46-year-old female with severe hearing loss in her left ear and profound hearing loss in her right ear. Ms. Snyder was born and grew up with typical hearing and developed appropriate listening and spoken language skills. One year ago, she began to experience hearing loss and became post-lingually deaf, which means that she became deaf after she acquired spoken language. Ms. Snyder recently received a cochlear implant in her right ear. She wears a hearing aid in her left ear. Although Ms. Snyder has typical expressive language skills, she has struggled with listening tasks since losing her hearing. As a bank teller, she interacts with clients who ask questions and make requests all day, and comprehending their speech has been very difficult. Ms. Snyder is hopeful that her new cochlear implant will improve her auditory comprehension at work and in her personal life. She has scheduled a series of speech therapy sessions with you in order to learn to listen with her new technology. She wants to work on functional activities that will help her listen in her daily life.

1. What is an appropriate LONG-TERM GOAL?

   _____

2. What are three appropriate SHORT-TERM OBJECTIVES? (Hint: Short-term objectives should correlate with the long-term goal listed above.)

   A.

   _____

   _____

   B.

   _____

   _____

   C.

   _____

   _____

3. List the TASK you would use to target the short-term objectives listed above. The task for 3A should pair with the short-term objective listed for 2A. Please list MATERIALS you plan to utilize.

A.

_____

_____

B.

_____

_____

C.

_____

_____

4. How would you introduce and explain the purpose of each short-term objective and task in the therapy session to the parent/caregiver?

A.

_____

_____

B.

_____

_____

C.

_____

_____

CHAPTER 3

Behavior Management

"You gotta accentuate the positive, eliminate the negative, latch on to the affirmative, but don't mess with mister in-between."

The lyrics of this old song suggest interesting and effective strategies for addressing challenging behaviors in young children and the promotion of appropriate social skills. Accentuating the positive may include environmental manipulations providing positive attention and feedback, and teaching social skills and emotional competencies to children. Even with these practices in place, there are times when behaviors may go awry, so careful and intentional response strategies are needed. A child's safety and emotional stability must always be of paramount importance when addressing environmental manipulations.

It is not unusual for children who have communication disorders to exhibit challenging behaviors. Behavior is a complex pattern of interaction. All behavior is a form of communication, and we all communicate through behavior. Behavior is purposeful, and we all continuously affect one another's behavior. Whether we recognize it or not, there is intention behind our actions. Challenging behavior is considered any behavior that hinders learning, engagement, and social interactions, and interferes with an individual's quality of life. When children display problematic behavior, they are communicating that something is not right. This chapter will address what challenging behavior is and principles for behavior management.

A child is considered to have problems with behavior if they are oppositional to the requests of adults, become frustrated easily, tantrum for longer periods than is typical, are aggressive, or don't respond to traditional behavioral strategies. A student may have difficulty with peer interaction or be rejected by their peers. As they get older, students may suffer from depression, anxiety, substance abuse, and suicide ideation. They may also engage in solitary activities and hobbies.

The impact of challenging behavior is far-reaching and can affect many aspects of the lives of children and their parents. In the short term, young preschool-aged children who demonstrate behavior challenges have fewer social interactions, poorer academic motivation, and increased occurrences of emotional and behavioral disorder diagnoses. Challenging behavior may lead to social isolation for not only affected children, but for their families as well, and may result in loneliness and depression from an early age. Early childhood behavior issues put children at risk for a lifetime of nonconforming social behaviors which include academic dropout, criminal behavior, drug use, and limited income and occupational success (Chazin & Ledford, 2016).

BEHAVIOR/LANGUAGE CONNECTION

Communication disorders can be a prime cause for challenging behaviors. If children do not possess the communication skills to express that they are upset or that something is not right, they may resort to inappropriate behaviors to get their point across (Buschbacher & Fox, 2003). Challenging behavior is a way of saying,

Some Common Functions of a Behavior:
• Obtain an item
• Communication
• Self-stimulation
• Fulfilling sensory need
• Avoidance
• Expression of emotion
• Boredom
• Attention seeking

"Something is not right; I am upset." Children may be hungry, tired, bored, or angry and may not have the ability to express how they feel or they may not be in tune with their emotional states to adequately relay their feelings to others using words. Also, if children feel unsafe or out of control, they resort more to kicking or hurting others as a means of feeling in control. It is the job of adults to figure out the meaning behind challenging behaviors and teach children more acceptable ways to communicate their feelings (Johnston & Reichle, 1993).

Language is thought to be central to the development of human personality. Understanding and correcting deficits in the area of expressive and reception language can improve behavior and help a child resolve emotional dilemmas. Reportedly, as many as 50–70% of all children exhibiting speech and language disorders also have diagnosable emotional and behavioral disorders (Prizant et al., 1990).

Many years ago, I worked with a middle-school-aged student who would become very distressed at school. She communicated her distress by hitting or kicking the other students or by throwing things. It took some trial and error, but it was soon discovered that she feared fire drills. The loud unexpected alarm was upsetting to her, and she would sit in fear each day dreading the rare, but inevitable, fire drill. Once the cause of her inappropriate behavior was discovered, school staff were able to work on a plan that would allay her fears. It was agreed that on fire drill days, the principal would come to this student's classroom and escort her to his office where she would be allowed to wear headphones and draw until the drill was over. This simple adjustment eased her concerns and resulted in more positive classroom interactions for not only the student, but her classmates as well.

Once we as adults understand the reason behind problematic behaviors, we can respond better and meet the needs of the child so that a behavioral outburst to communicate in unnecessary. Punishing a child for a behavior may stop it temporarily, but it does not meet the needs of the child or provide an alternate way for the child to act in a difficult situation. Also, adults who use punitive measures, when dealing with children, communicate to them that anger is an acceptable way to not only express oneself but also to solve problems—not a message that we wish to convey! When we as adults take the time to figure out what the child is trying to express, we are positioned to teach positive social skills and problem-solving abilities that will help the child respond to others in a constructive manner.

POSITIVE BEHAVIORAL SUPPORT (PBS)

Best practices for dealing with behavior issues are to look for the underlying cause of the misbehavior and teach prosocial skills rather than resort to punishment. Positive Behavioral Support (PBS) is a process grounded in Applied Behavioral Analysis (ABA) that seeks to discover the underlying cause of challenging behaviors rather than resorting to aversive punishment (Hieneman, 2015). PBS seeks to instill independence in individuals with behavioral concerns and improve their quality of life by teaching appropriate skills. If you wish to learn more about PBS, please visit the website: https://www.pbis.org/

The goal of a PBS plan is to help the child with emotion regulation. Eventually, we want our students to be able to understand and manage their own emotions and to be able to communicate their feelings to others in an appropriate manner. Emotional self-regulation helps children to work productively and get along with others which makes for a more positive learning experience for all those involved. Keep in mind that children's ability to regulate their emotions will be influenced by their developmental stage and life circumstances. These are two important factors to consider when developing an intervention plan of any type.

WHAT IS ABA?

Applied Behavioral Analysis (ABA) is a collection of principles which encourages practitioners to carefully observe and record behavior as it happens in order to understand the functional relationship between challenging behaviors and the environment in which they occur. ABA was designed to determine how to look at behavior as communication and understand why it's happening. The principles of ABA are frequently used to increase desired behaviors and decrease undesired behaviors (Park & Scott, 2009).

The ABC's of ABA
Behavior Formula: A → B → C
• A = Antecedent: Something in the environment that causes a behavior to happen or not to happen.
• B = Behavior: Response to the environment.
• C = Consequence: A reaction to the behavior that increases or decreases the probability of the behavior occurring again.

ABC Example:
A = Child enters a loud and brightly lit therapy room
B = Child becomes overstimulated and self-stimulated
C = Child finds relief from overstimulation but stigmatizes self from peers
ABC Example:
A = Child wants to play video game but is told it is time for bed
B = Child throws a tantrum
C = Child is allowed to continue to play video game

Consequences: The Terrific Trio!
• Positive reinforcement: something positive that is given to *increase* the frequency of a behavior
• Verbal praise
• Reward (candy, sticker, toy)
• Negative reinforcement: removing something negative to *increase* the frequency of a behavior
• Finishing a worksheet to be done with homework time
• Taking an aspirin which removes a headache
• Extinction—loss of attention to behavior

THE PROACTIVE PREVENTATIVE APPROACH TO BEHAVIOR MANAGEMENT

Principals of ABA and PBS can be successfully used to establish a proactive and preventative approach to behavior management. As we have discussed, children engage in challenging behavior as a form of communication. The first step is determining the function of the behavior. What is the child communicating? The child may be trying to gain the attention of adults. Whether interaction with adults is positive or negative, it is still attention. The child may be trying to avoid something. This could be an environment that is overstimulating or schoolwork that is too difficult or uninteresting to the child. We also need to describe the behavior itself. When describing the behavior, it is important to indicate its frequency, duration, and what it looks like. It is not enough to say that the child "appeared agitated" or "seemed angry." What exactly did the child do? "The child cried and pounded the floor for 15 minutes" is a much more useful description. Once the function of the behavior has been determined, the next step is for all involved adults to develop a common intervention strategy. Educating all adults in the child's life is important so that the behavior plan can be carried out in a consistent manner—consistency is the key to success. The resulting behavior plan should consider what skills should be taught to replace the problem behavior or what modifications to the environment should be made to make the behavior unnecessary (Smith & Fox, 2003).

TEACHING APPROPRIATE REPLACEMENT BEHAVIORS

One important aspect of the behavior intervention plan is to teach appropriate replacement skills for problem behavior. These skills are known as *functionally equivalent skills* and should be developmentally appropriate for the child and just as easy for the child to perform as the inappropriate behavior that is being replaced. For example, if kicking means "leave me alone," then teach the child a hand sign that means "leave me alone." It is also wise to teach the replacement skill, that is, functionally equivalent skills when the child is calm and not engaging in the challenging behavior. Another important aspect of the behavior intervention plan is to teach the child social skills, focusing on recognition of feelings and emotion, problem-solving skills, and self-regulation. Self-regulation is an important skill that allows the child to obtain, maintain, and modify emotion, behavior, attention, and activity levels suitable to particular tasks or situations.

The Proactive Preventative Approach to Behavior Management
Manage Antecedents and Consequences.
Teach Appropriate Skills.
Set Up Opportunities to Practice the New Behavior.
Reward Desirable Behavior.
Praise, Praise, Praise!

MANAGING ANTECEDENT AND CONSEQUENCES

One way to assure a proactive and preventative approach to behavior management is to control antecedents and consequences. Controlling the environment and our own actions may prevent challenging behavior from ever occurring in the first place. By assessing the common antecedents and consequences, it is easier to hypothesize the function of the behavior (Park & Scott, 2009). The antecedent must be carefully described. What is happening to the child or in the environment that is causing the behavior? For example, a child may engage in tantrums when asked to put a video game away so that school work can begin. You can control the environment and manage the antecedent (video game being discontinued) by giving the child a 10-minute warning or presenting the child with an If/Then chart. "If you complete five math problems, then you can play a video game" (Park & Scott, 2009). Be aware of the specific consequences that occur right after student behavior. Did the consequence increase the

Teaching New Behaviors
Important Techniques to Know:
• *Task Analysis*—Breaking down a complicated task and teaching individual parts.
• E.g., Getting dressed, making a bed.
• *Chaining*—Teaching each individual step of a task and then sequencing the steps.
• Forward—Teaching steps in a certain order.
• Backward—Reversing the order of the steps.
• *Prompting*—Helpful cues that help with task initiation.
• Vocal, physical, positional, gestural, attentional.
• *Shaping*—Different levels of reinforcement successive approximations of the target behavior ([bɑdo] vs. [bɑdəl]).

likelihood of the behavior or decrease it? Also, pay attention to the environment and what occurs before the behavior. Small signs can signal that "trouble is brewing."

The following information is adapted from Barkley (1990), Jensen (2005), Kauffman (2005), Meese (1996)) and displays disorders that are often characterized by challenging behaviors.

Anxiety Disorders
These are the most common mental health problems among children and adolescents. Children with emotional, behavioral disorders often have severe anxiety disorders. Primary Characteristics
Anxiousness occurs in problematic situations.
Avoidance of situations occurs due to being uncomfortable, nervous, and anxious.
Causes suggested include biological, genetic, and environmental influences; but still in question. Trauma experienced or witnessed may also cause symptoms. (e.g., dog bite, holiday costume)
• Generalized anxiety disorder (GAD)—always worries, frequent aches/pains with no physical evidence, easily tired but difficult to sleep, body constantly tense, may tremble, shake, have headaches
• Separation anxiety disorder (SAD)—excess anxiety and fear related to being separated from a significant individual; fear turns to panic; results in nightmares, distress, refusal to go to school, transition periods may increase anxiety
• Obsessive compulsive disorder (OCD)
Obsessions include intrusive, unwanted, repetitive, persistent thoughts. (e.g., thoughts of violence, fear of germs, lucky #s, symmetry, order, fear of harm to self or others, doubt if a behavior was done)
Compulsions are repetitive, purposeless behaviors that individuals feel compelled to perform. (e.g., excessive hand washing, grooming, cleaning, ordering, arranging, repeating rituals, hoarding)
May overlap with depression, Tourettes, substance abuse, eating disorders, and attention deficit disorder.
Medical research says there is a neurological basis for the disorder.
• Panic disorder
Panic attack is "an intense, discrete experience of extreme fear that seems to arise quickly and often without any clear cause." (Wicks-Nelson & Israel, 2003)
More common in girls and in adolescents. Fears dying, avoids social situations
Many physical symptoms occur such as shortness of breath, dizziness, heart palpitations, nausea, abdominal distress, being detached from oneself, numb tingling sensation, hot/cold flashes, chest pain/discomfort, choking, sweating

Mood disorders include *bipolar disorder* (lows/highs) and *depressive disorders (unipolar).*

- Depressive disorders are characterized by lack of motivation, extreme lethargy, lack of interest in past pleasurable activities, profound hopelessness (if severe with anxiety can lead to suicidal thoughts); mild symptoms may come and go with no long-term effects; severe can cause lifelong problems. In children, periods may occur episodically and then increase.

Symptoms of Childhood Depression

- Persistent sad or irritable mood

- Loss of interest in activities once enjoyed

- Significant change in appetite/body weight

- Difficulty sleeping or too much sleep

- Loss of energy

- Feelings of worthlessness or guilt

- Difficulty concentrating

- Recurrent thoughts of death/suicide

Why do they present with challenging behaviors?

- Frequent absences from school resulting in poor performance

- Outburst of shouting, complaining

- Lack of interest in playing with friends

- Social isolation

- Poor communication

- Difficulty with relationships

Attention Deficit Disorder (ADD)

- A neurobiological condition meaning the individual has a dysfunction in the central nervous system (CNS). The CNS consists of the brain, spinal cord, and all the nerves radiating throughout the body. Thoughts and movements are controlled by the CNS. ADD covers ADD and ADHD.

 - *ADD* is thought of as inattentiveness

 - *ADHD* implies inattentiveness compounded by hyperactivity.

Why do they present with challenging behaviors?

ADD causes difficulty with processing and producing expressive, receptive, and written language. Barkley (1990) classified behaviors associated with ADD into five categories:

1. Lack of persistence of effort to complete tasks

2. Behavioral impulsivity such as acting or talking before thinking

3. Hyperactivity

4. Failure to follow through on rules or directives

5. Fluctuation in the quality of the work output

ADD and Cognition: Messages are carried throughout the CNS and are required for transmitting cognitive messages and for motor activity. *Cognition* relates to the ability to think and process information such as memory, reasoning, comprehension, and judgment.

CONSIDER THE SENSES

As has been discussed, children exhibiting challenging behavior are communicating that they want to either get/access something or avoid/escape something. It is not uncommon for children to exhibit challenging behavior in order to seek sensory stimulation or to avoid sensory input. The accurate processing of sensory stimulation in the environment as well as in one's own body directly impacts behavioral reactions. Although not currently considered a stand-alone medical diagnosis, Sensory Processing Disorder (SPD) is thought to affect many children with developmental disabilities causing them to have issues receiving and/or responding to information through the senses. Although sensory processing issues are usually seen in children, adults, too, can have sensory processing concerns. It is also important to note that every child can respond negatively to certain sensory stimulation from time-to-time, but SPD is considered when responses to sensory information affect an individual's daily living skills. When determining the cause of misbehavior, sensory processing should be considered. *The Out-of-Sync Child* and *The Out-of-Sync Child*

Has Fun by Carol Stock Kranowitz and *Sensational Kids* by Jane Miller are excellent resources if you wish to learn more about how the processing of sensory information affects many children with developmental disabilities. Sensory processing issues occur on a spectrum. Children with sensory processing issues can be underresponsive to sensory information or "hyposensitive," or they can be overresponsive to sensory information or "hypersensitive." A hyposensitive child will exhibit less of a response to sensory information, may take longer to respond, or may require more intensive or longer-lasting sensory input. The hypersensitive child, on the other hand, may respond more intensely, more quickly, and/or for a longer period to sensory input. It is also possible for children to be hyposensitive to some sensory input, yet hypersensitive to other types of sensory stimuli. Dysfunctioning senses may lead to problems with attention and learning, sleep, eating, social interaction, health and safety, community living, and increased anxiety levels. It is also important to note the sensory input is most powerful when received through the mouth or groan—so pick your battles wisely (Miller, Fuller, & Roetenberg, 2014).

The Senses at a Glance: The following information is adapted from Kranowitz & Archer, 1998 and Moyes, 2010.
• Tactile: touch
• Proprioceptive: where our body parts are in relation to each other
• Vestibular: where our bodies are in space
• Auditory: sound
• Visual: sight

Proprioception	
Hypersensitive	**Hyposensitive**
Does not like being upside down	Moves constantly
Has trouble manipulating small objects	Bumps into or leans on people/objects
Avoids weight-bearing activities like running and jumping	Is unaware of bodily sensations (hunger/need for bathroom)
	Seeks out roughhousing

Tactile	
Hypersensitive	**Hyposensitive**
Dislikes certain textures	Doesn't seem to notice getting hurt
Dislikes having messy hands	Constantly touches objects
Dislikes having hair or nails cut	Mouths objects
Dislikes certain food textures	Likes pressure and tight clothes
Dislikes hugs or being touched	Enjoys hugs and roughhousing
Dislikes certain clothing	Is prone to self-injury (hand biting, head banging)
Visual	
Hypersensitive	**Hyposensitive**
Does not like bright lights	Fixates ("stims") on moving parts or fingers
Is distracted by irrelevant or small details	Stares at bright lights or reflections
Avoids direct eye contact	Experiences difficulty figuring out what or where objects are
Auditory	
Hypersensitive	**Hyposensitive**
Does not like loud noises	Likes high TV and music volume
Covers their ears	Does not respond to name
Is scared by unexpected noises (bells, sirens, alarms)	Creates sounds themselves for stimulations (tapping, banging, humming)
Is distracted by background noise in a classroom	
Makes repetitive noises to cover other disturbing noises	

Adaptation from "The Out-of-Sync Child" By Carol Stock Kranowitz.

SUMMARY AND CONCLUSION

According to Strain, Joseph, Hemmeter, Barton, and Fox (2017), prevention and promotion are the best ways to not only manage challenging behaviors but also to promote acceptable ways of interacting with others. Their 2017 *Tips for Responding to Challenging Behavior in Young Children* offers excellent suggestions for parents and interventionists to help children regulate their behavior and learn socially appropriate ways of behaving. The following is a summary of their suggestions:

1. Interactions with a misbehaving child should be kept to a minimum during troubling episodes. This recommendation is based on the two most common reasons for challenging behavior: (1) attempts to gain attention or (2) attempts to avoid or escape a nonpreferred activity.

2. When children are demonstrating problem behavior, interrupt and redirect their attention to the appropriate alternative action using minimal attention, discussion, and emotion. Redirection should start by explaining what should be done. For example, if the child has snatched a toy from another child, prompt a more appropriate social skill (e.g., "You can trade toys with Michael." Perhaps throwing blocks might be redirected to, "Let's build—you put one here!"). Notice that these recommendations involve minimal interaction and usually just one prompt.

3. Reinforce the nearest appropriate alternative behavior (e.g., "I see Jeff using his inside voice," or "Lori, I like how you share your toys with your friends."). Then, when the child uses the skill you are teaching, immediately use descriptive feedback to acknowledge the change.

4. It is a good idea to join in the child's play or have a conversation with the child concerning the child's interests or activity. Get on their level!

5. Most of your time and attention will be put into teaching alternate behaviors. Be sure to do this when the child is calm and not engaging in

inappropriate actions. If children are upset, it is likely that your teaching will not be effective.

6. Do not just wait until poor behavior occurs; continue to model appropriate modes of communication throughout the day.

7. Remember challenging behavior is a response to an antecedent. If challenging behavior seems to be reoccurring, consider what has been happening immediately following the challenging behavior and change it.

8. Find individualized reinforcers and do not be afraid to use them! Challenging behavior is easy and productive; your replacement behavior should be as well.

9. Find out what is motivating to your student. Find out what is attractive to the child and use these items and activities in your teaching. If what you are using is not motivating to the student, it will not work.

10. Make a plan, write it down, and teach all adults what to do! It is essential that all adults respond consistently to both appropriate and also challenging behavior.

11. Know that severe and persistent challenging behavior can require the use of individualized positive behavior support. Once challenging behavior is severe and persistent, it frequently necessitates the use of a process in which goals are set, data collected, and reason for the response is determined, so a comprehensive support plan can be developed and monitored to ensure success (Strain et al., 2017).

REFERENCES

Barkley, R. A. (1990). *Attention deficit hyperactivity disorder: A handbook for diagnosis and treatment*. New York, NY: Guilford Press.

Buschbacher, P. W., & Fox, L. (2003). Understanding and intervening with the challenging behavior of young children with autism spectrum disorder. *Language, Speech, and Hearing Services in Schools, 34*(3), 217–227.

Chazin, K. T., & Ledford, J. R. (2016). Challenging behavior as communication. In *Evidence-based instructional practices for young children with autism and other disabilities*. Retrieved from http://vkc.mc.vanderbilt.edu/ebip/challenging-behavior-as-communication

Hieneman, M. (2015). Positive behavior support for individuals with behavior challenges. *Behavior Analysis in Practice, 8*(1), 101–108.

Jensen, M. M. (2005). *Introduction to emotional and behavioral disorders*. Upper Saddle River, New Jersey: New Jersey & Ohio Pearson Merrill Prentice Hall.

Johnston, S. S., & Reichle, J. (1993). Designing and implementing interventions to decrease challenging behavior. *Language, Speech, and Hearing Services in Schools, 24*(4), 225–235.

Kauffman, J. M. (1997). *Characteristics of emotional and behavioral disorders of children and youth*. Upper Saddle River, NJ: Merrill/Prentice Hall.

Kranowitz, C. S. (2003). *The out-of-sync child has fun: Activities for kids with sensory integration dysfunction*. Newburyport, MA: Berkley Publishing Group.

Kranowitz, C. S., & Archer, E. (1998). *The out-of-sync child*. New York, NY: Berkley Publishing Group.

Meese, R. L. (1996). *Strategies for teaching students with emotional and behavioral disorders*. Pacific Grove, CA: Brooks/Cole Publishing Company.

Miller, L. J., Fuller, D. A., & Roetenberg, J. (2014). *Sensational kids: Hope and help for children with sensory processing disorder (SPD)*. New York, NY: Penguin Group.

Moyes, R. A. (2010). *Building sensory friendly classrooms to support children with challenging behaviors: Implementing data driven strategies!* Arlington, TX: Sensory World.

Park, K. L., & Scott, T. M. (2009). Antecedent-based interventions for young children at risk for emotional and behavioral disorders. *Behavioral Disorders, 34,* 196–211.

Prizant, B. M., Audet, L. R., Burke, G. M., Hummel, L. J., Maher, S. R., & Theadore, G. (1990). Communication disorders and emotional/behavioral disorders in children and adolescents. *Journal of Speech and Hearing Disorders, 55*(2), 179–192.

Smith, B., & Fox, L. (2003). *Systems of service delivery: A synthesis of evidence relevant to young children at risk of or who have challenging behavior*. Tampa, FL: University of South Florida, Center of Evidence-Based Practice; Young Children with Challenging Behavior.

Strain, P., Joseph, J., Hemmeter, M. L., Barton, E., and Fox, L. (2017). *Tips for Responding to Challenging Behavior in Young Children*. Retrieved from https://www.pbis.org/Common/Cms/files/pbisresources/2017-01%20PEP%20Tips.pdf

Wicks-Nelson, R., & Israel, A. C. (2003). Behavior disorders of childhood. Prentice Hall/Pearson Education. Upper Saddle River, New Jersey

CHAPTER 4

Speech Sound Disorders: Assessment and Intervention

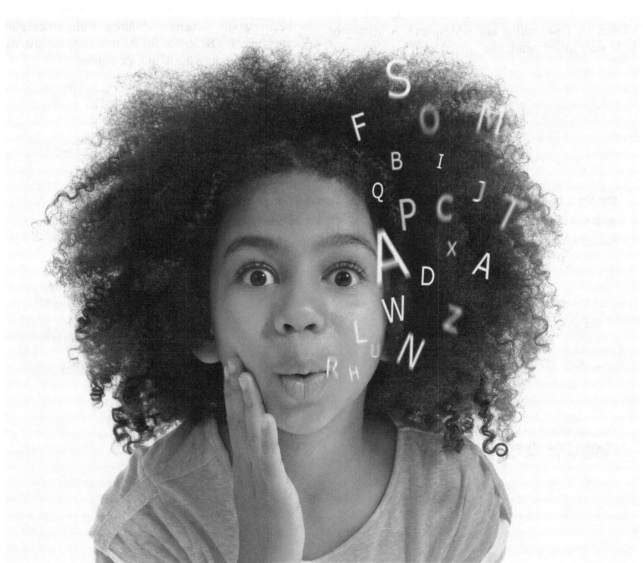

Africa Studio / Shutterstock.com

Speech Sound Disorder (SSD) is the most prevalent childhood communication disorder, comprising more than 70% of pediatric SLP's caseloads (Mullen & Schooling, 2010). Speech is not language, but it is the most common mode for expressing language due to its efficiency. Speech is the combination of articulated sounds—a series of complex motor movements which modify our voiced and unvoiced breath stream—and prosody, which is a general term referring to the acoustic characteristics of speech whose subtle variations alter the meaning of utterances and give indications about the talker's state on mind. SSD is an umbrella term that refers to any type of disorder that affects the intelligibility of speech at the sound level. These disorders may include difficulties with motor production, perception, or the phonological rules governing how sounds are used to form speech segment or any combination of the above. The effects of unintelligible speech are far-reaching and widespread. A history of SSD may affect academic, social, and psychological outcomes even into adulthood (Johnson, Beitchman, & Brownlie, 2010).

This chapter will focus on assessment and intervention of SSD in children and will describe and differentiate between disorders of articulation (phonetic) from those with a more phonological (phonemic) foundation. Use of the term "articulation disorder" emphasizes that speech is a motor activity, whereas, use of "phonological disorder" stresses that speech requires knowledge of language. Speech requires both knowledge of language (phonology) and speech production and perception skills. Children with phonological disorders may have difficulty using the rules of a language for putting sounds together to form words, while children with articulation disorders are thought to have difficulty with production and/or perceiving speech. To demonstrate, children with phonological impairment may not recognize /pl/ as an acceptable consonant cluster to begin words, whereas children with articulation disorder, may not be able to lift the tongue to the alveolar placement to produce the /l/ in a /pl/ cluster.

Speech Sound Development

The chart below illustrates the typical developmental progression of individual speech sounds. The sounds within each number indicate the age by which 85% of children have mastered production of that sound. For example, by age 6, 85% of children have mastered production of the "l" sound.

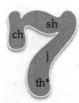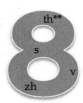

Chart adapted from the following sources: Sander (1972) and Goldman & Fristo (2000)

*Voiceless "th" as in "think" and "thing"
**Voiced "th" as in "the" and "those"

Goldman, R., & Fristoe., M. (2000). *Goldman-Fristoe 2 Test of Articulation*. Minneapolis, MN: Pearson Assessments.

Sander, E. K. (1972). When are speech sounds learned? Journal of Speech and Hearing Disorders, 37(1), 55–63.

Speech Sound Development

The following chart depicts typical speech sound development. The start of each bar indicates the age by which at least 50% of children have mastered a particular sound and the end of the bar indicates when 90% of children have mastered the sound. For example, by age 3, 50% of children will have mastered production of "r" and by 8 years 90% of children will have mastered the sound. Age in years is represented across the top and bottom. Adapted from Sander (1972), Grunwell (1981) and Smit et al. (1990).

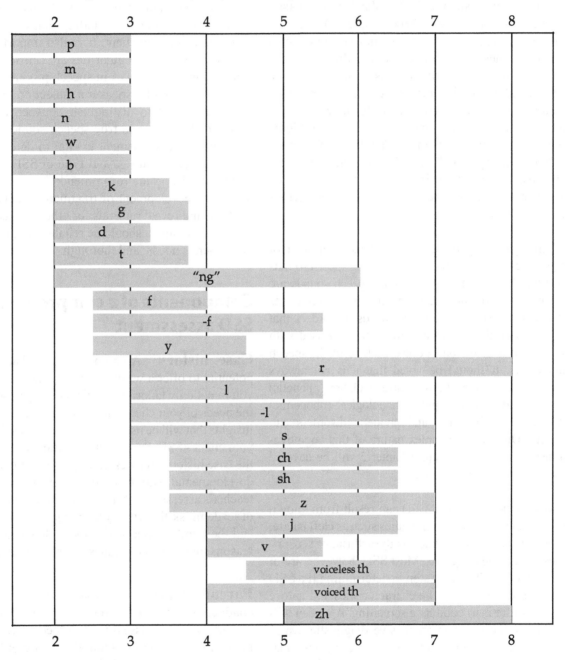

Grunwell, P. (1981). The development of phonology. First Language , iii, 161-191.

Sander, E. (1972). When are speech sounds learned? Journal of Speech and Hearing Disorders, 37, 55-63.

Smit, A., Hand, L., Freilinger, J., Bernthal, J., & Bird, A. (1990). The Iowa articulation norms project and its Nebraska replication. Journal of Speech and Hearing Disorders, 55, 779-798.

Chart designed by Rosie Prehoda, M.A. CCC-SLP. "Speech Sound Development Norms" chart is available for download at: https://www.teacherspayteachers. com/Store/Rosie-Prehoda

Articulation disorders are a type of SSDs that refer to errors in the production of phonemes which result from problems in speech motor control. These SSDs are sometimes referred to as "phonetic" disorders because they describe the way in which the sounds are being produced. These errors may be associated with structural issues (such as cleft palate), motor-based difficulties (such as dysarthria or apraxia), medical issues (such as recurrent otitis media), sensory issues (such as deafness), or intellectual disability. Children exhibiting articulation difficulties with the absence of structural anomalies, motor-based issues, or other concomitant disorders will usually have mild-to-moderate impairment characterized by problems producing certain phonemes (Van Riper & Smith, 1992). For example, a child with articulation disorder may have trouble coordinating the tongue for the correct production of the /r/ phoneme. These errors are typically consistent.

A phonological impairment is considered a disorder of language resulting in difficulty organizing speech sounds and using the rules that govern how speech sounds are combined and difficulties using the speech sound contrasts that aid in the discrimination of words. Disorders that are phonologically based are oftentimes confused with disorders of articulation because both result in speech sound errors. It should be noted that it is not always possible to differentiate between an articulation (phonetic) speech sounds disorder and a phonological (phonemic) one, and that phonemic and phonetic disorders can co-occur. Due to the complex nature of this cognitive-linguistic based impairment, Chapter 3 will be devoted solely to phonological disorders.

As was previously stated, SSD can result from known causes such as structural anomalies such as cleft palate, motor speech disorders, such as dysarthria, or sensory issues such as hearing loss. Most SSD, however, are of unknown cause. The first step in determining if a SSD exists and in describing the characteristics and nature of the disorder is to conduct a screening. A screen will help determine if a comprehensive diagnostic evaluation is warranted or if referral to other professional services is needed. The purpose is to identify those who may have a SSD, but not to diagnose or describe it. A screening will also guide you in determining the best course of action for the comprehensive assessment protocol, particularly if the SSD is not secondary to a known disability, such as cerebral palsy or structural abnormality.

COMPREHENSIVE ASSESSMENT

Once a screening has been conducted and a comprehensive assessment is indicated, it is the responsibility of the SLP to determine an appropriate assessment protocol which should take into account not only the areas of suspected need, but should also consider the cultural and linguistic, including dialect and accents, communities of the client. It is also important to note that not all speech irregularities are considered speech errors. Some differences in speech production may be due to a feature of a speaker's dialect or accent. SLPs must be careful to distinguish between dialectal or accent differences and true speech sound errors. The comprehensive assessment is vital in determining the nature, severity, causes, and type of SSD. An assessment will also guide recommendations for treatment, aid in the development of treatment targets for intervention, and reveal referrals for other needed services. A good assessment should be reliable, valid, tailored to your client's needs, and thorough.

Components of a comprehensive SSD assessment

Case history   A thorough case history has the potential to offer a wealth of information that will help you in not only tailoring the diagnostic protocol to meet the needs of your client, but it may also reveal important insights that will be useful in the differential diagnosis of your client's SSD. Specific information to be obtained in the case history includes: family background, birth and developmental histories, academic background including teacher's assessment of speech intelligibility and impact of academic skills, primary language spoken in the home, and the families concerns of the child's speech and the reasons for which they requested an evaluation.

Parent interview   It is natural to be nervous when conducting your first parent interview, but this vital portion of the assessment process can provide invaluable information about the nature of the client's speech issues and how they are perceived and handled by the family. It's important that you establish a goal and plan for the interview before you begin. Know in advance the information that you would like to obtain. The parent interview is a prime opportunity to clarify and confirm information or obtain missing elements in the case history. Start the interview by introducing yourself to the parents, including your title and credentials, discussing the purpose of the session and giving a brief description of the agenda, and providing an approximation of how long the evaluation should take. Next, transition by asking questions such as, "What brings you in today?" or "What are your concerns regarding your child's speech?" Then, discuss your client's history and current status of abilities, focusing on relevant communicative development, skills, concerns, and medical, developmental, and familial, social, and educational histories. When speaking with the parent, be warm, empathetic and engaging, avoid yes/no questions, choosing open-ended ones instead. Don't be afraid of pauses and give parents adequate response time. Be sure to write everything down! You will be happy that you have detailed notes to draw from when you are writing the diagnostic report.

Oral mechanism examination
It is conducted to evaluate the structural and functional integrity of the speech mechanism for the purposed of speech production.

Hearing screening
Either prior to or as part of the comprehensive assessment a hearing screening is conducted in a quiet environment and the typical protocol consists of screening each ear at a level of 20 dBHL at 500, 1000, 2000, and 4000 Hz. Results are recorded as "PASS" or "REFER."

Speech sound assessment
Speech sound attainment is a developmental process, and many children demonstrate "typical" errors and phonological patterns during this acquisition stage. It is the job of the SLP to differentiate between developmentally appropriate errors and patterns in order to distinguish age-appropriate errors from those that are uncommon or not age-appropriate. This portion of the examination should include both standardized measures and a variety of sampling procedures. Standardized measures provide standard scores which are often necessary to document for eligibility for services purposes. It is not appropriate to determine a standard score for any assessment that is not normed on a group representative of the client being assessed.

A thorough speech assessment should provide information about the child's speech sound system and should include an inventory of:

- phonemes used by the child
- different sound combinations
- syllable shapes produced (e.g., CV, VC, CVC, CCVC, CVCC)
- sound articulated in different word positions (e.g., initial, medial, and final word positions)
- speech sound errors, including type(s) (e.g., deletions, omissions, substitution, distortions, and additions)
- phonological processes (see Chapter 3 for more detail)

Single-Word Testing—Great starting point to determine number of phonemes in error. If the child is unintelligible, it provides a mechanism to know what the child is trying to say. It also allows for the elicitation of all phonemes in a variety of phonetic contexts. It may not accurately reflect production of the same phonemes in connected speech; that is why it is crucial that your testing protocol also contain a connected speech sample.

Sampling Procedures—These measures give an indication of speech in longer and connected utterances. Typically, as linguistic complexity increases, intelligibility will decrease. Sampling measures can be obtained during free-play activities or other mechanisms such as, retelling of a story, describing a picture, or conversing about a topic of interest. Also, sampling procedures can employ family members, peers, and siblings to help with elicitation. Sampling measures provide a more "natural" indication of the client's speech.

Important outcomes of the speech assessment portion of the evaluation include: severity, intelligibility, stimulibility, and speech perception.

Severity—A qualitative judgment rating that indicates the significance of the speech disorder. There are various measures, but an easy and frequently used one is Percentage Consonants Correct (PCC) which determines severity on a continuum from mild to severe.

Intelligibility—a subjective determination on how intelligible the child's speech is to the listener. Intelligibility judgments range from "intelligible" to "unintellible." This measure is often used to determine the need for intervention and to evaluate progress in therapy. A 3-year-old or older child, who is unintelligible is usually recognized as a candidate for treatment.

Stimulibility—This refers to the degree in which the child is able to imitate error speech sounds in different contexts and with different models and levels of cueing. This measure helps determine prognosis for treatment, determine if error sound(s) are likely to be acquired without intervention, and select appropriate therapy targets.

Speech Perception—This is used to establish if the client can differentiate between an error production and the standard production of a phoneme.

Phonetic Inventory—Also called "Independent Analysis" this is a listing of the speech sounds that a client can produce. The phonetic inventory does not compare the child's production to the adult standard. This is an important measure particularly if the child has a limited repertoire and is unintelligible. For example, a child can be so unintelligible that a single-word articulation measure cannot be obtained. In this instance, the SLP can transcribe all utterances produced by the child and complete the phonetic inventory to gain an idea of the types of phoneme the child is able to produce.

Phonemic Inventory—Also called "Relational Analysis" this is a listing of the phonemes that the child uses contrastively, in other words, sounds that the child uses correctly and conform to the adult standard. Standardized tests are an efficient way to obtain the phonemic inventory.

Receptive and Expressive Language Assessment— Because speech and language are intricately connected, it is recommended that a screening of receptive and expressive language skills be a part of any assessment of speech. If a screening of these abilities reveals concerns, more thorough testing may be conducted.

Phonological Processing—If the child has numerous errors that appear to follow a pattern, phonological testing may be warranted. Phonological SSDs are covered in detail in Chapter 3.

It is important to document speech sound errors using phonetic transcription so that an analysis may be performed in order to determine diagnosis. Phonetic transcription is a powerful tool to document the clinically relevant aspects of disordered speech. It is usually recommended that square brackets be used in phonetic transcription.

There are a number of different types of speech errors and ways to notate the errors: substitutions, omissions, distortions, and additions (Van Riper & Erickson, 1996). The following is a description of speech error types:

Substitution: Substitutions are the most common type of speech errors and occurs when one sound is substituted for another sound. An example would be [tek] for [kek]; the /t/ is substituted for the /k/. There are different ways to denote a sound substitution:

x→y means "x becomes y."

y/x means "y for x."

x→y/z means "x becomes y in the environment of z." This symbolization describes how a phonetic or word context influences speech production.

The above notations provide a convenient mechanism to describe speech sound changes.

Omission: An omission occurs when a speech sound in a target word is not produced. An example would be [bʌ] for [bʌs].

Distortion: An allophone (phoneme variation) is produced for the intended phoneme. An example would be the dentalized or frontal /s/, in the word [s̪op].

Addition: The insertion of an extra sound in a word. An example would be the /ə/ in the word [bəlæk].

TARGET SELECTION

Selecting appropriate treatment target is extremely important in the remediation of SSD. There are a number of considerations to help with this vital task:

Intelligibility considerations: use targets that would bring about the most gains in overall speech intelligibility.

Developmental considerations: use speech acquisition norms of typically developing children to determine target selection.

Complexity considerations: use more complex, linguistically marked targets that are not present in the child's repertoire to bring about the generalization of less marked phonemes.

Relevancy considerations: use targets that are meaningful to the client and family (e.g., sound in the child's name).

Once treatment targets have been identified, the following are treatment strategies proposed by Fey (1986) that may be employed to facilitate acquisition of therapy goals:

Vertical—Intense practice on one or two targets are chosen and are drilled intensely until a specific criterion level (usually conversational level) is achieved before proceeding to additional targets.

Horizontal—Multiple targets are addressed less intensely during the same session, which is thought to provide exposure to more aspects of the sounds system.

Cyclical—Elements of both horizontal and vertical strategies are employed to provide practice on a specific target or targets for a predetermined period before moving on to additional target(s).

STIMULUS WORDS SELECTION

Like choosing treatment targets, identifying appropriate stimulus words is an important aspect of treatment planning. Points to consider when choosing words for a treatment session:

Facilitating contexts—certain co-articulatory context conditions may aid the client's production of a target sound. For example, for some clients high back vowels provide a facilitating context for correct placement of /s/, therefore *suit /sut/* would be a good stimulus word. Contextual tests or "deep tests" can help in identifying facilitating contexts.

Stimulible contexts—words identified during stimuliability testing make good stimulus words particularly when first beginning treatment.

Semantically potent words—choose words that the client knows and uses. *Polka* may be a great word to target a velar [L], but it is unlikely that it is a word meaningful to a young child. *Milk* would be a much better choice to target velar [L].

How many stimulus words are enough? It depends. It is better to have fewer words with facilitating contexts that are meaningful to the client than to have more words that don't meet the above criteria for target selection.

TREATMENT TECHNIQUES

There are many low-cost techniques that may help in the establishment of phonemes to increase awareness of the target phoneme and/or to give feedback about placement and movement of the articulators. The following is a list of these budget-friendly yet effective methods:

- *Use a mirror*—Many children find this visual feedback of placement and movement of the articulators very helpful.

- *Use gestures*—Hand gestures cueing placement and movement of the articulators are simple yet helpful.

- Use www.talktools.com

- *Use amplification*—Amplifying target phonemes may improve attention, reduce distractibility, and increase sound awareness and discrimination.

- Use tactile feedback—place tools, devices, or substances within the mouth (e.g., tongue depressors, peanut butter) to provide feedback on appropriate tongue position and coordination.

- *Use metaphors*—Compare some aspect of speech to something the child is familiar with (e.g., the [ʃ] sound is the "sleeping baby" sound). Visit the websites www.promptinstitute.com and www.talktools.com for more suggestions for eliciting speech sounds.

Feedback is Fundamental

Pragmatics should be the focus of all therapy sessions. Keep feedback to the client relevant to impact on communication. Phrases such as, "It was so easy to understand that word when you say it with a clear /s/!" or "I like the way you fixed that word to make it clearer—way to go!" Visit websites https://www.asha.org/students/mentoring/feedback/ and https://www.opencolleges.edu.au/informed/features/giving-student-feedback/ for more information on providing pragmatically appropriate feedback.

TREATMENT APPROACHES

Treatment approaches for disorders of articulation (phonetic) disorders typically target each sound error individually. These approaches are often chosen for clients whose errors are thought to be motor-based. There is usually a 3-phase sequence (fhttps://www.asha.org/PRPSpecificTopic.aspx?folderid=8589935321&section=Treatment) for most articulation-based treatment approaches:

Establishment—involves both the elicitation and stabilization of the target sounds/behaviors.

Generalization—involves facilitating the use of established sounds in progressively more complex linguistic levels (e.g., syllables, words, phrases/sentences, conversational speech).

Maintenance—involves stabilizing target sounds/behaviors by encouraging self-monitoring of speech and self-correction of sound errors to make correct productions more automatic.

The following is a brief description of some popular articulation approaches. More information can be found at https://www.asha.org/PRPSpecificTopic.aspx?folderid=8589935321&section=Treatment

VAN RIPER (TRADITIONAL) APPROACH

This approach, which focuses on correction of individual phonemes, was developed by Charles Van Riper and relies on clinician modeling. The recommended procedure begins with sensory perceptual training or "ear training" (Van Riper, 1939) and proceeds through a set sequence of production training goals. The sequence of intervention is as follows: Ear training → Sound taught in isolation → sound taught in increasing complexity (i.e., sound, syllable, word, phrase, sentences, conversation) → sound generalized into multiple settings and contexts (Brumbaugh & Smith, 2013). Stimulation method and phonetic placement method are two recommended strategies for teaching the correct production of error sounds. The stimulation method uses direct imitation of an auditory-visual model of the error phoneme, while the phonetic placement method uses various devices to attain jaw, lip, and tongue position for correct production of the phoneme.

PAIRED-STIMULI APPROACH

This highly structured approach, based in operant conditioning, uses a "keyword," which is a word in which production of the target phoneme is articulated correctly. Keywords are paired with misarticulated words in order to generalize through maximum opportunities. Keywords are used as a bridge to facilitate more consistent productions across various words with the target phoneme. It is theorized that because behaviors are being built upon skills already in the client's repertoire, sounds establishment should be more time efficient. Typically, one keyword is paired with 10 training words. There are three productions levels: word, sentence, and conversational levels.

MULTIPLE PHONEME APPROACH

This approach outlines the targeting of all misarticulated sounds at the same time. The clinician uses whatever techniques are necessary to elicit each error sound in isolation. This approach is very similar to the Traditional Approach with the exceptions that auditory discrimination is not used and that every misarticulated sound is treated during each session.

CORE VOCABULARY APPROACH

The Core Vocabulary Approach focuses on whole-word production and was developed for children with inconsistent speech sound productions for whom more traditional types of therapy approaches were not successful This therapy approach uses functional whole words typically used by the child as reported by caregivers and teachers. The words are targeted until child is able to produce them consistently and intelligibly. The rationale for the approach is that inconsistent speech disorder results from a phonological planning problem rather than a cognitive-linguistic deficit. This approach is thought to target the underlying speech-processing deficit operating in the child's speech and therapy is structured in order to produce system wide change (Dodd, Holm, Crosbie, & McIntosh, 2006).

NONSPEECH ORAL-MOTOR THERAPY

These tasks are used prior to teaching speech sounds or as a complement to speech sound training. It is thought that immature or inadequate oral-motor control or strength may contribute to unintelligibility and that there may be benefits to teaching the control of the articulators prior to teaching the production of individual phonemes.

Nonspeech oral-motor strategies are controversial within our field due to lack of an evidence-base. Nonspeech-oral-motor tasks are used to supplement treatment and are rarely used as a primary approach to remediation.

CONSIDERATIONS FOR SERVICES IN PUBLIC SCHOOLS

The Individuals with Disabilities Education Act (IDEA, 2004) outlines eligibility criteria for services in a school setting. Following these criteria, the SLP must conclude:

- that a SSD exists,
- that an adverse effect on educational performance occurs resulting from the disability,
- that specially designed instruction and/or related services and supports are required to assist the student in making progress in the general education curriculum.

The student's resulting individualized education program (IEP) documents eligibility for speech-language pathology services as well as the student's goals and dismissal process.

REFERENCES

Fey, M. E., & Stalker, C. H. (1986). A hypothesis-testing approach to treatment of a child with an idiosyncratic (morpho) phonological system. *Journal of Speech and Hearing Disorders*, *51*(4), 324–336.

Van Riper, C., & Erickson, R. (1996). *Speech correction: An introduction to speech pathology and audiology* (9th ed.). Boston, MA: Allyn & Bacon

The Individuals with Disabilities Education Act retrieved from: https://sites.ed.gov/idea/

Mullen R., & Schooling T. (2010). The national outcomes measurement system for pediatric speech-language pathology. *Language, Speech, and Hearing Services in Schools*, *41*, 44–60.

Johnson C, Beitchman J, & Brownlie E. (2010). Twenty-year follow-up of children with and without speech-language impairments: Family, educational, occupational, and quality of life outcomes. *American Journal of Speech-Language Pathology*, *19*(1), 51–65.

Brumbaugh, K. M., & Smit, A. B. (2013). Treating children ages 3–6 who have speech sound disorder: A survey. *Language, Speech, and Hearing Services in Schools*, *44*(3), 306–319.

Van Riper, C. (1939). Ear training in the treatment of articulation disorders. *Journal of Speech Disorders*, *4*(2), 141–142.

Van Riper, C. G., & Smith, D. E. (1992). *An introduction to general American phonetics* (3rd ed.). Prospect Heights, IL: Waveland Press.

Dodd, B., Holm, A., Crosbie, S., & Mcintosh, B. (2006). A core vocabulary approach for management of inconsistent speech disorder. *Advances in Speech Language Pathology*, *8*(3), 220–230.

Chapter 4   Activities

NAME: _____   **DATE:** _____

The following 10 therapy goals are missing vital details. Apply the skills you learned in Chapter 1 to correct these goals and make them *SMART* goals.

ARTICULATION:

1. The patient will produce initial /b/ in single syllables during therapy as measured by observation, with 80% accuracy without using PROMPT cues.

2. By the end of the IEP, the patient will produce /r/ in the final position of words during therapy with 80% accuracy in imitated speech.

3. By the end of the IEP, the patient will produce /r/ in all positions of words with 90% accuracy as measured by observation or language sample.

4. In six months, the patient will discriminate correct production of /p/ in single syllables as measured by observation, when given 8/10 opportunities.

5. Over 5 consecutive sessions, the patient will produce /r/ blends in words with 80% accuracy as measured by observation, given verbal prompts.

6. By the end of the IEP, the patient will produce /m/ in the initial position with 80% accuracy as measured by observation, given no tactile cues.

7. By the end of the IEP, the patient will produce /h/ in the initial position of words with 80% accuracy as measured by observation.

8. By the end of the IEP, will produce /l/ in the final position of single syllables with 80% accuracy as measured by observation, during imitated speech.

9. The patient will identify the presence of /r/ in speech with 80% accuracy as measured by observation from 4/5 trials, given 2 cues or less.

10. By the end of the IEP, the patient will spontaneously produce /s/ in the final position of words with 80% accuracy as measured by observation.

Report Writing Practice

Use the following case history and diagnostic information along with skills learned in this Chapter and Chapter 1 to write a diagnostic report (See Appendix F for a diagnostic report example).

Report Writing Activity: ARTICULATION

SPEECH/LANGUAGE/HEARING Case History/CHILD SPEECH AND HEARING CLINIC

TO THE PARENTS OR GUARDIAN:

You have requested an appointment for an evaluation of your child's speech, language, hearing problem. To plan ahead for this interview, we need certain information. Please complete this form to the best of your ability.

All information will be held confidential.

I. General Information

Child's Name: **Sally Sue Smith**

Phone: **123-4567**

Birth Date: **June 6, 2010**   Age: **8 years**   Sex: **Female**   Grade: **3rd grade**

Address: **354 WestPoint Drive**   City: **Fayetteville**   State: **Arkansas**   Zip: **72701**

School: **WestPoint Elementary**   Teacher: **Mrs. Carter**

School District: **Fayetteville School District**

Father's Name: **Samuel Smith**   Age: **38**

Address: **354 WestPoint Drive**   City: **Fayetteville**   State: **Arkansas**   Zip: **72701**

Occupation: **Construction Worker**   Business Phone: **768-7980**

Place of Occupation: **Hard Hat Construction**

Education; number of years completed: **13; high school diploma**

Mother's Name: **Susan Smith**   Age: **36**

Address: **354 WestPoint Drive**   City: **Fayetteville**   State: **Arkansas**   Zip: **72701**

Occupation: **Hairdresser**   Business Phone: **721-5362**

Place of Occupation: **Great Cuts Hair Salon**

Education; number of years completed: **13; high school diploma**   **2; beauty school**

If mother is employed, who cares for the child? **When not in school, Sally is watched by older sibling(s).**

Who will be responsible for payment of charges?   **Medicaid**

Brothers and/or sisters of the child:

Name: **Samantha Smith**   Age: **12**   School: **WestPoint Middle School**   Grade: **7th grade**

Name: **Scotty Smith**   Age: **4**   School: **WestPoint Preschool**   Grade: **N/A**

FORM B 05

Relatives or others living in the home:

Name: **N/A**   Relationship: **N/A**

Who referred you to the University of Arkansas Speech and Hearing Clinic?

Name: **Dr. Bill**   Relationship: **Sally's pediatrician**

Address: **900 Wellness Street**   City: **Fayetteville**   State: **Arkansas**   Zip: **72703**

II. Statement of the Problem:

Describe the problem:
Sally has difficulty saying 'r' in words

When was the problem first noticed?
Sally has always had trouble with 'r', but we really started noticing it become a problem the end of last year when she was in 2nd grade.

What has been done about it?
We asked our Pediatrician if he thought it was a problem that she still can't really say 'r' well and he recommended us to get a speech evaluation done.

What is the child's reaction to the problem?
Sally has become shy and doesn't want to talk because she has noticed that she can't say 'r' very well. She now doesn't want to ask the teacher questions while at school because she has trouble saying the teacher's name (Carter).

III. Pregnancy and Birth History:

During this pregnancy did the mother experience any unusual illness, condition or accident? If so, describe:
No

Were there any complications during the delivery such as caesarean, extremely long labor, or use of instruments?
No

IV. Developmental History:

At what age did the following occur?

Sat alone unsupported: **6 months**   Crawled: **9 months**   Walked alone: **12 months**

Maintained bowel and bladder control while awake: **3 years**   asleep: **4 years**

Does the child seem awkward or uncoordinated?   **No**

V. Medical History:

Does your child have any long-term medical conditions for which they are now being or have been treated?   **No**

Does your child take any medication regularly?   **No**

Has your child had a speech examination prior to this time? **No**

Where? _____

When? _____

What were the results?

Has your child had a hearing test prior to this time? **Yes**

Where? **School** When? **Last year**

What were the results?
Results were normal

Has your child had a neurological examination prior to this time? **No**

Where? _____

When? _____

What were the results?

Has your child had a psychological examination prior to this time? **No**

Where? _____

When? _____

What were the results?

Has your child had an eye examination prior to this time? **Yes**

Where? **School** When? **Last year**

What were the results?
Results were normal

Has your child had a recent medical examination? **No**

Where? _____

When? _____

What were the results?

Name of child's pediatrician/physician: **Dr. Ronald Bill**

Address: **900 Wellness Street**

City, State, Zip: **Fayetteville, Arkansas 72703**

Phone #: **846-9005**

Check the following illnesses this child has had:

_____ Measles_____ Influenza_____ Draining Ears_____ Head Injury

_____ Mumps_____ Meningitis_____ Chronic Colds_____ Heart Disease

_____ Whooping Cough_____ Encephalitis **X** Allergies_____ Kidney Disease

X Chicken Pox_____ Epilepsy_____ Sinus Problems_____ High Fever

_____ Scarlet Fever_____ Tonsillitis_____ Excessive Ear Wax

Has this child ever had earaches or ear infections? _____ Yes **X** No. If yes, how often and in

which ear(s)? _____

How was it treated? _____

Has this child ever had a PE tubes, tonsillectomy and/or adenoidectomy? _____ Yes **X** No.

If yes, when _____ Physician _____

Is there a history of hearing loss in the family? _____Yes **X** No If yes, indicate which relative and at
what age the hearing loss was diagnosed. _____

_____

_____

Has your child ever worn a hearing aid? _____ Yes **X** No If yes, what kind of aid and in which
ear(s)? _____

_____

_____

VI. <u>Daily Behavior:</u>

Has your child been harder to manage than other children?   **Not really**

Describe any unusual behavior:

Describe your child's interests:

Sally loves outdoor activities like swimming and going to the beach. She also really likes to draw, especially when it's drawing on the sidewalk with chalk. She has a love for animals and says she wants to be a veterinarian when she grows up.

VII. <u>Speech and Hearing History:</u>

Does your child talk? **Yes**   If not, how does your child communicate?

When did your child first use words meaningfully? **Around a year old**

When did your child begin to use two-word sentences? **Around 18 months**

Does your child understand what you say to him/her? **Yes**

How well is s/he understood by parents? **We understand her well. We know what she is trying to say, even though she can't say 'r'**

By others? **Others seem to also understand Sally pretty well**

Do you think your child hears adequately? **Yes**

If not, what do you feel is the reason?

Has your child had frequent colds or ear problems? **No**

VIII. <u>Educational History:</u>

Has your child repeated any grades? **No**   If so, which ones?

With what subjects has your child had particular difficulties? **None**

Has your child ever had special help through the school? **No**

If so, please describe:

How does your child feel about school? **Sally really enjoys school and being with her friends. Recently though, she's told us that she doesn't like going because she's afraid of talking in front of her classmates, especially when she has to say her teacher's name.**

After receiving Sally's case history, a date was scheduled for an evaluation. During the evaluation, an OME and hearing screening were performed as well as two standardized tests. The results of each of those are as follows:

Summary of Findings:

ORAL MECHANISM EVALUATION: Observation of oral-facial structures was done to assess the structure and function of Sally's oral mechanism. Facial features were judged to be symmetrical. No drooling, anterior tongue carriage or open mouth posture were observed. Tongue size and shape as well as mobility appeared to be normal. No concerns with shape and contour of hard and soft palates were noted. No deviation or bifid in the uvula was noted and no concerns with velopharyngeal closure were noted. Overall, oral motor structures/ functioning appeared to be adequate to support continued speech and language development.

<u>**VOICE AND FLUENCY:**</u> All parameters were considered to be appropriate for her chronological age and gender.

<u>**HEARING SCREENING:**</u> Sally passed a hearing screening, bilaterally.

The two Assessment tests that Mrs. Allen used to evaluate Sally were:

1. The Goldman-Fristoe Test of Articulation-3rd Ed (GFTA-3)

The Goldman-Fristoe Test of Articulation, Third Edition (GFTA-3) assesses articulation of the consonant and consonant cluster sounds of Standard American English. The following scores were obtained:

Sounds in Words

Raw Score	Standard Score	Confidence Interval (95%)	Percentile Rank
11	71	67–79	3

Sounds in Sentences

Raw Score	Standard Score	Confidence Interval (95%)	Percentile Rank
26	64	61–75	1

2. Photo Articulation Test-3rd Ed (PAT-3)

The Photo Articulation Test, Third Edition (PAT-3) was administered in order to assess articulation. The following scores were obtained:

Raw Score	Percentile	Age Equivalent	Standard Score
8	1	4-6	68

Sally ranked in the 1st percentile based on her age group demonstrating articulation errors in the following phonemes:

	Productions
Initial	s/z, w/r, -p, v/b
Medial	d/s, j/l, -m
Final	ch/sh,

3. Clinical Evaluation of Language Fundamentals-Fifth Edition (CELF-5) Screener

The Clinical Evaluation of Language Fundamentals-Fifth Edition (CELF-5) Screener was also administered to Sally. Her scores were within normal limits.

Given the case history, and results from the oral-mech, hearing screening and standardized assessments, Mrs. Allen believes the prognosis for Sally to improve her articulation is good and recommends that Sally come in for speech therapy once a week for 8 weeks.

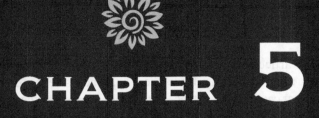

CHAPTER 5

Phonological Disorders: Assessment and Intervention

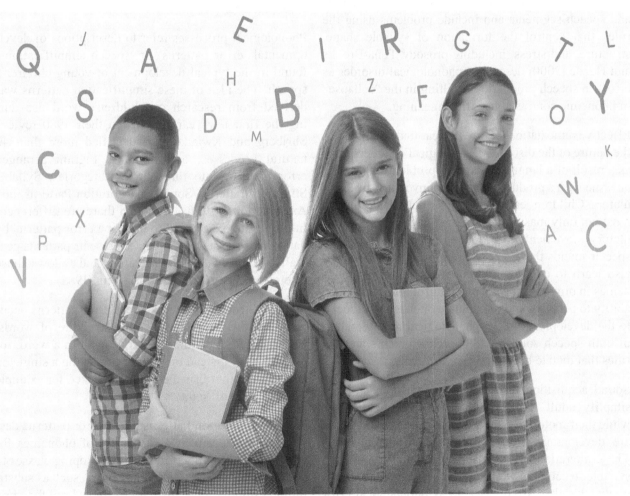

Africa Studio / Shutterstock.com

The previous chapter dealt with articulation disorders which involve speech sounds errors resulting from imprecise articulatory contact that can be due to structural errors, sensory impairments or cognitive delays. These deficits are often referred to as "phonetic disorders" because they deal with the way in which the sounds are produced by the vocal tract. Phonological disorders may appear to sound similar to disorders of articulation; however, the underlying cause is different and the treatment recommended for remediation of phonological disorders is different from what is typically recommended for articulation disorders.

Phonological (phonemic) disorders have a cognitive-linguistic origin in which children have difficulty developing and using the language rules that underlie speech. Phonological disorders refer to difficulties with the phonological representation of speech sounds and speech segments and include problems using the rules that control the formation of syllable shape, structure, and stress, including prosody. Peña-Brooks and Hegde (2000) describe a phonological disorder as errors in speech production resulting in the "collapse" of phonemic contrasts that affect meaning.

Effective remediation requires a clear understanding of the nature of the disorder. Phonological disorders arise as a result of a language learning problem rather than an issue with a production problem involving the articulators. Children learning to speak American English must not only master the different and complex articulatory movements to produce the approximately 44 speech sounds that comprise our language, they must also learn to contrast and combine these same phonemes in order to produce meaningful utterances. The ability to perceive and manipulate phonemes is crucial to the development of the phonological representation of both speech sounds and speech segments and the rules that dictate how words are formed.

Sound acquisition research has shown that children simplify adult forms of words in consistent ways, while their motoric systems and language rule systems are developing to make speech easier to produce. These alterations affect classes of sounds and/or the syllable structure of words and because the changes are predictable they are referred to as phonological error patterns. There are many error patterns described in the literature, and while some are a normal or "natural" part of development, others are not.

When remediating a phonologically based speech disorder, instead of targeting phoneme errors one-at-a-time, as is typically the case for articulatory errors, phonological approaches seeks to determine similarities among error phonemes and the error pattern that is being demonstrated. The goal of phonological approaches is to target these similar error patterns. It is theorized that children will internalize phonological rules and apply these rules to other sounds with the targeted pattern.

PHONOLOGICAL ERROR PATTERNS

One of the most important aspects of a diagnostic evaluation is establishing if a child is indeed using phonological error patterns. This requires careful assessment and analysis of the child's speech. Speech-language pathologists analyze speech by reviewing errors to determine if commonalities exist among them that form patterns.

Phonological processes refer to descriptions of developmental 'error patterns' or 'speech simplifications' found in the typical development of young children's speech. The idea of these simplification patterns was derived from research on children's word use during the first few years of life. In their 1980 review, Shriberg and Kwiatkowski identified more than 40 natural processes, and in 1981, Ingram arranged error patterns into three broad categories: Syllable Structure Patterns, Sounds Substitution Patterns, and Assimilation Patterns. Although there are differences in the terminology used to describe error patterns by various researchers, this chapter presents patterns generally established in the literature and follows those offered by Stoel-Gammon and Dunn (1985).

Syllable Structure Patterns: these error patterns occur when children alter the syllabic structure of words, such as leaving off the final consonant in a word, for example [ko] instead of /kot/, or producing a singleton consonant rather than a consonant cluster, for example [pun] instead of /spun/.

Sound Substitution Patterns: these error patterns describe the replacement of one class of phonemes for another. It is common for earlier developing classes to be exchanged for later developing ones, such as substituting a stop for a fricative, for example [top] for /sop/.

Assimilation Patterns: these error patterns are sometimes referred to as "consonant harmony" because they describe the child's attempt to make the target word easier to produce by making all the consonants in a word similar, for example [lɛlo] for /jɛlo/.

Speech Sound Development

The chart below illustrates the typical developmental progression of individual speech sounds. The sounds within each number indicate the age by which 85% of children have mastered production of that sound. For example, by age 6, 85% of children have mastered production of the "l" sound.

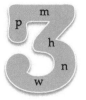 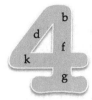 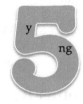 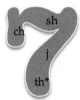 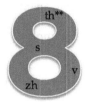

Chart adapted from the following sources: Sander (1972) and Goldman & Fristo (2000)
*voiceless "th" as in "think" and "thing"   **voiced "th" as in "the" and "those"

The following chart illustrates examples of speech sound patterns or phonological processes. These errors are often seen during typical speech development; however, should be phased out by the following ages:

Process/Pattern	Example	Developed out by...
Initial Consonant Voicing	Pat→bat	3;0
Final Consonant De-Voicing	Big→bick	3;0
Stopping of "f" & "s"	Fish→tish, soap→doap	3;0
Final Consonant Deletion	Duck→du, Bus→bu	3;3
Fronting	Cat→tat, Goat→doat	3;6
Stopping of "v" & "z"	Vote→tote, zoom→boom	3;6
Weak syllable deletion	Elephant→efant, Banana→nana	4;0
Cluster Reduction	Spoon→poon, Clap→cap	4;0
Deaffrication	Chore→shore, Jug→dug	4;0
Stopping of "sh" "j" & "ch"	Shop→dop, jump→bump, choo→too	4;6
Gliding	Run→wun, Leg→weg	5;0
Stopping of voiced and voiceless "th"	Them→dem, thing→ting	5;0
Prevocalic Voicing	Came→game, tag→dag	6;0

Chart adapted from Bowen (1998)

Chart designed by Rosie Prehoda, M.A. CCC-SLP. "Speech Sound Development Norms" chart is available for download at: https://www.teacherspayteachers.com/Store/Rosie-Prehoda

PHONOLOGICAL ERROR PATTERN PRACTICE

The exercises below are designed to help you identify the different types of patterns and understand the nature of phonological disorders.

1. **Syllable Structure Patterns:** the syllable structure of a word is changed to make it easier to say. There will either be alterations in the number of syllables of a multisyllabic word or a change the syllable shape of the word.

Weak Syllable Deletion   This pattern can only occurs on multisyllabic words. Typically, the unstressed or "weak" syllable of a word is omitted. Usually, the unstressed syllable will be at the beginning of a word or in the middle of the word. You may recall a young family member requesting [gɛti] for dinner rather than /spəgɛti/.

Examples:

"elephant" /ɛləfənt/ → [ɛfənt]
"potato" /pəteto/→[teto]
"television" /tɛləvɪʒɪn /→[təvɪʒɪn]

Final Consonant Deletion   This pattern is very common and results when a CVC target word is produced with open syllable because the final singleton consonant is omitted.

Examples:

"boot" /but/→[bu]
"run" /rʌn/→[rʌ]
"set" /sɛt/→[sɛ]

Initial Consonant Deletion   This pattern is not as common as Final Consonant Deletion and it is not considered a natural pattern or one that is seen in normal development. As the name implies, the initial singleton consonant is deleted.

Examples:

"show" /ʃo/→[o]
"hug" /hʌg/→[ʌg]
"wet" /wɛt/→[ɛt]

Epenthesis   This pattern is characterized by the insertion of a vowel, usually the schwa, between a consonant cluster, which results in an extra syllable in the target word. The addition of a vowel, such as the schwa, between a consonant cluster simplifies the production of the cluster. Epenthesis actually occurs when any extra phoneme, be it consonant or vowel, is inserted in a word, but most occurrences involve insertion of the schwa.

Examples:

"claw" /klɔ/→[kəlɔ]
"glass" /glæs/→[gəlæs]
"spy" /spaɪ/→[səpaɪ]

Reduplication   This pattern, sometimes referred to as "doubling," occurs when a syllable is completely or partially repeated. Typically, it is the first syllable of a bisyllabic word that is repeated.

Examples:

"table" /tebəl/→[tata]
"water" /wɑtɚ/→[wɑwɑ]
"basket" /bæskət/→[bæbæ]

Diminutization   This pattern describes the insertion of [i] at the end of a word resulting in an extra syllable in a word.

Examples:

"boot" /but/→[buti]
"dog" /dɑg/→[dɑgi]
"horse" /hɔrs/→[hɔrsi]

Cluster Reduction or Deletion   These patterns occur when children attempt to simplify a consonant cluster by omitting a part of it or the whole cluster. Typically, the most difficult to produce consonant will be the one that is omitted from the cluster.

Examples:

"spot" /spɑt/→[pɑt] (cluster reduction)
"bring" /brɪŋ/→[rɪŋ] (cluster reduction)
"great" /gret/→[et] (cluster deletion)

Substitution Patterns   This is the most common type of simplification and occurs when one sound is substituted for another sound independent of phonetic context, i.e., the sound change is not due to assimilation. In order to be considered a substitution pattern, there must be a systematic sound change that affects classes of sounds or sound sequences.

Stopping   This error pattern occurs when a stop phoneme replaces a fricative or an affricate sound. Most often, the substituted stop will have the same manner of articulation and voicing as the target sound that it replaces.

Examples:

"fish" /fɪʃ/→[tɪʃ]
"soap" /sop/→[pop]
"jump" /dʒʌmp/→[dʌmp]

Exercise 5.1   Transcribe the following words showing weak syllable deletion.

1. supposed to _____

2. caravan _____

3. octopus _____

4. tomato _____

5. nursery _____

6. photograph _____

7. butterfly _____

8. computer _____

9. banana _____

10. tomorrow _____

Exercise 5.2 Transcribe the following words showing the effect of final consonant deletion (FCD) or initial consonant deletion (ICD). If one of these error patterns is not possible, write NP.

Target	FCD	ICD
1. shut	_____	_____
2. right	_____	_____
3. Jim	_____	_____
4. fat	_____	_____
5. buy	_____	_____
6. dime	_____	_____
7. whack	_____	_____
8. king	_____	_____
9. mow	_____	_____
10. lake	_____	_____

Exercise 5.3 Transcribe the following words showing epenthesis.

1. plastic	_____		6. slap	_____
2. class	_____		7. glove	_____
3. brush	_____		8. cross	_____
4. brick	_____		9. snow	_____
5. prince	_____		10. plate	_____

Exercise 5.4 Transcribe the following words showing reduplication.

1. copy	_____		6. bottle	_____
2. picture	_____		7. water	_____
3. sister	_____		8. brother	_____
4. cupcake	_____		9. stomach	_____
5. burger	_____		10. soda	_____

Stridency Deletion This simplification pattern occurs when a strident phoneme is replaced with a non-strident sound or when a strident sound is deleted.

Examples:

> "soap" /sop/→[θop]
> "soap" /sop/→[top]
> "soap" /sop/→[op]

Fronting This pattern involves a change in place of articulation. Palatal and velar sounds /ʧ ʤ ʃ ʒ k g ŋ/ are replaced with sounds with a more anterior placement, most commonly the stops /t/ and /d/.

Examples:

> "cop" /kɑp/→[tɑp]
> "gate" /get/→[tet]
> "key" /ki/→[ti]

Depalatalization For this pattern, a palaltal obsturent sound is replaced by a more anterior nonpalatal obstruent sound.

Examples:

> "shoe" /ʃu/→[tu]
> "beige" /beʒ/→[bed]
> "chin" /ʧɪn/→[sɪn]

Alveolarization This pattern describes a minor shift in the place of articulation from the lips or teeth to the alveolar ridge. The sound substitution will only involves obstruents.

Examples:

> "bee" /bi/→[di]
> "thick" /θɪk/→[tɪk]
> "fast" /fæst/→[tæst]

Labialization This pattern also describes a minor shift in the place of articulation from the alveolar ridge or teeth to the lips. Similar to alveolarization, labialization only involves obstruents.

Examples:

> "doll" /dɑl/→[bɑl]
> "thank" /θeŋk/→[peŋk]
> "sit" /sɪt/→[pɪt]

Exercise 5.5 Transcribe the following words showing diminutization.

1. bird _____   6. feet _____

2. fish _____   7. leg _____

3. book _____   8. sheep _____

4. bell _____   9. boat _____

5. pig _____   10. rain _____

Exercise 5.6 Transcribe the following words showing cluster reduction or deletion. If cluster reduction or deletion is not possible for the word, write NP.

1. bread _____   6. stew _____

2. trip _____   7. tick _____

3. frog _____   8. glue _____

4. crawl _____   9. cloak _____

5. floor _____   10. flea _____

Exercise 5.7   Transcribe the following words showing stopping.

1. fat   _____
2. love   _____
3. sun   _____
4. calf   _____
5. shop   _____

6. see   _____
7. wish   _____
8. puzzle   _____
9. dress   _____
10. face   _____

Exercise 5.8   Transcribe the following words showing stridency deletion.

1. beach   _____
2. moose   _____
3. cheese   _____
4. castle   _____
5. fold   _____

6. shape   _____
7. cliff   _____
8. file   _____
9. beef   _____
10. ace   _____

Exercise 5.9   Transcribe the following words showing fronting.

1. cookie   _____
2. ship   _____
3. chair   _____
4. game   _____
5. cake   _____

6. shop   _____
7. kite   _____
8. shy   _____
9. cheap   _____
10. goose   _____

Gliding   This is a very common error pattern among young children and involves the replacement of liquids with glides.

Examples:

"rocket" /rɑkɪt/→[wɑkɪt]
"leak" /lik/→[wik]
"listen" /lɪsɪn/→[jɪsɪn]

Vowelization   This error pattern occurs when syllabic liquids or nasals, rhotic diphongs, rhotic central vowels, or velar [L] sounds are replaced with vowels.

The vowels most commonly substituted are [ə], [o], and [ʊ]. This pattern is sometimes referred to as "vocalization."

Examples:

"apple" /æpəl/→[æpo]
"color" /kʌlɚ/→[kcʌlə]
"hair" /hɛr/→[hɛə]

Assimilation Simplification Patterns   These simplification patterns describe a sound becoming more like a neighboring sounds, i.e., the sound change is due to the influence of phonetic context (Mackay, 1987).

These simplification patterns are sometimes called "consonant harmony."

Labial Assimilation

This assimilation occurs when a child changes a non-labial phoneme to a labial phoneme due to the presence of a neighboring labial phoneme in a word. Can be complete or partial and progressive or regressive.

Examples:

"bug" /bʌg/→[bʌb] (complete, progressive)
"pen" /pɪn/→[pɪb] (partial, progressive)
"cop" /kɑp/→[bɑp] (partial, regressive)

Alveolar Assimilation

This assimilation occurs when a sound changes to a alveolar due to the influence of another alveolar in the word. Can be complete or partial and progressive or regressive.

Examples:

"goat" /got/→[tot] (complete, regressive)
"toss" /tɑs/→[tɑt] (complete, progressive)
"kid" /kɪd/→[tɪd] (partial, regressive)

Exercise 5.10   Transcribe the following words showing depalatalization.

1. rush   _____
2. shape   _____
3. jar   _____
4. brush   _____
5. coach   _____

6. wrench   _____
7. enjoy   _____
8. change   _____
9. share   _____
10. dish   _____

Exercise 5.11   Transcribe the following words showing alveolarization.

1. the   _____
2. make   _____
3. pony   _____
4. vote   _____
5. third   _____

6. think   _____
7. thief   _____
8. pie   _____
9. bunny   _____
10. feet   _____

Exercise 5.12   Transcribe the following words showing labialization.

1. teeth   _____
2. tall   _____
3. dime   _____
4. desk   _____
5. thaw   _____

6. thunder   _____
7. thorn   _____
8. time   _____
9. soft   _____
10. safe   _____

Velar Assimilation This assimilation occurs when a sound changes to a velar due to the influence of another velar in the word. Can be complete or partial and progressive or regressive.

Examples:

"keep" /kip/→[kig] (partial progressive)
"goat" /got/→[gog] (complete progressive)
"rug" /rʌg/→[kʌg] (partial regressive)

Nasal Assimilation This assimilation occurs when a sound changes to a nasal due to the influence of another nasal in the word. Can be complete or partial and progressive or regressive.

"fan" /fæn/→[næn] (complete regressive)
"mode" /mod/→[mon] (partial progressive)
"ring" /rɪŋ/→[nɪŋ] (partial regressive)

Prevocalic Voicing This pattern results when a voiceless obstruent preceding a vowel becomes voiced.

Examples:

"cat" /kæt/→[gæt]
"sad" /sæd/→[zæd]
"cheap" /ʧip/→[ʤip]

Exercise 5.13   Transcribe the following words showing gliding.

1. lamp _____
2. list _____
3. radio _____
4. late _____
5. rip _____

6. wrist _____
7. walrus _____
8. lazy _____
9. lot _____
10. leaf _____

Exercise 5.14   Transcribe the following words showing vowelization.

1. paper _____
2. people _____
3. pencil _____
4. mail _____
5. bird _____

6. brother _____
7. power _____
8. letter _____
9. muscle _____
10. flower _____

Exercise 5.15   Transcribe the following words showing labial assimilation.

1. wax _____
2. moss _____
3. bean _____
4. Mike _____
5. wrap _____

6. rope _____
7. zoom _____
8. bike _____
9. maze _____
10. pet _____

Postvocalic Devoicing The pattern occurs when a voiced obstruent in the final position of a word becomes voiceless.

Examples:

"pig" /pɪg/→[pɪk]
"dad" /dæd/→[dæt]
"give" /gɪv/→[gɪf]

Children with speech sound production issues that appear to be phonologically based, may have a broader phonological processing problem. Phonological processing is just as it sounds—the ability to use the sounds of your language to process both spoken and written language (Wagner & Torgesen, 1987). There are three distinct components of phonological processing: phonological awareness, phonological working memory, and phonological retrieval—all three play a part in not only the development of speech production but also in reading and writing skills, therefore, these abilities will all be discussed in more detail later in the literacy chapter. Children with an expressive speech disorder that is phonological in nature, should be screened for broader phonological processing issues and spoken and written language development should be closely monitored. It may also be necessary to incorporate goals related to phonological awareness, phonological working memory, and phonological retrieval

---

Exercise 5.16 Transcribe the following words showing alveolar assimilation.

1. bat	_____	6. duck	_____
2. team	_____	7. coat	_____
3. body	_____	8. fruit	_____
4. kite	_____	9. road	_____
5. root	_____	10. ride	_____

Exercise 5.17 Transcribe the following words showing velar assimilation.

1. cone	_____	6. neck	_____
2. gas	_____	7. twig	_____
3. gold	_____	8. cap	_____
4. kid	_____	9. hike	_____
5. rock	_____	10. cave	_____

Exercise 5.18 Transcribe the following words showing nasal assimilation.

1. mess	_____	6. toxin	_____
2. lung	_____	7. zoom	_____
3. bum	_____	8. much	_____
4. pain	_____	9. knock	_____
5. nest	_____	10. Molly	_____

Exercise 5.19   Transcribe the following words showing prevocalic voicing.

1. tide _____
2. peach _____
3. sock _____
4. shake _____
5. salt _____

6. turkey _____
7. kite _____
8. pass _____
9. chase _____
10. poke _____

Exercise 5.20   Transcribe the following words showing postvocalic devoicing.

1. wig _____
2. bread _____
3. loud _____
4. ride _____
5. tube _____

6. Doug _____
7. frog _____
8. prize _____
9. knob _____
10. played _____

into treatment plans as deficits in these areas can hinder the development of literacy skills (Anthony et al., 2011; Leitão & Fletcher, 2004;) Bishop and Adams (1990) found that children who exhibit unintelligible speech at 5½ years of age will oftentimes also exhibit problems with decoding and spelling.

TREATMENT APPROACHES

Phonological approaches are chosen in hopes that children will internalize phonological rules and generalize these rules to other sounds with similar error patterns (e.g., stridency deletion, cluster reduction). In therapy minimal pairs (i.e., pairs of words that differ by a single phoneme) are used and emphasis is placed on the function of sounds and the internalizing of phonemic rules and contrasts.

There are several popular treatment approaches for remediation of phonological speech sound disorder. Please refer to https://www.asha.org/PRPSpecificTopic.aspx?folderid=8589935321&section=Treatment for additional information on treatment of phonological disorders. Many of them focus on "contrasting" word pairs and

differentiating the sound properties among phonemes that produce different words. For example, the words "bat" and "pat" differ by the feature of voicing. Minimal Pairs, Maximal Oppositions, and Multiple Oppositions are examples of contrast therapy approaches.

Maximal Oppositions—This approach uses pairs of words with one of the words containing a speech sound produced correctly by the child. The correctly produced sound is contrasting with a maximally opposing sound that is not produced correctly by the child. For example, the child is unable to produce the /s/ phoneme, but is able to produce /m/. Words such as meat and seat would be chosen to contrast the maximally opposed /s/ and /m/ (Gierut, 1989, 1990, 1992).

Multiple Oppositions—This approach is highly useful for children with moderate to severe phonological disorder and is a linguistic approach to speech therapy. It is similar to the Minimal Pair approach, but differs in that more sounds errors are targeted. The rational is that children who produce a significant number of speech sound errors may substitute or "collapse" several sounds into one single sound. Several speech sound errors are targeted and contrasted during the same session (Williams), 2000a, 2000b). An example of phoneme collapse would be the replacement of the sounds /k/, /p/, /h/, and /tr/ with /t/. This may possibly result in the words *Kay* /ke/, *pay* /pe/, *hay* /he/, and *tray* /tre/ all being produced [te].

Cycles Approach—Designed for highly unintelligible children, the Cycles Approach was developed in 1983 by Barbara Hodson and Elaine Paden. The approach is based on the theory that normal phonological development is gradual and that easier to produce or "primary" patterns are obtained before more complex "secondary" ones. The aim of each "cycle" is to simulate the emergence of sounds and/or patterns, therefore increasing the child's intelligibility in a brief timeframe. Once target patterns are identified through phonological assessment, each pattern is trained for a total of 60 minutes before moving onto subsequent patterns. All primary phonological patterns are targeted each cycle of treatment before moving onto secondary targets and a different cycle. After once cycle has been completed another cycle begins. Cycles continue until all targeted patterns are correctly produced in the child's conversational speech. Treatment is discontinued when the children reaches a specified criteria level (e.g., 100% production across three consecutive sessions) (Hodson, 2010; Prezas & Hodson, 2010).

Metaphon Therapy—The rationale behind this approach is that children with phonological issues have not acquired the rules of the phonological system properly; therefore, metaphonological awareness (i.e., the awareness of the phonological structure of language is taught by contrasting sound properties). For example, for children who consistently "stop" continuant speech sounds, the concept of "short" (stops) versus "long" (continent) sounds are presented. It is recommended that patterns that will have the most impact on intelligibility, are stimulable, or are not seen in typically developing children of a similar age be targeted first (Howell & Dean, 1991).

REFERENCES

Anthony, J. L., Williams, J. M., Durán, L. K., Gillam, S. L., Liang, L., Aghara, R., ... & Landry, S. H. (2011). Spanish phonological awareness: Dimensionality and sequence of development during the preschool and kindergarten years. *Journal of Educational Psychology, 103*(4), 857.

Dean, E., & Howell, J. (1991). *Treating phonological disorders in children: metaphon: theory to practice*. Far Communications

Leitão, S., & Fletcher, J. (2004). Literacy outcomes for students with speech impairment: long-term follow-up. *International Journal of Language & Communication Disorders, 39*(2), 245–256.

Peña-Brooks, A., & Hegde, M. N. (2000). *Assessment and treatment of articulation and phonological disorders in children: A dual level text*. Austin, TX: Pro-Ed.

Ingram, D. (1981). *Procedures for the phonological analysis of children's language*. Baltimore, MD: University Park Press.

Shriberg, L. D., & Kwiatkowski, J. (1980). *Natural process analysis: A procedure for phonological analysis of continuous speech samples*. New York, NY: Wiley.

Stoel-Gammon, C., & Dunn, C. (1985). *Normal and disordered phonology in children*. Baltimore, MD: University Park Press.

Newman, David. *Multiple Oppositions Therapy*. N.p., Sept. 2014. Web. 24 Apr. 2016

Wagner, R. K., & Torgesen, J. K. (1987). The nature of phonological processing and its causal role in the acquisition of reading skills. *Psychological Bulletin, 101*(2), 192–212.

Bishop, D. V., & Adams, C. (1990). A prospective study of the relationship between specific language impairment, phonological disorders and reading retardation. *Journal of Child Psychology and Psychiatry, 31*(7), 1027–1050.

Williams, A. L. (2000). Multiple oppositions: Theoretical foundations for an alternative contrastive intervention approach. *American Journal of Speech-Language Pathology, 9*(4), 282–288.

Williams, A. L. (2000). Multiple oppositions: Case studies of variables in phonological intervention. *American Journal of Speech-Language Pathology, 9*(4), 289–299.

Chapter 5   Activities

NAME: _____   DATE: _____

The following 5 therapy goals are missing vital details. Apply the skills you learned in Chapter 1 to correct these goals and make them *SMART* goals.

PHONOLOGY:

Expressive:

1. In six months, the patient will imitate syllables during therapy as measured through observation, with 90% accuracy given visual models and verbal prompts.

2. By the end of the IEP, the patient will communicate in utterances with 80% intelligibility, as measured by observation, within structured tasks and given picture and verbal cues.

3. Over five consecutive sessions, the patient will produce words with appropriate syllabic stress with 80% accuracy, as measured by observation during a structured task and given limited verbal prompts.

4. By the end of the IEP, the patient will correctly produce final consonants with 80% accuracy as measured by observation when engaged in a structured activity.

5. By the end of the IEP, the patient will produce continuant speech sounds in words without stopping with 80% accuracy as measured by observation.

Report Writing Practice

Use the following case history and diagnostic information along with skills learned in this chapter and in Chapter 1 to write a diagnostic report (See Appendix F for a diagnostic report example).

Report Writing Activity: PHONOLOGY

SPEECH/LANGUAGE/HEARING Case History/ CHILD

I. General Information Child's Name: Carson Jones Phone: 453-6780

Birth Date: January 19, 2013   Age: 5 years   Sex: Male   Grade: Kindergarten

Address: 870 Stapleton Street   City: Orlando   State: Florida Zip: 32004

School: Orlando Primary School   Teacher: Mrs. Franklin   School District: Orlando School District

Father's Name: William Jones   Age: 32   Address: 870 Stapleton Street   City: Orlando
State: Florida   Zip: 32004   Occupation: Sales Representative Business   Phone: 213-5900
Place of Occupation: AT&T Education;   number of years completed: 13;   high school diploma

Mother's Name: Tammy Jones   Age: 32   Address: 870 Stapleton Street   City: Orlando
State: Florida   Zip: 32004   Occupation: Dental Assistant Business   Phone: 233-4506
Place of Occupation: Smiles Dental Education;   number of years completed: 13;
high school diploma + on the job training

If mother is employed, who cares for the child?   When not in school, Carson is watched by older brother

Who will be responsible for payment of charges?   Medicaid

Brothers and/or sisters of the child: Name: Louis Jones   Age: 12 School: Orlando Middle
School   Grade: 7th grade

Relatives or others living in the home: Name: N/A   Relationship: N/A

Who referred you to the University of Arkansas Speech and Hearing Clinic?

Name: Mrs. Franklin   Relationship: Carson's school teacher   Address: 100 Learning Ave.
City: Orlando   State: Florida   Zip: 32005

II. Statement of the Problem:

Describe the problem: Instead of Carson saying "THank you", he says "ank you". He also can't say his name very well, he leaves out the 's' in both his first and last name.

When was the problem first noticed? Carson has always had this problem, but we didn't think anything of it because we figured he would grow out of it.

What has been done about it? Carson's kindergarten teacher recommended we get his hearing checked and a speech evaluation because she thought he may be a little behind his other kindergarten classmates.

What is the child's reaction to the problem? Carson doesn't seem to notice his speech problems.

III. Pregnancy and Birth History:

During this pregnancy did the mother experience any unusual illness, condition or accident? If so, describe: No

Were there any complications during the delivery such as caesarean, extremely long labor, or use of instruments? No

IV. Developmental History:

At what age did the following occur?

Sat alone unsupported: 7 months Crawled: 9 months Walked alone: 11months

Maintained bowel and bladder control while awake: 4 years asleep: 5 years

Does the child seem awkward or uncoordinated? No

V. Medical History:

Does your child have any long-term medical conditions for which they are now being or have been treated? No

Does your child take any medication regularly? No

Has your child had a speech examination prior to this time? No

Has your child had a hearing test prior to this time? Only when he was born — his newborn hearing screen

Where? Hospital When? 2013

What were the results? It took him a while to pass but his results came back normal.

Has your child had a psychological examination prior to this time? No

Has your child had an eye examination prior to this time? No

Has your child had a recent medical examination? No

Name of child's pediatrician/physician: Dr. Courtney Wood

Address: 14 Checkup Ave.

City, State, Zip: Orlando, Florida 32009 Phone #: 571-3400

Check the following illnesses this child has had:

_____ Measles _____ Influenza __ X __ Draining Ears _____ Head Injury

_____ Mumps _____ Meningitis _____Chronic Colds _____ Heart Disease

_____ Whooping Cough _____ Encephalitis _____ Allergies _____ Kidney Disease

_____ Chicken Pox _____ Epilepsy _____ Sinus Problems _____ High Fever

_____ Scarlet Fever _____ Tonsillitis _____ Excessive Ear Wax

Has this child ever had earaches or ear infections? __ X __ Yes ____ No. If yes, how often and in

which ear(s)? __ Carson had them frequently ear infections when he was younger, mainly in his right ear

_____

How was it treated? _____ Carson got tubes put in his ears to help with draining the fluid

_____

Has this child ever had a PE tubes, tonsillectomy and/or adenoidectomy? __ X ____ Yes ____ No.

If yes, when __ Carson got his tubes when he was around 2–3 years _____ Physician _____ Dr. Wood
_____

Is there a history of hearing loss in the family? __ X __ Yes __ No If yes, indicate which relative and at what age the hearing loss was diagnosed. ____ Carson's older brother, Louis was born with hearing loss

Has your child ever worn a hearing aid? _____ Yes _ X _ No If yes, what kind of aid and in which ear(s)?

VI. Daily Behavior:

Has your child been harder to manage than other children? Not typically.

Describe any unusual behavior:

Describe your child's interests: Carson loves racecars and remote-control cars. Because his brother is a number of years older, Carson usually plays well by himself. He likes building towers with blocks and other toys he can find.

VII. Speech and Hearing History:

Does your child talk? Yes If not, how does your child communicate?

When did your child first use words meaningfully? Around 18 months

When did your child begin to use two-word sentences? Around 24 months

Does your child understand what you say to him/her? Yes, I seem to think so

How well is s/he understood by parents? It takes some concentration, but I think my husband and I can understand Carson pretty well

By others? Others sometimes have a hard time understanding Carson

Do you think your child hears adequately? I think so

If not, what do you feel is the reason? He may have trouble hearing because of his frequent ear infections as a small child

Has your child had frequent colds or ear problems? Yes

VIII. Educational History:

Has your child repeated any grades? No If so, which ones?

With what subjects has your child had particular difficulties? Even though Carson is only in kindergarten, he doesn't seem to like reading or spelling

How does your child feel about school? So far, Carson really enjoys school. He doesn't care for spelling or when he is made to sit and practice reading, but he likes going and being social with his friends!

After receiving Carson's case history, a date was scheduled for an evaluation. During the evaluation, an OME and hearing screening were performed as well as two standardized assessments. The results of each of those are as follows:

Summary of Findings:

<u>**ORAL MECHANISM EVALUATION:**</u> Observation of oral-facial structures was done to assess the structure and function of Carson's oral mechanism. Facial features were judged to be symmetrical. No drooling, anterior tongue carriage or open mouth posture were observed. Tongue size and shape as well as mobility appeared to be normal. No concerns with shape and contour of hard and soft palates were noted. No deviation or bifid in the uvula was noted and no concerns with velopharyngeal closure were noted. Overall, oral motor structures/functioning appeared to be adequate to support continued speech and language development.

<u>**VOICE AND FLUENCY:**</u> All parameters were considered to be appropriate for her chronological age and gender.

<u>**HEARING SCREENING:**</u> Carson passed a hearing screening, bilaterally.

The two Assessment tests that Mrs. Edwards used to evaluate Carson were:

1. Khan-Lewis Phonological Analysis 3rd Ed. (KLPA-3)

	Phonological Process	**Number of Occurrences**	**Total Possible Occurrences**	**Percent of Occurrences**
Manner	Affrication	102	of 151 =	68%
	Frication	0	of 111 =	0%
	Gliding	46	of 81 =	56%
	Glottal replacement	0	of 159 =	0%
	Liquidization	0	of 124 =	0%
	Stopping	32	of 59 =	54%
Place	Backing to velars of /h/	0	of 134 =	0%
Reduction	Deletion of initial consonant	0	of 58 =	58%
	Deletion of medial consonant	0	of 27 =	0%
Voicing	Initial devoicing	0	of 41 =	0%
	Medial devoicing	0	of 22 =	0%
	Medial Voicing	0	of 11 =	0%

Carson demonstrated errors in stopping, gliding, and affrication. Stopping occurs when a stop consonant (b/p/t/d/g) is placed at the beginning of a word. For example, the word "soap" may sound like the word "dope". Gliding is when a liquid consonant (/l, r/) is replaced with a glide consonant (/w, y/). An example of gliding would be saying the word "wabbit" for "rabbit". Affrication is where a non affricate consonant is replaced with an affricate (/ch/ /j/). For example, the word "door" may be pronounced at "joor".

2. Comprehensive Test of Phonological Processing (CTOPP)

Subtest	Raw Score	Scaled Score	%ile Rank (mean = 50%)	Descriptive Term
Elision	3	13	37%	Average
Blending Words	8			
Sound Matching	5			
Memory for Digits	12	10	50%	Average
Non-word Repetition	13			
Rapid Digit Naming	51	10	50%	Average
Rapid Letter Naming	63	10	50%	Average
Rapid Color Naming	56	10	50%	Average
Rapid Object Naming	60			

3. Developmental Indicators for Assessment of Learning, Fourth Edition:

Total Score	Standard Score	Percentile Rank	Decision	
			Cutoff level	OK/Potential Delay
30	82	11%	7%	OK

Given the case history, and results from the oral-mech, hearing screening and Assessment tests, Mrs. Edwards believes the prognosis for Carson to improve his phonology is good. Mrs. Edwards recommends that Carson comes in for speech therapy once a week for an hour.

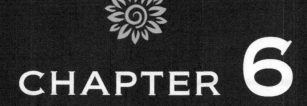

CHAPTER 6

Early Intervention for Language Skills

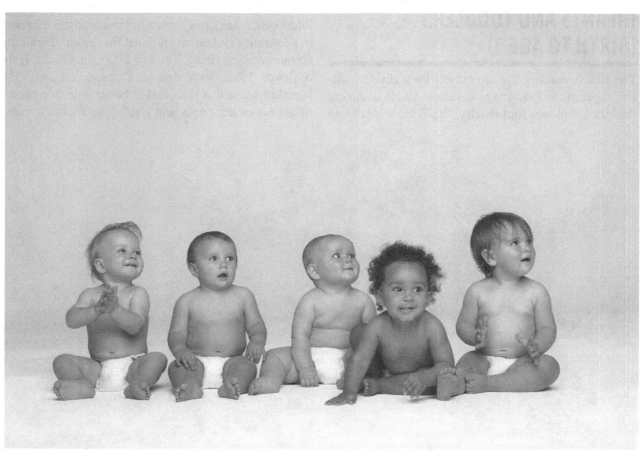

"Play gives children a chance to practice what they are learning."

—Fred Rogers

OVERVIEW

The purpose of this chapter is to provide a review of early language development milestones and to discuss how interventionists can facilitate these skills with infants and toddlers. Play skills are of the utmost importance for this age group. It is critical for parents to understand not only what milestones are appropriate for their child, but also how to utilize play so that interactions are purposeful and communicative learning opportunities for their child. It is often the role of the interventionist to provide parents and caregivers with this information as well as to demonstrate how to facilitate these skills.

LANGUAGE MILESTONES FOR INFANTS AND TODDLERS (BIRTH TO AGE 3)

The first 3 years of life are critical for a child's auditory, speech, and language development. It is during this time that **neuroplasticity**, the brain's ability to reorganize itself and form unique neural connections, is at its highest capacity (Sharma & Nash, 2009). The human brain has the ability to reorganize throughout the entire lifespan; however, the rate at which neural connections take place significantly slows after the age of three. This knowledge can help to validate that humans can continue to learn throughout their life. There is no "cut-off" age for learning, but rather a reduced rate of neural reorganization. Research has well-supported the notion that early intervention is effective and important, especially for children with developmental delays and for those from disadvantaged backgrounds (Bryant & Ramey, 1987; Guralnick, 1997; Guralnick & Bricker, 1987; Olson, 1987; Rossetti, 2001; Shonkoff & Hauser-Cram, 1987).

Children with communication delays are not the only beneficiaries of early intervention. Family-focused early intervention has been shown to have a positive impact in the family system and not just for the child with the communication delay (Bruder, 2000; Innocenti, Huh, & Boyce, 1992; Orr, Cameron, Dobson, & Day, 1993). It makes sense that if a child is better able to communicate his or her needs and wants, the frustration and

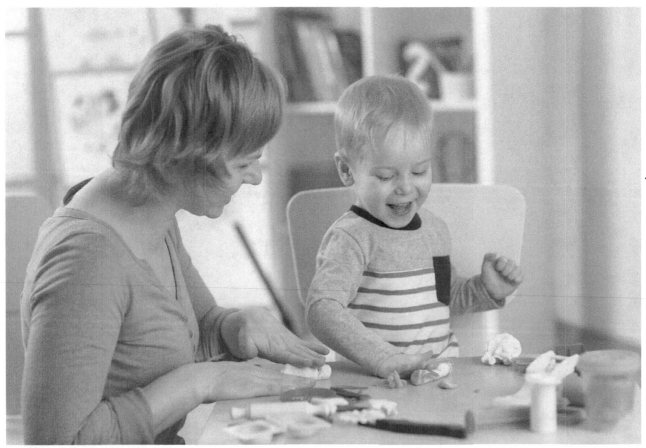

Oksana Kuzmina/Shutterstock.com

potential source of stress from the frustration both subside. This creates an improved environment for all involved in the child's life.

For language intervention to be effective, the interventionist and parent need to be aware of what skills are normal for both the child's **chronological age** and the child's **developmental age**. A child's chronological age is the age that is measured from the time of his or her birth. The developmental age is measured based on the child's development. For example, if a 3-year-old boy produced language skills at an 18-month-old level, his chronological age would be 3 years; however, his developmental age would be 18 months. This information is critical for an interventionist to consider when developing an intervention plan. It is inappropriate for an interventionist to utilize activities in therapy sessions that are far beyond the child's developmental age. For example, "play-doh" is a great toy to facilitate language skills; however, it would be inappropriate to use this toy with a 6 months old (in chronological age or developmental age), who is likely to put the toy in his or her mouth.

That being said, interventionists are to be aware of the need to explain communication developmental milestones as they relate to both the child's chronological age and developmental age. The treatment plan (a.k.a. plan of care) for a child with a language delay should be designed based on the child's current developmental skills (developmental age) and the interventionist's desired outcomes (skills appropriate for chronological age or an improvement in developmental skills). See Table 6.1 *Communication and Play Milestones* for a reference of communication and play skills developmental milestones based on *chronological* age.

Clear and concise resources that are both easy to understand and informative for service providers and families are needed. A couple of parent resources recently developed by the American Speech Language Hearing Association (ASHA) include the *"Identify the Signs"* campaign (www.identifythesigns.org) and *"Communicating with Baby: Tips and Milestones from Birth to Age 5"* (www.identifythesigns.org/communicating-with-baby-toolkit/).

As previously mentioned, play skills are critical for children because structured, semi-structured, and free play are the primary means of education for infants and toddlers. A solid knowledge base in age-appropriate play skills is needed by interventionists. Refer to Table 6.1

for a reference of play skill development based on chronological age. Clinicians are also encouraged to reference and use the Westby Developmental Playscale, Revised (Westby, 2000) when determining a child's play skills and generating a developmentally appropriate plan of care. First document what skills a child is exhibiting and in what matter the child is attempting to communicate before documenting everything the child is unable to do or goals the child has yet to achieve.

CAREGIVER COACHING

There may be times that, even when powered with excellent training, resources, and references, an interventionist may feel that a child with whom he or she is working is not making progress at expected rates. An interventionist is with the child only a small amount of time each week so it is the child's family that is the most important factor in facilitating language development. It is imperative that parents/caregivers be involved in the intervention process (Odom & Wolery, 2003). Caregiver coaching has been shown to be an effective means by which to facilitate communication as part of an early intervention program (Kaiser & Hancock, 2003; Woods, Kashinath, & Goldstein, 2004; Yoder & Warren, 2002). As a young interventionist, it may be intimidating to talk to parents/caregivers. Gaining knowledge in caregiver coaching strategies can help to ease the intimidation factor. In 1991, Stonestreet, Johnson, and Acton developed a list of recommendations to set the standard for developing a functional and efficient relationship with parents. Recommendations included creating a positive atmosphere, recognizing that each family has specific and individual needs, ensuring that caregivers have a feeling potential for positive change and success, developing active listening skills (see chapter 2 for information on auditory skill development), educating families on all potential communication and intervention options, facilitating and encouraging parent interaction and involvement in the intervention process, explaining all medical terminology used (including terminology in evaluation reports) in a way that is easy for parents to understand, understating and allowing time for a grieving process following a diagnosis, providing parents peer support if possible, ensuring parents play active roles in the development of the plan of care, and focusing on outcomes and progress (rather than lack of skill or delay).

A commonly used model for caregiver training in early intervention is the *Hanen Early Language Parent*

Table 6.1 Communication and Play Milestones

0–3 Months			
Receptive Language	**Expressive Language**	**Cognition**	**Social Communication (Pragmatics) and Play**
• Startles to sudden noises • Quiets to familiar voice • Sensitive to prosodic and rhythmic noises • Responds to speaker's face • Responds to talking by quietening or smiling	• Cries to express hunger and anger • Begins to vocalize to express pleasure • Occasionally vocalizes in response (especially to primary caregiver's voice) • Attempts to imitate noises heard by three months	• Awareness of familiar people/situations • Looks at objects/faces briefly • Anticipates certain events, e.g., being fed	• Appears to listen to speaker • Regularly looks directly at speaker's face by three months • Watches mouth of speaker rather than whole face • Smiles/coos in response, in particular to mother/primary caregiver • Emerging ability to imitate facial expressions
4–6 Months			
Receptive Language	**Expressive Language**	**Cognition**	**Social Communication (Pragmatics) and Play**
• Usually stops crying in response to familiar voice • Frequently localizes sound source with head or eye turn • Discriminates between angry and friendly vocal tones • Demonstrates understanding for the meaning of "no" by 6 months • Understands names associated with primary caregivers by 6 months	• Vocalizes for needs and wants • Vocalizes in response to singing, to speech, and during play activities • Blows raspberries, coos, yells, gurgles • Starts to use a variety of vocalizations to express happiness, contentment, and displeasure • Vocalizes when alone or with others	• Demonstrates joint attention • Reaches for desired items/objects • Starts to learn about cause and effect (e.g., plays with rattle) • Recognizes familiar people • Mouths objects/toys in play	• Maintains eye contact • Loves games such as "Peek-A-Boo", "Patty Cake" • Produces differentiated vocalizations for different reasons • Imitates facial expressions • Initiates communication interactions • Emerging understanding of vocal turn taking
7–9 Months			
Receptive Language	**Expressive Language**	**Cognition**	**Social Communication (Pragmatics) and Play**
• Responds with appropriate arm gestures when prompted with familiar phrases: "up up, hi, bye bye"	• Babbles consistently • Imitates CV syllables in babble [pa pa] • Vocalizes in response to name	• Imitates physical actions • Recognizes familiar objects • Places object in one hand and then the other	• Desires communication interactions • Emerging anticipation of familiar activities • Nods, waves and claps

7–9 Months			
Receptive Language	**Expressive Language**	**Cognition**	**Social Communication (Pragmatics) and Play**
• Enjoys music or singing • Consistently stops activity when name is called • Identifies names of a few familiar objects by localizing them when they are named • More regularly stops activity in response to "no" • Will sustain interest up to a minute while looking at pictures or books with adults • Emerging ability to follow simple commands	• Emerging ability to initiate communication interaction games, e.g., Pat-a-cake, Peek-a-Boo, hand clapping, etc. • Emerging ability to "sing" • Vocalizes for greetings and requests (often in the form of babbles) • Vocalizes to get attention • Uses some gestures and language appropriately, e.g., shakes head for "no"	• Holds one cube and takes another • Smiles at self in mirror • Loves hiding and finding games • Gives, points, shows • Pulls rings off peg	• Enjoys interactive play • Emerging turn-taking skills
10–12 Months			
Receptive Language	**Expressive Language**	**Cognition**	**Social Communication (Pragmatics) and Play**
• Emerging ability to follow commands involving giving familiar toys and objects to an adult on verbal request • Dances to music • Demonstrates understanding of approximately 50+ words • Consistently completes simple commands when provided gestural cues • Enjoys pointing to pictures when they are named	• Produces jargon of 4 or more syllables with adult-like intonation • Inconsistently pairs babbling with pointing • Inconsistently produces words in jargon • Inconsistently communicates to toys/objects using longer verbal patterns • Frequently responds to songs or rhymes by vocalizing (seeming to sing/rhyme along) • Imitates action paired with sound • Produces word approximations inconsistently • May use first words, e.g., bye bye, mama • Vocalizes to protest	• Enjoys building 2-block towers • Resists when toy is taken away • Imitates laughter and growls • Identifies two objects as being the same	• Initiates activity transitions by vocalizing or gesturing for desired activities • Inconsistently directs others by tugging, pushing • Stacks toys in play • Places objects in containers • Turns knobs, wheels • Explores parts of objects, nesting objects and mean end objects (e.g., Jack-in-the-Box)

(Continued)

Table 6.1 Communication and Play Milestones (Continued)

13–15 Months			
Receptive Language	**Expressive Language**	**Cognition**	**Social Communication (Pragmatics) and Play**
• Consistently completes one step directions during play • Understands simple "where" questions • Consistently identifies a variety of familiar objects in functional and non-functional contexts • Emerging ability to identify body parts (e.g., eyes, nose) • Understands 150–250 words • Demonstrates understanding of pronouns: you, me • Emerging ability to point to familiar items/objects in pictures	• Produces 1–7 words consistently • Produces vocalization and gesture to obtain desired object(s) • Imitates new words • Sings	• Participates in play for 2 minutes • Enjoys playing shape-sorter games • Builds a tower with two cubes • Emerging ability to make marks on paper with thick crayon • Demonstrates functional use of objects • Emerging object permanence (e.g., removes lid of box to find hidden toy)	• Engages in turn-taking involving back and forth vocalizations • Plays fetching game • Initiates play and communication by showing things (e.g., toy food items during play)

16–18 Months			
Receptive Language	**Expressive Language**	**Cognition**	**Social Communication (Pragmatics) and Play**
• Emerging ability to match familiar items in appropriate categories • Emerging ability to follow 1-step commands • Understands more simple questions • Emerging ability to identify body parts in pictures • Understands 50 or more words (understands 150–250 words by 18 months) • Consistently responds when name is called • Identifies some clothing items, toys and food	• Produces more word approximations and jargon significantly fades • Imitates words • Consistently vocalizes to request • Increases vocabulary, 10 or more meaningful words (25–100 different words by 18 months) • Decreases use of gesture—relies on talking to communicate	• Imitates circular scribble • Places 3–6 pegs in pegboard • Picks up small objects • Turns bottle/container upside down to obtain toy • Points to pictures in a book and begins to turn pages • Demonstrates consistent object permanence: finds familiar object not in sight	• Requests object or help from adult by gesturing and vocalizing • Initiates vocal interaction • Prefers to be with familiar people • Shows caution with strangers • Imitates other children • Role plays simple actions previously seen • Imitates a pretend play action (e.g., giving a drink) • Relates objects functionally • Uses one simple imaginative action in play • Uses play themes related to child's body (e.g., sleeping, eating)

19–24 Months			
Receptive Language	**Expressive Language**	**Cognition**	**Social Communication (Pragmatics) and Play**
• Completes two requests with one object • Listens to reason (logic) • Chooses two familiar objects upon request • Comprehends action phrases • Understands familiar action words in pictures • Points to a range of body parts, (e.g., hands, toes, elbow, back) • Begins to understand personal pronouns—my, mine, you • Understands 200–500 words by 24 months • Understands simple "wh" questions • Completes three to four separate directions	• Occasionally imitates 2–3 word phrases • Increases expressive vocabulary to 30 words or more (100 to 300 different words by 24 months) • Attempts "stories"— longer utterances in jargon to get message across • Uses his or her own name when talking about self • Uses "mine" • May use 2–3 word phrases with nouns, some verbs and some adjectives by 24 months • Asks, "What's that?"	• Uses one object as symbol for another (e.g., hair brush for microphone) • Places triangle, circle, square in shape board • Imitates vertical strokes on paper • Imitates symbolic play, (e.g., cleaning house) • Stacks blocks/builds tower • Threads three beads • Begins to tear paper • Imitates ordering of nesting cups or boxes • Begins to categorize objects in play • Uses two toys together • Activates mechanical toy	• Begins to develop more self-confidence and is happy to be with other people • Initiates pretend play • Responds to requests from adults • Practices adult-like conversation about familiar themes • Uses words to interact • Requests information, (e.g., What is this?) • Develops turn taking in conversation • Imitates an adult using an object • Uses similar looking object as the needed object (e.g., paper for blanket) • Sequences two or three similar actions • Uses play themes that reflect daily activities in the home (e.g., feeding a doll)

25–30 Months			
Receptive Language	**Expressive Language**	**Cognition**	**Social Communication (Pragmatics) and Play**
• Responds appropriately when asked for "just one" • Begins to understand prepositions, (e.g., in, on, under) • Begins to understand concept of quantity (e.g., one, all) • Understands subject pronouns (e.g., he, she, they, we) • Emerging ability to understand size differences • Understands the conjunction: "and" • Understands plural /-s/ and present progressive /-ing/	• Uses 2–3 word phrases more consistently • Uses some personal pronouns (e.g., me, you) • Produces approximately 150–400 different words by 30 months • Recites nursery rhymes and favorite songs • Uses negation (e.g., don't, no) • Asks for help using two or more words (e.g., help please, want more, milk please) • Begins to name primary colors • Repeats 2 numbers counting	• Performs related activities in play • Turns one page of a book at a time • Matches identical picture to picture and shape to shape • Puts two parts of a whole together • Understands number concept of one and two • Uses toys appropriately • Imitates vertical, horizontal and circular lines when drawing/ coloring	• Enjoys talking (e.g., pretends to have a conversation on the phone) • Shares toys • Uses play themes that reflect daily life in and out of the home (e.g., fixing the car, shopping) • Uses play actions that are simple, logical, and sequential • Uses inanimate objects in play (e.g., table as a car) • Imitates another child in play

(Continued)

Table 6.1 Communication and Play Milestones (Continued)

31–36 Months			
Receptive Language	**Expressive Language**	**Cognition**	**Social Communication (Pragmatics) and Play**
• Understands 500–1,500 words by 36 months • Understands time concepts (e.g., today, yesterday, tomorrow) • Understands "What is missing?/Which one does not belong?" • Identifies familiar object use in pictures • Consistently takes conversational turns • Understands most common verbs • Understands articles: "the, a" • Carries out 2–3 verbal requests in single command • Identifies parts of an object • Demonstrates interest in learning "why" and "how"	• Uses some regular plurals • Uses possessives • Uses present progressive /-ing/ • Imitates up to a 7-syllable sentence • Consistently recalls 3 words, letters, or numbers • Begins to use conjunctions (e.g., and, because) • Names three or more colors • Labels gender vocabulary • Gives both first and last name when asked • Produces 3–4 word simple sentences • Produces questions (e.g., who, what, where, why • Uses subject pronouns (e.g., he, she, they, we, you, me) • Uses some semi-auxiliary verbs (e.g., wanna, gotta) • Speaks primary language fluently	• Adds missing body parts to a drawing • Completes 2–3 interlocking puzzle pieces • Shares toys and takes turns • Develops parallel play • Begins to develop interest in writing and drawing • Begins fantasy play • Sorts and categorizes (e.g., blocks and pegs) • Names object when part of it is shown in a picture	• Takes turns and shares • Engages in make believe activities • Begins to ask permission of others • Expresses feeling • Uses questions for a variety of reasons (e.g., to obtain information, to request) • Indicates role playing someone else, but only for a short period of time • Uses same inanimate objects for two or more functions • Uses play actions that are detailed and logical with no planned story line • Uses play events that are reflective of less frequent experiences in life events (e.g., doctor)

Adapted from a variety of sources.

Program (Girolametto, Greenburg, & Manolson, 1986). A primary component of this program is that caregivers are active participants in the intervention process for their child. For young clinicians, this program is easy to use and work through with caregivers. The interventionist helps the adult learn to respond to their child's communication attempts in ways that best facilitate language growth. Key skills learned in this program include: observing communication attempts, learning to let the child lead activities, responding to communication attempts in ways to facilitate language growth, taking turns in communication interactions, helping caregivers learn how to facilitate more language in their communication interactions with their child, and encouraging parents to be intentional about their child's language development by pre-planning materials and activities to facilitate specific skills. It

is difficult for a caregiver to determine what and how his or her child is attempting to communicate if he or she is not sure of the communications attempts produced by the child. The foundational skill of knowing what communication attempts are being observed, and knowing what the child is attempting to do is critical in determining next steps in the intervention plan (Seifer, Clark, & Sameroff, 1991; Hanft, Rush, Shelden, 2004).

INTRODUCTION TO IFSPS

Most often a child is referred for a language evaluation at the recommendation of his/her primary care physician (PCP). Families can of course request an evaluation; however, it is best practice to notify the child's PCP and request permission to complete a language evaluation.

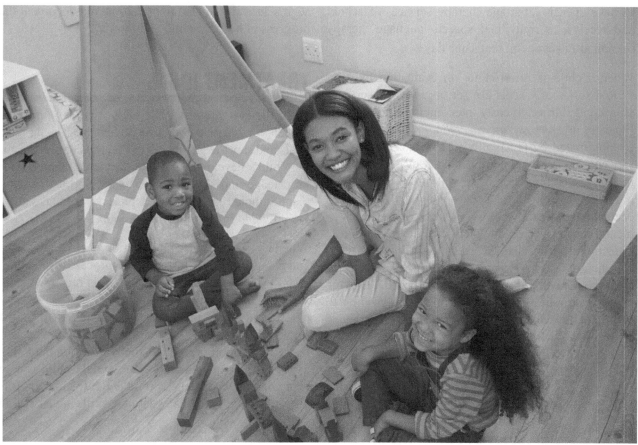

Monkey Business Images/Shutterstock.com

After completing the evaluation of a young child, it is time to determine the child's plan for intervention. Family involvement in the evaluation process as well as utilizing parents as informants in the development of the child's treatment plan can be beneficial. There may be communication interactions that are happening (or not happening) at home that a formal assessment may not pick up on (but could be a developmentally appropriate objective on the child's plan of care). Involving parents in the evaluation also allows them to feel their concerns are being addressed and helps establish a foundation that parents play an integral role in the development of their child's communication skills.

In 1975, Public Law 96.142 the Education of All Handicapped Children Act was passed. This initial legislation did not include early intervention services; however, it was landmark legislation in that it was the first time school-age children, regardless of skill level, were recognized as needing *free and appropriate education* (*FAPE*). When the bill was reauthorized in 1986 as the Education of the Handicapped Amendments Act (PL 99-475), early intervention services were included in Part H. Then, in 2004, the Individuals

with Disabilities Education Improvement (IDEA) (PL 108-446) was passed. This legislation incorporated the unique recognition that the first 3 years of life involved significant brain development and documented the need to enhance state and local agencies to better serve children with special needs. Early intervention services that were initially covered under Part H were now covered under Part C of IDEA. This legislation, reauthorized in 1997 and continuing to present day, is important because it sets the foundation for intervention services for speech–language pathologists, and stipulates that services should be provided based on the concept of *family-centered care* (based on the needs of the child and family) and in a *naturalistic environment* (e.g., a location where the child will feel most comfortable. Often this is the child's home.). Early intervention is one funding source for children birth through the age 2 years, 11 months. Speech therapy services could also potentially be funded through a local, state, private insurance, or out-of-pocket funding source for this age group as well. Families and interventionists need to be aware of guidelines and requirements for funding sources as well as what funding sources are available. For example, in some states, a child is unable to have speech–language therapy services at school and receive an individual speech–language therapy session after school on that same day.

When a child is referred for an evaluation by their PCP, a series of wheels are set in motion if services are provided through early intervention funding. This typically involves an *interdisciplinary evaluation* that is coordinated by the family's early intervention service coordinator. An interdisciplinary evaluation could include the combination of several professions including but not limited to: speech–language pathology, occupational therapy, physical therapy, or developmental therapy. Upon completion of the evaluation, a transition meeting that involves the early intervention coordinator, parent(s), and service providers is typically the next step in the process. A speech–language pathologist may be asked to sit in on this meeting to help explain evaluation results and help to establish appropriate goals for intervention with the family and the child's educators and caregivers. From this meeting, the child's *individualized family service plan (IFSP)* is developed. This is a comprehensive document that is updated periodically by the intervention team and serves as a way to plan intervention and document the progress of both the child and family.

TREATMENT IDEAS

After the evaluation is completed, it is then up to the speech–language pathologist to establish long-term goals and short-term objectives that are appropriate for the child's developmental age. Review Chapter 1 for knowledge and skills needed to develop a treatment plan. Sample receptive and expressive language goals are provided in the following sections.

When working in early intervention, including parents and caregivers in each step of the process (evaluation, goal development, and intervention) is recommended. As that relationship is established, it is also recommended that the speech–language pathologist implement therapy tasks (activities) that are both developmentally appropriate and motivating for the child. Typical developmental milestones and the child's are to be compared when developing the treatment plan. It is also important to review what play skills are emerging

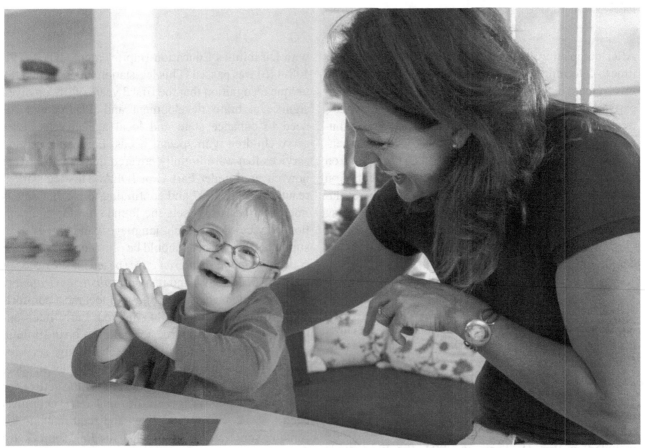

Monkey Business Images/Shutterstock.com

and what play skills are mastered by the child as this will guide the development of therapy session lesson plans. For example, it would be inappropriate to use 'Plah Doh' as a therapy material with a child who has the developmental age of 6 months who likely would want to put the dough in his or her mouth to explore the toy. More appropriate toys to incorporate in therapy sessions would include (but not be limited to): blocks, stackable toys, or touch-and-feel books.

GOALS AND OBJECTIVES

When writing treatment goals and objectives, remember the definition of each component of professional documentation. The *evaluation* is the document that summarizes the child's strengths and weaknesses in speech and language skills. It is from the evaluation that a *treatment plan or plan of care (POC)* is developed. Goals and objectives listed on the POC must correlate with the weaknesses listed on the evaluation report. For example, if a child has been diagnosed with only an expressive language delay, it would not be appropriate for that child's treatment plan to have goals and objectives listed that target receptive language skills. POC documents typically consist of long-term goals and short-term objectives. *Long-term goals* are broad goals that aim to change a facet of communication within a pre-determined allotment of time. *Short-term objectives* (Also sometimes termed "behavioral objectives" or "objectives") are the specific steps by which the interventionist plans to achieve the long-term goals. Short-term objectives must be specific, measurable, and time-driven. For additional information on how to generate long- and short-term goals, please refer to Chapter 1. Sample goal and objectives for early intervention follow. There are a variety of ways to write goals and objectives and treatment plans are to be developed with each child's unique skill set and needs for improvement in mind. The list provided below is not a comprehensive list, but is meant to provide emerging clinicians with a foundation upon which to further develop the skill of goal writing in the future.

SAMPLE LONG-TERM GOALS

1. Child will improve receptive language skills to be commensurate with same-aged peers.

2. Child will improve expressive language skills to be commensurate with same-aged peers.

3. Child will improve receptive language skills to enhance communication.

4. Child will improve expressive language skills to enhance communication.

SAMPLE *DO* AND *CONDITION* STATEMENTS FOR SHORT-TERM OBJECTIVES

For the objectives below to be complete, a *criterion* statement for mastery would need to be added. For example, if a clinician chose to use the same objective, "The child will vocalize in response to speech" the clinician would also need to add a *condition* and *do* statement. See the example provided below.

During semi-structured play activities,	= Condition Statement
the child will vocalize in response to speech	= Do Statement
5 times during a single session for 3 consecutive sessions.	= Criterion Statement

The final draft of the short-term objective would be:

During semi-structured play activities, the child will vocalize in response to speech 5 times during a single session for three consecutive sessions.

For additional information on the development of criterion statements, please see Chapter 1. Table 6.2 provides sample language goals for early intervention. Take note that goals are divided based on *chronological age* and this may not match a child's *developmental* age. Treatment plans (also referred to as Plan of Care (POC) documents are to reflect a baseline of the child's developmental age and goals to help bridge the gap between the child's developmental age and chronological age if applicable. Bridging the developmental and chronological age gap may not be possible in all cases. If achieving developmental skills commensurate with chronological age is not judged to be realistic in the reporting period, goals should be developed to help the child improve language skills.

Table 6.2 Early Intervention Language Goals

0–3 Months	
Receptive Language	**Expressive Language**
• The child will demonstrate awareness of strangers. • The child will demonstrate awareness of unfamiliar situations.	• The child will produce differentiated cries (tired, hungry, in pain). • The child will produce coos and vocal play. • The child will engage in oral-motor play through imitation (i.e., tongue protrusion, smile, open/close mouth).
3–6 Months	
Receptive Language	**Expressive Language**
• The child will experiment with cause-effect toys: shakes rattle, bang toys, bang drum/music toy. • The child will demonstrate desire for objects out of reach.	• The child will vocalize for pleasure/ displeasure/ excitement. • The child will produce babble to comment to self and when playing alone. • The child will vocalize in response to speech.
6–9 Months	
Receptive Language	**Expressive Language**
• The child will (give, point, show) a familiar item/object upon request. • The child will search for partially hidden objects. • The child will respond to 'no'. • The child will wave hi/bye-bye in imitation. • The child will search for familiar person when named. • The child will imitate familiar actions.	• The child will produce a variety of syllable shapes (CV, VCV, CVCV) in structured and free play activities. • The child will imitate sound/object associations (i.e., bear growl, monkey sound etc.,) • The child will produce a variety of vocalizations to express emotions- anger, contentment, and frustration. • The child will produce an approximation to "sing" along with familiar songs.
9–12 Months	
Receptive Language	**Expressive Language**

• The child will demonstrate knowledge of cause-and-effect by repeating pleasurable action (i.e., squeezing squeaky duck toy, tapping light-up toy).
• The child will demonstrate object permanence by searching for objects out of sight.
• The child will demonstrate comprehension of specific games by responding to verbal requests (i.e., "play peek-a-boo")
	• The child will produce variegated babble (dageedagee) in free and structured play activities.
	• The child will produce adult-like intonation to:
	  • scold
	  • exclaim
	  • greet
	• The child will produce "uh-oh" and "ow" in appropriate contexts.
	• The child will use a consistent verbal approximation for a familiar person or familiar object

12–18 Months	
Receptive Language	**Expressive Language**
• The child will demonstrate functional use of objects. • The child will match objects by association/function. • The child will readily participate in rhymes and finger plays. • The child will understand 50 words. • The child will choose 2 familiar objects on request.	• The child will use 1–10 words. • The child will use jargon (words mixed with babble and adult-like sentence intonation). • The child will produce approximations to ask question.

18–24 Months	
Receptive Language	**Expressive Language**
• The child will group objects to make collections. • The child will pretend play about familiar situations. • The child will receptively identify 100 words.	• The child will name 5–7 familiar items/objects. • The child will expressively use 20–75 words (60% nouns, 25% verbs).

18–24 Months	
Receptive Language	**Expressive Language**
• The child will understand "you" or "your". • The child will understand the prepositions "in" and "on". • The child will understand questions: "Where? What's that?" • The child will choose the correct picture from set of five familiar items/objects. • The child will respond to commands with 4 meaningful units without pointing or eye cues. • The child will follow 2-step, related commands without cues.	• The child will occasionally use some word endings (-ing, -s). • The child will use negation + verb phrase. • The child will produce 2–3 word phrases. • The child will use: "my, me, or mine." • The child will use: "in, on, over (there), up." • The child will use "more" + noun phrase to request.

(Continued)

Table 6.2 Early Intervention Language Goals (Continued)

24–36 Months	
Receptive Language	**Expressive Language**

• The child will demonstrate an understanding of item/object function.
• The child will demonstrate an understanding of the following functional language concepts:
  Size (big/little)
  Quantity (one/all)
  Time (today, yesterday, tomorrow)
• The child will understand subject pronouns ("he, she, we, they, I").
• The child will understand part/whole relationships.
• The child will understand "What's missing?" "What doesn't belong?"
	• The child will conjoin nouns with "and".
	• The child will use adjectives (e.g., color, size, quantity)
	• The child will use subject pronouns: "you, I, it."
	• The child will use object pronouns: "you, me, it."
	• The child will use possessive pronouns: "my, your."
	• The child will use possessive noun: "mine."
	• The child will use prepositions.
	• The child will use contractions: "don't, can't."
	• The child will use time-related adverbs.
	• The child will take 2 turns in conversations.
	• The child will verbally introduce and change topics.
	• The child will use words to express emotion.
	By 30–36 months:
	• The child will use definite article: "the"
	• The child will use quantifiers: "many, all".
	• The child will use double adjectives in sentences.
	• The child will use a variety of prepositions.
	• The child will use "and" to conjoin verbs.
	• The child will use adverbs to indicate how and when an action took place.
	• The child will ask "Why not?" and "What happened?"

Adapted from a variety of sources including but not limited to: ASHA (2018), Bzoch, League, and Brown (2003), Estabrooks, MacIver-Lux, and Rhoades (2016), Fenson, Marchman, Thal, Dale, Reznick, and Bates (2007), NIDCD (2017), Owens (2015), Pathway (2018), Rossetti (2006), Singleton and Shulman (2018), and Wiig, Secord, and Semel (2004).

SUMMARY

This chapter was intended to provide a brief review of communication development from birth through 3 years of age. Reviews of pertinent laws and relevant resources for this age group were also provided. Functional ideas for how to implement therapy objectives were discussed as well as sample goals and objectives to implement in therapy sessions. This chapter would be beneficial as a foundational measure for emerging clinicians who would like guidance for where to start in their attempt to apply the content they have learned in the classroom. This chapter may also be useful for parents working with children who have communication delays. Ultimately, this chapter is most beneficial for children who have communication delays whom the early interventionist serves.

REFERENCES

American Speech Language Hearing Association (ASHA). (2018). *How does your child hear and talk?* Retrieved from https://www.asha.org/public/speech/development/chart/

Bryant, D. M., & Ramey, C. T. (1987). An analysis of the effectiveness of early intervention programs for environmentally at-risk children. In M. J. Guralnick & F. C. Bennett (Eds.), *The effectiveness of early intervention for at-risk and handicapped children* (pp. 33–78). San Diego, CA: Academic Press.

Bruder, M. B. (2000). Family-centered early intervention: Clarifying our values for the new millennium. *Topics in Early Childhood Special Education, 20*(2), 105–115.

Bzoch, K. R., League, R., & Brown, V. L. (2003). *Receptive-expressive emergent language test third edition (REEL-3)*. St. Antonio, TX: Pearson.

Estabrooks, W., MacIver-Lux, K., & Rhoades, E. A. (Eds.). (2016). *Auditory-verbal therapy: for young children with hearing loss and their families, and the practitioners who guide them.* San Diego, CA: Plural Publishing.

Fenson, L., Marchman, V. A., Thal, D. J., Dale, P. S., Reznick, J. S., & Bates, E. (2007). *MacArthur-Bates communicative development inventories* (2nd ed.), Baltimore, MD: Paul H. Brookes.

Girolametto, L. E., Greenberg, J., & Manolson, H. A. (1986). Developing dialogue skills: The Hanen early language parent program. *Seminars in Speech and Language, 4*(7), 367–382.

Guralnick, M. J. (1997). Effectiveness of early intervention for vulnerable children: A developmental perspective. *American Journal on Mental Retardation, 102*(4), 319–345.

Guralnick, M. J., & Bricker, D. (1987). *The effectiveness of early intervention for children with cognitive and general developmental delays.* New York, NY: Academic Press.

Hanft, B. E., Rush, D. D., & Shelden, M. L. L. (2004). *Coaching families and colleagues in early childhood.* Baltimore, MD: Brookes Publishing Company.

Individuals with Disabilities Education Improvement Act or IDEA (2004), PL 108–446, 20 U.S.C. §1400.

Innocenti, M. S., Huh, K., & Boyce, G. C. (1992). Families of children with disabilities: Normative data and other considerations on parenting stress. *Topics in Early Childhood Special Education, 12*(3), 403–427.

Kaiser, A. P., & Hancock, T. B. (2003). Teaching parents new skills to support their young children's development. *Infants and Young Children, 16,* 9–21.

Law, P. (1975). Law 96.142 (November 29, 1975). *Education for All Handicapped Children Act.*

National Institute on Deafness and Other Communication Disorders (NIDCD). (2017). *Speech and Language Developmental Milestones.* Retrieved from https://www.nidcd.nih.gov/health/speech-and-language

Odom, S. L., & Wolery, M. (2003). A unified theory of practice in early intervention/early childhood special education: Evidence-based practices. *The Journal of Special Education, 37*(3), 166.173.

Olson, M. (1987). Early intervention for children with visual impairments. In Guralnick MJ, Benneu FC (Eds.). *The effectiveness of early intervention for at-risk and handicapped children* (pp. 297–324). New York, NY: Academic Press.

Orr, R. R., Cameron, S. J., Dobson, L. A., & Day, D. M. (1993). Age-related changes in stress experienced by families with a child who has developmental delays. *Mental Retardation, 31*(3), 171.

Owens Jr, R. E. (2015). *Language development: An introduction.* St. Antonio, TX: Pearson.

Pathway (2018). *Communication.* Retrieved from https://pathways.org/topics-of-development/communication/milestones/.

Rossetti, L. M. (2001). *Communication intervention: Birth to three.* Boston, MA: Cengage Learning.

Rossetti, L. M. (2006). *The Rossetti infant-toddler language scale.* East Moline, IL: LinguiSystems.

Seifer, R., Clark, G. N., & Sameroff, A. J. (1991). Positive effects of interaction coaching on infants with developmental disabilities and their mothers. *American Journal on Mental Retardation, 96*(1), 1–11.

Sharma, A. & Nash, A. (2009). Brain maturation in children with cochlear implants, *ASHA Leader, 14*(5), 16.17.

Shonkoff, J. P., & Hauser-Cram, P. (1987). Early intervention for disabled infants and their families: a quantitative analysis. *Pediatrics, 80*(5), 650–658.

Singleton, N.C., & Shulman, B. B. (2018). *Language development: foundations, processes, and clinical applications* (3rd ed.). Burlington, MA: Jones & Bartlett Publishers.

Stonestreet, R. H., Johnston, R. G., & Acton, S. J. (1991). Guidelines for real partnerships with parents. *Infant-Toddler Intervention, 1*(1), 37–46.

Westby, C.E. (2000). A scale for assessing development of children's play. In K Gitlin-Weiner, A. Sandgrun & C. Schaefer (Eds.), *Play diagnosis and assessment.* New York, NY: Wiley.

Wiig, E. H., Secord, W., & Semel, E. M. (2004). *CELF preschool 2: Clinical evaluation of language fundamentals preschool* (2nd ed.). New York, NY: Pearson/PsychCorp.

Woods, J., Kashinath, S., & Goldstein, H. (2004). Effects of embedding caregiver-implemented teaching strategies in daily routines on children's communication outcomes. *Journal of Early Intervention, 26,* 175–193.

Yoder, P. J., & Warren, S. F. (2002). Effects of prelinguistic milieu teaching and parent responsivity education on dyads involving children with intellectual disabilities. *Journal of Speech, Language, and Hearing Research, 45,* 1158–1174.

PRACTICE

This purpose of this section is to provide emerging clinicians an opportunity to practice utilizing the information provided in the aforementioned chapter. Case scenarios provided are meant to facilitate discussion between emerging clinicians and educators to provide a foundation for competent clinical practice. There is often more than one way to answer the case scenario questions provided in this section. Long-term goals are meant to be over-arching goals for therapy during the current reporting period. Short-term objectives are to correlate with long-term goals and are to be utilized as steps to achieve the long-term goal. Emerging clinicians need always be mindful that short-term objectives are to be clearly stated, measurable, and time driven. Tasks are to be developmentally appropriate for the child (which may not necessarily correlate with the child's chronological age).

Case Scenario 6-1 Worksheet

NAME: _____   DATE: _____

Brain is an 18 month-old male with a diagnosis of Down syndrome. His recent evaluation indicated he is currently receiving occupational therapy for fine motor weakness. He started walking at 15 months of age and is also receiving physical therapy. His father reported he currently has two words, "dada" and "ball." The evaluation reported receptive language skills within the average range of performance for his chronological age. A severe delay in expressive language (*Strengths: babbling in long syllable strings, gestures to communicate, appropriate joint attention, vocalizes in response to speech, vocalizes for needs and wants, and vocalizes to greet a familiar adult. Weaknesses: less than 10 words, inconsistent imitation on demand, minimal attempts to "sing" along, minimal sound/object associations, and limited vocalization to protest, comment, and request.*) was reported. There are currently no concerns with feeding and swallowing and Brain has age-appropriate play skills. Hearing and vision were also determined to be within normal limits at this time.

1. What is an appropriate LONG-TERM GOAL?

   _____

2. What are <u>three</u> appropriate SHORT-TERM OBJECTIVES? (Hint: Short-term objectives should correlate with the long-term goal listed above.)

   A.

   _____

   _____

   B.

   _____

   _____

   C.

   _____

   _____

3. List the TASK you would use to target the short-term objectives listed above. The task for 3A should pair with the short-term objective listed for 2A. Please list MATERIALS you plan to utilize.

A.

_____

_____

B.

_____

_____

C.

_____

_____

4. How would you introduce and explain the purpose of each short-term objective and task in the therapy session to the parent/caregiver?

A.

_____

_____

B.

_____

_____

C.

_____

Case Scenario 6-2 Worksheet

NAME: _____   DATE: _____

Kendra is a 2-year-old female with a diagnosis of a severe mixed (both receptive and expressive) language delay. Her family reported they have no concerns with other developmental milestones at this time. Her most recent evaluation report indicated that she started sitting unassisted at 6 months, walking at 12 months, has recently shown an interest in toilet training, can feed herself and currently utilizes both a sippy cup and standard cup for drinking. Kendra was reported to have the following strengths in receptive language: inconsistently follows simple commands with gestural cues and able to attend to a game or book for one minute. The following weaknesses were reported for receptive language: following commands with no gestural cues, understanding "where" questions, receptively, identifying body parts, receptively identifying clothing, and comprehending action phrases. *Kendra was reported to have the following strengths in expressive language: producing jargon and babble of up to 4 syllables, initiates communication interactions, imitates single words, produces 5 words, and enjoys singing approximations. The following weaknesses were reported for expressive language: imitating new words spontaneously, using voicing + gesture for requests, using words to request, using words to protest, using words to comment during free play, and asking questions.* There are currently no concerns with feeding, swallowing, or play skills. Hearing and vision were also determined to be within normal limits at this time.

1. What is an appropriate LONG-TERM GOAL?

    _____

2. What are <u>three</u> appropriate SHORT-TERM OBJECTIVES? (Hint: Short-term objectives should correlate with the long-term goal listed above.)

    A.

    _____

    _____

    B.

    _____

    _____

    C.

    _____

    _____

3. List the TASK you would use to target the short-term objectives listed above. The task for 3A should pair with the short-term objective listed for 2A. Please list MATERIALS you plan to utilize.

A.

_____

_____

B.

_____

_____

C.

_____

_____

4. How would you introduce and explain the purpose of each short-term objective and task in the therapy session to the parent/caregiver?

A.

_____

_____

B.

_____

_____

C.

_____

_____

CHAPTER 7

Introduction to Augmentative and Alternative Communication

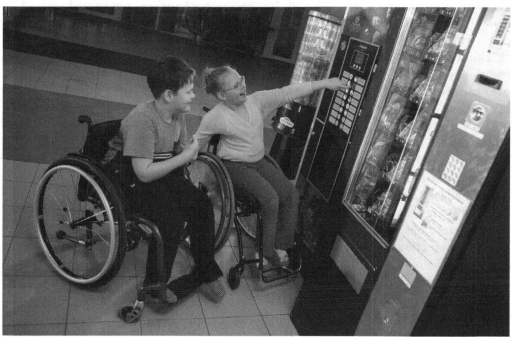

Zoja Hussainova/Shutterstock.com

Sarah and Dan are middle schoolers with cerebral palsy. Secondary to their cerebral palsy, Sarah and Dan do not have speech that other people can easily understand. Instead of speech, Sarah and Dan use computer devices to communicate. Using these devices, Sarah and Dan participate in their classes, complete their homework, talk to friends in the hallway and after school, and order their favorite meals when they go to eat at restaurants with their families.

—Christine Holyfield

Sarah and Dan use augmentative and alternative communication (AAC) to interact with others and participate in life. AAC is a term that includes technologies and strategies that allow for individuals to communicate through means other than speech (Beukelman & Mirenda, 2013). Some individuals use AAC to supplement limitations in speech. Some individuals have no speech at all, and AAC is their only form of communication. In addition to compensating for limitations in speech, AAC can also be useful for compensating for and building language in individuals who experience language limitations in conjunction with speech limitations.

WHO REQUIRES AAC?

Individuals of any age may require AAC to fully communicate and participate in life's interactions (Beukelman & Mirenda, 2013). Young children with intellectual and developmental disabilities (IDD) who are at risk for limited speech development, for instance, benefit from AAC intervention (Romski, Sevcik, Barton-Hulsey, & Whitmore, 2015). For these young children, it is never too early to start AAC intervention. Access to AAC can help young children develop interaction skills (e.g., turn taking) as well as expressive and receptive language. Even if it is unknown if the child will develop speech or not, AAC intervention should be used. Clinicians should not wait to determine if speech will eventually develop, because during this time opportunities for language and interaction growth will have passed. Even if only used for a short amount of time until speech fully develops, AAC offers important opportunities for interaction. And, there is no evidence that using AAC slows a child's speech development (Millar, Light, & Schlosser, 2006; Schlosser & Wendt, 2008). In fact, the research evidence suggests AAC intervention can even promote speech development (Millar et al., 2006; Schlosser & Wendt, 2008).

On the other end of the age spectrum, adults who used speech successfully throughout their life may face changes in which they begin to require AAC to fully communicate (Beukelman & Mirenda, 2013). For example, adults may experience conditions in which their speech deteriorates over time, such as amyotrophic lateral sclerosis (ALS). For adults with speech that becomes limited, AAC can allow for continued communication (Beukelman, Fager, Ball, & Dietz, 2007). Continued access to communication through AAC can allow continued connectedness with loved ones, opportunities at work, and involvement in the community. Other adults may develop conditions that affect not only their speech, but their language as well. For instance, some adults who experience strokes may develop limitations to speech and language in result. For these individuals, in addition to supporting expressive communication in compensation for speech limitations, AAC can also promote receptive and expressive language.

TYPES OF AAC

There are a wide variety of AAC options available. One way to think about the different options is to organize them by the level of technology involved (Beukelman & Mirenda, 2013). AAC options can vary greatly in the level of technology they utilize, with some AAC using no technology whatsoever and some AAC relying on high-tech computers.

Often, individuals who require AAC employ a variety of technology options across multiple technology levels (Loncke, Campbell, England, & Haley, 2006). Together, use of these multiple AAC technology options encompasses the individual's comprehensive *AAC system*. For instance, an AAC user may require no technology whatsoever to communicate effectively with a close loved one. That same AAC user may use computer technology to interact with a stranger effectively. However, when interacting with a stranger at the beach, the user may use printed paper to communicate.

Various levels of technology have related benefits and drawbacks. Different options can be useful in different contexts or for different individuals. Below, the different levels of AAC technologies are discussed.

No-Tech

Some AAC options require nothing external to the person communicating. The level of technology of these options is: *no-tech* (Beukelman & Mirenda, 2013). No-tech AAC includes gestures, facial expressions, body movements, and manual signs. For instance, some children and adults with IDD and limited speech

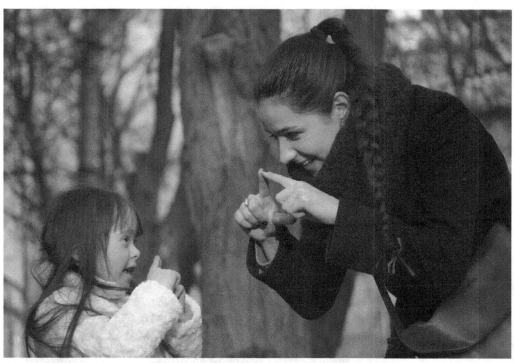

Denis Kuvaev/Shutterstock.com

are taught words in American Sign Language (ASL) to communicate a variety of concepts to family and other communication partners (e.g., Thompson, Cotnoir-Bichelman, McKerchar, Tate, & Dancho, 2007). The photo above shows a young girl with Down syndrome is learning a new sign from her mother. When the young girl communicates using this sign, she is using no-tech AAC.

Low-Tech

Some AAC options involve the use of technology beyond the person communicating that requires no batteries. The level of technology of these options is: *low-tech* (Beukelman & Mirenda, 2013). Low-tech AAC includes printed photos, drawings, printed words, and paper and pencil for writing. Many individuals who use AAC have low-tech AAC as one aspect of their AAC system. For instance, adults who have experienced stroke may use pen and paper to write messages when they cannot retrieve the spoken word. They may also use booklets filled with words and sentences and photos of their life to support their communication with others (Fried-Oken, Beukelman, & Hux, 2012; Iacono, Lyon, Johnson, & West, 2013). The first photo on the next page shows a man pointing to printed sentences and photos to share with his

grandson about a recent trip he took. When the man communicates using these printed supports, he is using low-tech AAC.

Mid-Tech

Some AAC options involve the use of technology with a battery component, but no computer component. The level of technology of these options is: *mid-tech* (Beukelman & Mirenda, 2013). Mid-tech AAC includes the use of laser pointers to select printed material and recording machines to play prerecorded words or phrases. Talking photo albums are one mid-tech AAC option that be used by adults with limited speech and language (e.g., Bourgeois, Fried-Oken, & Rowland, 2010). For instance, a family member of an adult with dementia and related speech and language loss may record messages about family members and major family events (e.g., weddings) onto a talking photo album. Then, the adult with dementia can use the talking photo album to share with other individuals about his or her family—a major aspect of his or her life. The second photo on the next page shows a woman using a talking photo album to share with her granddaughter about her life when she was a young woman, her siblings, her career, and her wedding. When the woman communicates using these printed supports, she is using mid-tech AAC.

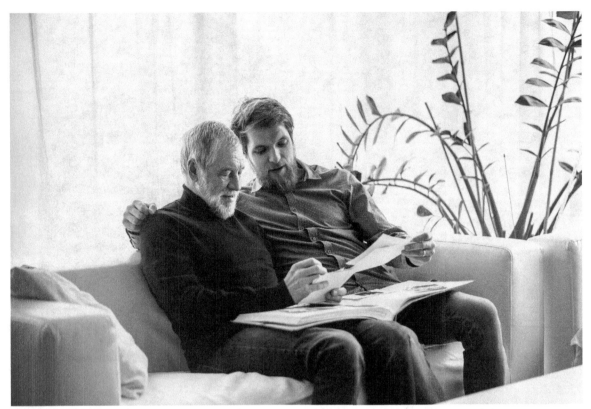

Halfpoint/Shutterstock.com

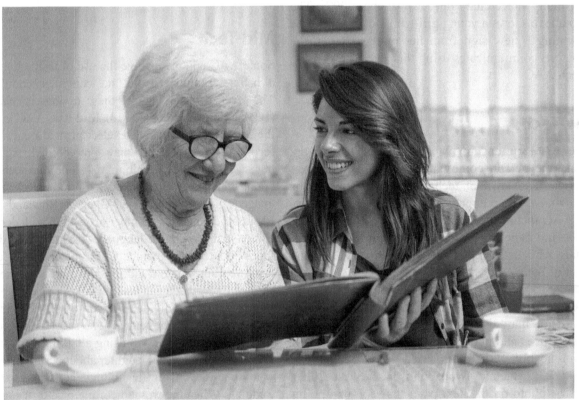

Bojan Milinkov/Shutterstock.com

HIGH-TECH

Some AAC options involve the use of a computer component. The level of technology of these options is: *high-tech* (Beukelman & Mirenda, 2013). High-tech AAC includes the use of smartphones, tablets, and computer devices designed specifically for AAC. For instance, children and adults with limited speech can benefit from communication applications (apps) on mobile technology to communicate (Alzrayer, Banda, & Koul, 2014). The photo below shows a young child using a communication app on a tablet to answer a question in the classroom. When she communicates using this app, she is using high-tech AAC.

SKILLS FOR USING AAC

Individuals across the lifespan and across a range of diagnoses (e.g., autism spectrum disorder, cerebral palsy, Alzheimer's disease) can successfully use AAC to communicate and more fully participate in life (Beukelman & Mirenda, 2013). However, a number of skills are involved in using AAC to communicate. The skills required for using AAC vary across technology options.

Regardless of the particular skills required, any individual introduced to AAC technology to communicate will require some form of intervention related to learning the technology (Beukelman & Mirenda, 2013). Of course, intervention for a young child who is developing expressive language through use of AAC will look quite different than intervention for an adult with ALS who has typical language but no longer has functional speech. In fact, intervention for young children may focus largely on language building while language building is an unneeded intervention for adults with typical language.

Yet, while skills targeted in AAC intervention will vary from individual to individual and from AAC technology to AAC technology, all skills related to AAC intervention can be organized under four overarching categories. Those categories are skills for: linguistic competence, social competence, operational competence, and strategic competence (Light, 1989).

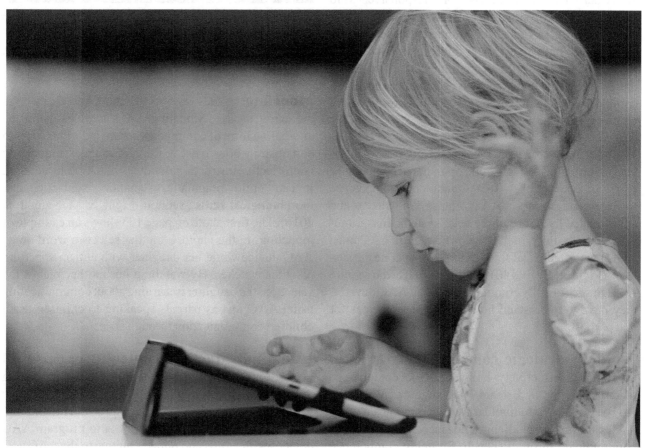

CroMary/Shutterstock.com

Building linguistic competence AAC intervention can effectively build linguistic competence (e.g., Caron, Light, Holyfield, & McNaughton, 2018; Holyfield, Caron, Drager, & Light, 2018; Soto & Dukhovny, 2008). "Linguistic competence refers to an adequate mastery of the linguistic code, including phonological, morphological, syntactic, and semantic aspects" (Light, 1989, p. 139). In addition to building language skills, building linguistic competence for individuals who use AAC also means learning language information specific to the AAC technology. For instance, linguistic competence for learning sign language includes learning to recognize hand shapes and their meanings. Linguistic competence for learning an app with picture symbols includes learning the meaning of each picture symbol (e.g., that a green arrow means "go").

Building social competence AAC intervention can effectively build social competence (e.g., Caron et al., 2018; Trottier, Kamp, & Miranda, 2011). Social competence for a person who uses AAC involves the pragmatic use of communication through AAC. It also includes relational skills including "a positive self-image, an interest in others and a desire to communicate, active participation in conversations, responsiveness to partners, and the ability to put partners at ease" (Light, 1989, p. 140). In order to communicate successfully using AAC, individuals must understand how to use language for effective communication and must understand that they themselves can be successful communicators with important information to share with others.

Building operational competence AAC intervention can effectively build operational competence (e.g., Achmadi et al., 2012). Operational competence for communication via AAC requires knowledge and skills related to the use of the AAC system. To communicate successfully, individuals who require AAC must "develop the technical skills required to operate the system" (Light, 1989, p. 140). For individuals who require AAC to successfully communicate using AAC devices, they have to understand how to use those devices for that purpose.

Building strategic competence AAC intervention can effectively build strategic competence (Rackensperger, Krezman, McNaughton, Williams, & D'Silva, 2005). Individuals who communicate using AAC face unique challenges not faced by individuals communicate through speech. Strategic competence involves developing "compensatory strategies to allow them to communicate effectively within restrictions" (Light, 1989, p. 141). For example, individuals communicating by pointing to printed words or photos must make sure to get communication partners to look at the paper before pointing to communicate. Individuals communicating using a tablet may need to learn to adjust the volume up when entering a loud area, then turn the volume back down when leaving for a quieter area.

GOALS AND OBJECTIVES

All skills required for successful communication through AAC can be organized as building either linguistic, social, operational, and strategic competence (Light, 1989). Therefore, all goals and objectives in AAC intervention should relate to one (or more) of the four competences. The table below outlines example AAC intervention goals for each of the four areas of competence for successful AAC use.

TREATMENT IDEAS

A number of strategies have been shown to be effective in AAC intervention (Beukelman & Mirenda, 2013). A few common and useful instructional strategies in AAC intervention are outlined below.

Modeling One way to teach AAC is through modeling its use. Modeling AAC involves using the alternative form of communication an individual uses to demonstrate how to use it. Research suggests modeling is an effective instructional strategy in AAC intervention; it can build pragmatic, semantic, syntactic, and morphological skills (Sennott, Light, & McNaughton, 2016). The first photo on page 103 shows an example of modeling. In the photo, a mother selects a word on an AAC device while her daughter with autism spectrum disorder watches. By watching her mother makes the selection, the daughter is learning about communicating using AAC just as parents speaking to children teach children communication through speech.

Using individualized content Another useful instructional strategy for AAC intervention is relating teaching to the individual's life. This can improve learning by making it more meaningful and motivating. One way to individualize content is to program AAC devices with words and phrases unique to the AAC user

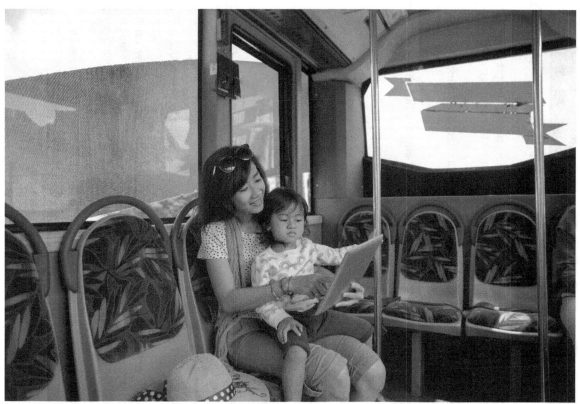

Odua Image/Shutterstock.com

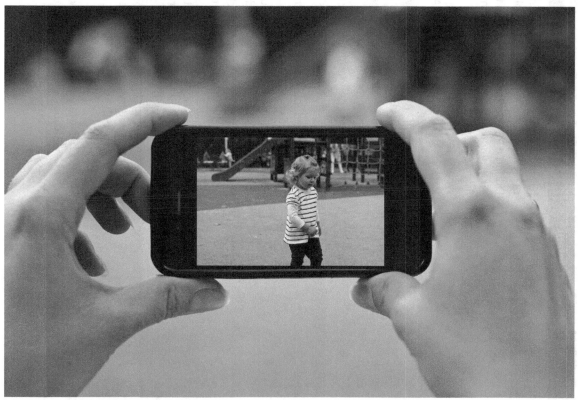

Michal Staniewski/Shutterstock.com

Table 7.1 Example Goals for AAC Intervention across Each Area Skills Required for Communicative Competence

Area of Communicative Competence	Example Goals
Linguistic	• [Client] will accurately identify 18/20 picture symbols from his/her AAC app by pointing to printed versions of them presented out of a field of four choices across three consecutive sessions.
	• During a 5-minute interaction with the clinician, [client] will use his/her AAC device to express present progressive –ing, plural –s, and past tense –ed morphemes accurately in 80% of obligatory contexts across three consecutive interactions.
	• When presented with 26 letter sounds (e.g., "mmmmm") orally from the clinician, [client] will select the corresponding letter on the keyboard on his/her AAC device with 90% accurately.
Social	• Using his/her AAC device, [client] will independently greet his/her medical support staff member when the staff member enters his/her house on 5 of 7 consecutive days.
	• During a group interaction with peers, [client] will take an average of two communicative turns per minute using his/her communication device.
	• [Client] will independently identify five attributes about himself/herself that make him/her an interesting and desirable communication partner.
Operational	• [Client] will independently locate the placement of 27/30 vocabulary words on his/her AAC app when presented with the words orally by the clinician.
	• [Client] will demonstrate accurate use of a laser pointer attached to his/her head to select 8/10 words printed and placed on the wall when presented with each word orally by the clinician.
	• When prompted by the clinician, [client] will effectively use his/her AAC device to send a message while interfacing with each of the following: e-mail, texting, and social media across two consecutive sessions.
Strategic	• Across five situations with different levels of background noise and distraction, the client will effectively use no-tech communication strategies to capture the attention of a communication partner before using low-tech AAC to communicate with that partner.
	• While on outings in the community, [client] will point to a notecard that says "I understand everything you say. I will respond to you by pointing to letters on a board. It may take me a minute. Please watch and be patient." to begin an interaction in the community (e.g., asking a question about a product before purchasing it) across five consecutive outings.
	• [Client] will reselect a vocabulary word on his/her low-tech AAC display following a selection that was not seen by a communication partner in order to resolve the communication breakdown in 3/5 obligatory contexts across two consecutive sessions.

and his or her life. Such unique vocabulary can make it more likely for AAC to be relevant and supporting in an individual's life (Beukelman & Mirenda, 2013). These high relevance words can be programmed on a high-tech AAC device in response to the context in which they occur. For instance, clinicians can use a tablet to take photos of an individual in a particular life context and then use those photos to represent vocabulary on an AAC device. Doing so in the moment is considered "just-in-time" programming (Schlosser et al., 2016). For instance, in the second photo on page 103, a clinician takes a photo of a child playing on the playground. She will show program the photo to say "play" and then offer it for the child to use to communicate.

Training communication partners In addition to teaching the individuals who require AAC to use it successfully, it is also important to train communication partners on using AAC as well (Kent-Walsh & McNaughton, 2005). Communication partner intervention is a highly effective approach to AAC intervention (Kent-Walsh, Murza, Malani, & Binger, 2015). In order to provide effective communication partner training, clinicians should consider incorporating the following

eight stages outlined by Kent-Walsh and McNaughton (2005):

1. Pretest and commitment to instructional program (e.g., discussing skills the communication partners want to learn and how the training can help them do so),

2. Strategy description (e.g., a definition of the skills related to supporting AAC use the communication partners will learn in the training),

3. Strategy demonstration (e.g., the clinician showing how to use the skill to support the individual who uses AAC),

4. Verbal practice of strategy steps (e.g., helping the communication partner in listing every step involved in the skills to support AAC use),

5. Controlled practice and feedback (e.g., role playing the skill with the communication partner, offering praise and advice throughout the role play),

6. Advanced practice and feedback (e.g., offering guidance while the communication partner is using the skills with the individual who requires AAC),

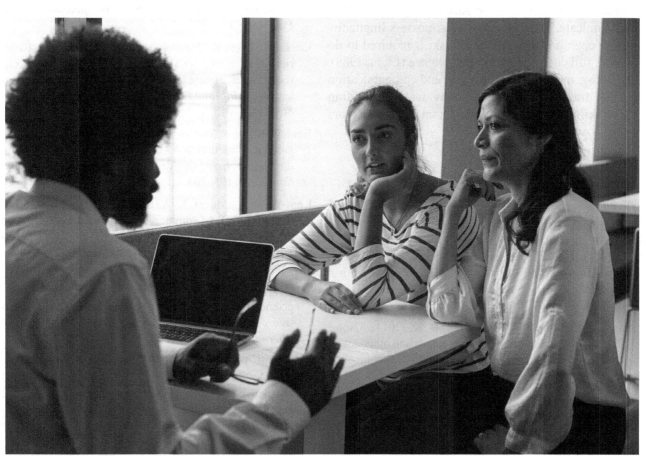

Monkey Business Images/Shutterstock.com

7. Posttest and commitment to long-term strategy use (e.g., reviewing all the learning the communication partner did throughout the training and how it can benefit the individual who uses AAC), and

8. Generalization of targeted strategy use (e.g., guiding the communication partner when practicing skills for supporting the AAC user in new contexts).

For instance, in the photo on page 105, a teacher provides initial training to a mother and sister of an adolescent with autism spectrum disorder who communicates using an app on a tablet about how to use modeling to support the child in building language and communication using AAC.

SUMMARY

AAC intervention can benefit individuals of any age who—temporarily or permanently—experience limited functionality of speech (Beukelman & Mirenda, 2013). Many different AAC options exist, ranging from options that require no technology (e.g., sign language) to options that use mobile technology (e.g., an app on a tablet). In order to successfully use AAC to communicate, and individual must possess linguistic, social, operational, and strategic skills required to do so with full communicative competence (Light, 1989). Modeling, individualized content, and communication partner training can support individuals in building these skills for becoming competent communicators using AAC.

REFERENCES

Achmadi, D., Kagohara, D. M., van der Meer, L., O'Reilly, M. F., Lancioni, G. E., Sutherland, D., . . . Sigafoos, J. (2012). Teaching advanced operation of an iPod-based speech-generating device to two students with autism spectrum disorders. *Research in Autism Spectrum Disorders, 6*(4), 1258–1264.

Alzrayer, N., Banda, D. R., & Koul, R. K. (2014). Use of iPad/iPods with individuals with autism and other developmental disabilities: A meta-analysis of communication interventions. *Review Journal of Autism and Developmental Disorders, 1*(3), 179–191.

Beukelman, D., & Mirenda, P. (Eds.). (2013). Augmentative and alternative communication: Supporting children and adults with complex communication needs (4th ed.). Baltimore, MD: Paul H. Brookes Publishing Co.

Beukelman, D. R., Fager, S., Ball, L., & Dietz, A. (2007). AAC for adults with acquired neurological conditions: A review. *Augmentative and Alternative Communication, 23*(3), 230–242.

Bourgeois, M., Fried-Oken, M., & Rowland, C. (2010). AAC strategies and tools for persons with dementia. *The ASHA Leader, 15*(3), 8–11.

Caron, J., Holyfield, C., Light, J., & McNaughton, D. (2018). "What Have You Been Doing?": Supporting displaced talk through augmentative and alternative communication video visual scene display technology. *Perspectives of the ASHA Special Interest Groups, 3*(12), 123–135.

Caron, J., Light, J., Holyfield, C., & McNaughton, D. (2018). Effects of dynamic text in an AAC app on sight word reading for individuals with autism spectrum disorder. *Augmentative and Alternative Communication, 34*(2), 143–154.

Fried-Oken, M., Beukelman, D. R., & Hux, K. (2012). Current and future AAC research considerations for adults with acquired cognitive and communication impairments. *Assistive Technology, 24*(1), 56–66.

Holyfield, C., Caron, J. G., Drager, K., & Light, J. (2018). Effect of mobile technology featuring visual scene displays and just-in-time programming on communication turns by preadolescent and adolescent beginning communicators. *International Journal of Speech-Language Pathology, 1*–11.

Iacono, T., Lyon, K., Johnson, H., & West, D. (2013). Experiences of adults with complex communication needs receiving and using low tech AAC: An Australian context. *Disability and Rehabilitation: Assistive Technology, 8*(5), 392–401.

Kent-Walsh, J., & McNaughton, D. (2005). Communication partner instruction in AAC: Present practices and future directions. *Augmentative and Alternative Communication, 21*(3), 195–204.

Kent-Walsh, J., Murza, K. A., Malani, M. D., & Binger, C. (2015). Effects of communication partner instruction on the communication of individuals using AAC: A meta-analysis. *Augmentative and Alternative Communication, 31*(4), 271–284.

Light, J. (1989). Toward a definition of communicative competence for individuals using augmentative and alternative communication systems. *Augmentative and Alternative Communication, 5*(2), 137–144.

Loncke, F. T., Campbell, J., England, A. M., & Haley, T. (2006). Multimodality: A basis for augmentative and alternative communication–psycholinguistic, cognitive, and clinical/educational aspects. *Disability and Rehabilitation, 28*(3), 169–174.

Millar, D. C., Light, J. C., & Schlosser, R. W. (2006). The impact of augmentative and alternative communication intervention on the speech production of individuals with developmental disabilities: A research review. *Journal of Speech, Language, and Hearing Research, 49*(2), 248–264.

Rackensperger, T., Krezman, C., Mcnaughton, D., Williams, M. B., & D'silva, K. (2005). "When I first got it, I wanted to throw it off a cliff": The challenges and benefits of learning AAC technologies as described by adults who use AAC. *Augmentative and Alternative Communication, 21*(3), 165–186.

Romski, M., Sevcik, R. A., Barton-Hulsey, A., & Whitmore, A. S. (2015). Early intervention and AAC: What a difference 30 years makes. *Augmentative and Alternative Communication, 31*(3), 181–202.

Schlosser, R. W., Shane, H. C., Allen, A. A., Abramson, J., Laubscher, E., & Dimery, K. (2016). Just-in-time supports in augmentative and alternative communication. *Journal of Developmental and Physical Disabilities, 28*(1), 177–193.

Schlosser, R. W., & Wendt, O. (2008). Effects of augmentative and alternative communication intervention on speech production in children with autism: A systematic review. *American Journal of Speech-Language Pathology, 17*(3), 212–230.

Sennott, S. C., Light, J. C., & McNaughton, D. (2016). AAC modeling intervention research review. *Research and Practice for Persons with Severe Disabilities, 41*(2), 101–115.

Soto, G., & Dukhovny, E. (2008). The effect of shared book reading on the acquisition of expressive vocabulary of a 7 year old who uses AAC. In *Seminars in speech and language* (Vol. 29, No. 02, pp. 133–145). © Thieme Medical Publishers.

Thompson, R. H., Cotnoir-Bichelman, N. M., McKerchar, P. M., Tate, T. L., & Dancho, K. A. (2007). Enhancing early communication through infant sign training. *Journal of applied behavior analysis, 40*(1), 15–23.

Trottier, N., Kamp, L., & Mirenda, P. (2011). Effects of peer-mediated instruction to teach use of speech-generating devices to students with autism in social game routines. *Augmentative and Alternative Communication, 27*(1), 26–39.

Case Scenario 7-1 Worksheet

Angela is a 58-year-old woman experiencing early-onset dementia. She lives at home with her husband and dog. Her two daughters live in nearby towns. Angela works as a media specialist in her city's historical library. Lately, she has been using speech less and less. When she does use speech, it often does not seem to make sense given the context of the interaction.

1. List an AAC technology that could benefit Angela.

   _____

2. Describe an interaction in which Angela would use the above AAC technology, and how it would help her be more successful.

   _____

3. Create an appropriate AAC intervention goal for Angela. State whether the goal addresses linguistic, social, operational, or strategic competence.

   _____

4. Choose an instructional strategy that could support Angela in reaching this goal and how it could be used in intervention.

   _____

Case Scenario 7-2 Worksheet

Clay is a 3-year-old with autism spectrum disorder. He makes a few select vocalizations in response to words from others, but he has not yet spoken a word to communicate. His parents know he has a lot of skills, and he is very interested in books and trains. However, they are worried about him going to preschool next year. They are worried he will have no way to show his teachers how much he knows or to interact with other children.

1. List an AAC technology that could benefit Clay.

   _____

2. Describe an interaction in which Clay would use the above AAC technology, and how it would help him be more successful.

   _____

3. Create an appropriate AAC intervention goal for Clay. State whether the goal addresses linguistic, social, operational, or strategic competence.

   _____

4. Choose an instructional strategy that could support Clay in reaching this goal and how it could be used in intervention.

   _____

Case Scenario 7-3 Worksheet

Jordyn is a 16-year-old high schooler with an intellectual disability and no speech due to a physiological difference in her brain. For most of her life, Jordyn has been using photos and objects to communicate. However, this option is really limiting her language as she has a large receptive vocabulary she does not have access to communicate expressively. Jordyn would likely benefit from a new AAC option to have access to more sophisticated communication.

1. List an AAC technology that could benefit Jordyn.

   _____

2. Describe an interaction in which Jordyn would use the above AAC technology, and how it would help her be more successful.

   _____

3. Create an appropriate AAC intervention goal for Jordyn. State whether the goal addresses linguistic, social, operational, or strategic competence.

   _____

4. Choose an instructional strategy that could support Jordyn in reaching this goal and how it could be used in intervention.

   _____

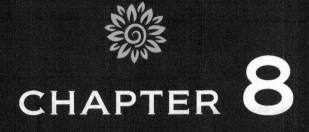

CHAPTER 8

Early Childhood Intervention for Language Skills

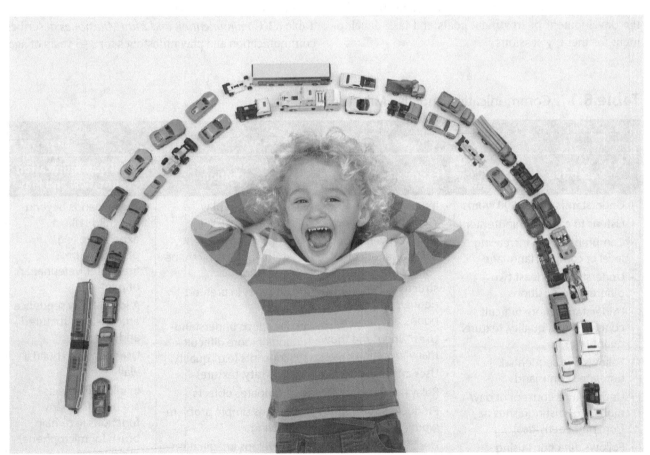

FamVeld / Shutterstock.com

"The more that you read, the more things you will know. The more you learn, the more places you'll go."

—Dr. Seuss

OVERVIEW

The purpose of this chapter is to provide a review of early childhood language milestones and to discuss how interventionists can facilitate these skills. The preschool age is critical for developing early pragmatic skills as well as setting the foundation for literacy and academic success. Parents and caregivers are not to be forgotten when providing intervention for this age group as they continue to serve as the child's primary teacher. Interventionists must be able to articulate goals, objectives and tasks well so that parents are easily able to carry over objectives in a variety of contexts in the child's functional settings. This chapter serves as a review of language development in early childhood and provides an opportunity for discussion among educators and emerging clinicians regarding the development of treatment goals and task development for therapy sessions.

LANGUAGE MILESTONES FOR EARLY CHILDHOOD

The efficacy of early intervention programs is well established in the literature (Anderson et al., 2003; Hajizadeh et al., 2017; Rolnick & Grunewald, 2003) and crosses cultural divides (Lazar & Darlington, 1982; Schweinhart, Weikart, & Larner, 1986; Sklerov, 1974; Zigler, Abelson, Trickett, & Seitz, 1982). Research has demonstrated that language development in early childhood can have long-lasting implications later in life (Barnett, 1995; Halfon & Hochstein, 2002). As is the case in early intervention, a child's developmental age, as well as their chronological age, must be taken into account during assessment and intervention planning. To determine a child's developmental age. It is important that examiners and interventionists are familiar with communication milestones. Table 8.1 *Communication and Play Milestones* describes communication and play milestones for 3–5 years of age.

Table 8.1 Communication and Play Milestones

37–42 Months			
Receptive Language	**Expressive Language**	**Cognition**	**Social Communication (Pragmatics) and Play**
• Understands 500–1,500 words • Listens to a 10–15 minute story • Comprehends an increasing level of complex language • Understands at least two different prepositions • Understands more difficult concepts (e.g., quality, texture, quantity) • Follows two sequential, unrelated commands • Understands concept of day/night (e.g., distinguishes day from night activities) • Follows directions using concepts of empty/full, same/different • Understands locational prepositions (e.g., next to) • Understands regular past tense verbs • Begins to understand comparatives (e.g., "I am taller than you.")	• Imitates a 5- to 7-syllable sentence • Holds conversations using a variety of correct grammatical structures (e.g., plural nouns, possessive nouns, and pronouns) • Uses "when" and "how many" questions • Uses articles: a, an, the • Relays a message • Produces 900–1,000 words • Describes what objects can be used for • Starts to answer "what if?" questions • Answers "What is missing?" • Answers "Which one does not belong" and "Why?"	• Imaginative play emerges • Consistently sorts items/objects by shape and color • Engages in pretend play • Develops understanding of more difficult concepts (e.g., quality, quantity, texture) • Compares objects • Begins simple problem solving • Develops imagination • Identifies common objects in pictures	• Play expands beyond the child's direct experience (e.g., pretend to be a firefighter, veterinarian, or pilot) • A logical play sequence emerges in structured and free play • Uses blocks to build a wall • Inanimate objects are used for many functions (e.g., hair brush for microphone) • Play association is consistent (e.g., if one child is playing "house" in a center, the other assumes additional "house" roles to play along) • Role play is fluid

43–48 Months			
Receptive Language	**Expressive Language**	**Cognition**	**Social Communication (Pragmatics) and Play**
• Understands 4,000–6,000 words • Continues to expand vocabulary comprehension • Understands singular vs. plural nouns • Completes sequential command with three parts/steps • Understands difference between past/present/future verb tenses • Answers final word analogies • Identifies objects missing from scene • Understands time phrases (e.g., "all the time, next week) • Understands day/morning/afternoon/night • Demonstrates understanding of comparisons of speed/weight • Emerging understanding of opposites • Understands higher level prepositions (e.g., between, above/below)	• Logically answers questions about simply stories • Uses possessive pronouns • Uses of plurals—irregular and regular • Talks about pictures and story books • Uses more sophisticated imaginative play • Uses negatives (e.g., shouldn't/won't/ can't) • Uses comparisons and makes inferences • Uses variations of to be (e.g., am, was) • Uses "How much?" and "How?" Questions • Spontaneous utterances are mostly grammatically correct • Communicates easily with adults and peers • Engages others in conversation easily	• Draws simple objects • Concentrates to complete problem solving tasks • Understands time concepts (e.g., today/tomorrow/ yesterday/ morning/afternoon/night) • Associates an object with an occupation, (e.g., stethoscope to doctor, badge to police officer) • Continues to develop imagination • Copies simple picture line drawings • Matches patterns • Emerging ability to recognize familiar words (e.g., "stop" on sign) • Emerging ability to recall address and phone number • Recalls parts of stories	• Enjoys new things • Prefers to play with peers • Role play continues to be fluid • Play themes expand and begin to be more complex (more characters/roles) • A play strategy is present in free play activities • Uses body parts as objects. • Imaginary objects start to be referred to in play • A doll's house is fully utilized in play. Characteristics begin to be attributed to the doll. • Emerging ability to discern fantasy from reality

49–60 Months			
Receptive Language	**Expressive Language**	**Cognition**	**Social Communication (Pragmatics) and Play**
• Understands function of body parts • Understands opposites • Engages and understands most concepts in stories (e.g., enjoys humor and surprise) • Understands comparatives and superlatives • Consistently identifies the difference between real and fantasy in stories • Understands: first, next, last • Appropriately responds to complex sentences	• Consistently uses 4–6 word sentences in spontaneous utterances • Produces complete sentences • Consistently produces the following grammatical markers (e.g., subject pronouns, object pronouns, possessive pronouns, plural –s, possessive –s, regular past/present/future tense verbs) • Uses conjunctions to begin a sentence (e.g., so, but)	• Identifies some letters • Emerging ability to write his/her name • Identifies some symbol/number correspondences • Tells jokes and enjoys humor • Enjoys counting and can count to a minimum of 10 objects at one time • Emerging ability to reason and argue with peers and adults	• Play is pre-planned and organized with complex sequences and sub-plots • Narrates object function and use is present during play • Cooperates and negotiates during play • Maintains role throughout play session • When playing with a doll, the child narrates the child's character and activities

(Continued)

Table 8.1 Communication and Play Milestones (Continued)

49–60 Months			
Receptive Language	**Expressive Language**	**Cognition**	**Social Communication (Pragmatics) and Play**
• Understands most of what is communicated by peers, family, and educators in familiar settings • Inconsistently identifies indefinite pronouns (e.g., few, many, both, every)	• Consistently answers "what if" questions • Emerging ability to ask for permission • Uses conjunctions (e.g., and, or) • Generates lengthy stories • Emerging use of adverbs • Uses irregular plural nouns (e.g., children, teeth, etc.) and irregular verbs (e.g., found, swam, ran, etc.)		• Adapts talking style based on communication partner and location of communication interaction • Consistently able to engage in competitive games • Establishes topic maintenance during conversations and play

Adapted from a variety of sources.

It is important to note that pre-literacy skills (the foundation of learning to read) start during this developmental period as well. For additional information on literacy skill development, see chapter 9.

Tracking development and progress can sometimes be difficult for this group of children. Parent report measures such as the *MacArthur-Bates Communication Developmental Inventories (CDIs)* (Fenson et al., 2006) or the *Communication and Symbolic Behavior Scale* (Wetherby & Prizant, 2002) can be beneficial in establishing language baselines and treatment plans. There are times that standardized testing does not provide the rich data needed to establish language goals that would be most useful and functional for the child (Price, Hendricks, & Cook, 2014). This is when communication sampling or narrative analysis may be beneficial.

Communication sampling is a means by which to gather a *representative* sample of a child's speech or language production in an effort to establish a baseline skill level. See Chapter 4 for additional information regarding speech sampling (documentation of phonology, articulation, prosody, voice, and fluency). For the purpose of this chapter, language sampling, documentation of syntax, semantics, and pragmatics, will be briefly discussed.

Cultural and linguistic diversity are important considerations when preparing to gather a language sample. It is unlikely that a clinician will be familiar with the culture of all clients he or she serves. Thankfully, there

are resources available to help clinicians gain insights in to their cultural biases and how they can better serve culturally and linguistically diverse individuals. (ASHA, 2002, 2010). It is important that clinicians gather as much information as possible regarding personal biases as well as the client's cultural preferences *prior* to gathering the language sample. If a child is not comfortable and motivated to communicate, the language sample gathered may not be truly representative of his/her abilities.

When gathering the language sample, non-verbal communication is important to document as well. This might include gaze shifts, behavioral outbursts, changes in demeanor given different settings, or even documentation of communicative intent. Some children are able to communicate quite efficiently without ever uttering a word. Some children use *American Sign Language or an Augmentative and/or Alternative Communication* (AAC) device to communicate. See chapter 7 to learn more about augmentative and alternative communication. If a child does not use his or her voice, clinicians are not to assume he or she is not attempting to communicate. Language samples can be completed regardless of the child's communication approach. It is just as important to note nonverbal language and communicative attempts as it is to note verbal expressive language.

When collecting the language sample, it is important to be in a setting that creates interest for the child so that he or she is motivated to communicate. Depending on the child and his or her language skills, a language sample generally includes a minimum of 20 purposeful or functional communication attempts. For children with higher level language skills, a language sample may be collected in 20 minutes or less. Ultimately, the clinician wants to collect a representative sample of the child's language skills in an effort to establish relevant and functional goals for the child's plan of care. It is recommended that clinicians audio and video record language samples if possible. After language samples are collected, the sample is transcribed. Speech samples are transcribed using the *International Phonetic Alphabet* (IPA), however, language samples are transcribed orthographically because the goal is to evaluate language content (semantics - word meanings), use (pragmatics - social communication), and form (syntax - grammar, morphology, and phonology).

After language samples are transcribed, the analysis begins. This can be done manually or via computer-based software programs such as *Computerized Language Analysis (CLAN)* and *Systematic Analysis of Language Transcripts (SALT)*. Software typically analyzes the data, but it is up to the examiner or interventionist to complete the final step of comparing outcomes to normative data. Language samples do not have to be completed as part of a comprehensive assessment and can be completed anytime during treatment in an effort to document progress. Early clinicians need keep in mind that open-ended questions (those that are unable to be answered with a simple "yes" or "no" response) and statements such as "I wonder what will happen if. . ." are good strategies to use with young children to encourage expressive language.

There are a variety of options for those interested in completing language sample analysis manually. One of the most common analysis procedures used is to determine the *Mean Length of Utterance* (MLU). This analysis was first conceptualized in the research of Roger Brown (1973) and is meant to serve as a way to develop morphological development as well as syntax in children. A *morpheme* is a meaningful unit of language. To compute the MLU, divide the total number of morphemes produced by the number of utterances counted. It is important to use only completely intelligible utterances in the final count. Bowen (2011) provides a good description and breakdown of a language sample. After determining the client's MLU, it can be compared it to normative data for the child's chronological age

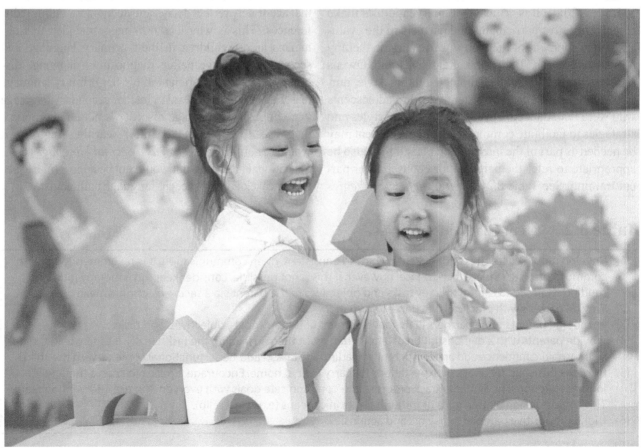

Dragon Images/Shutterstock.com

(Miller, Freiberg, Holland, & Reeves, 1992; Owens, 2004; Paul & Norbury, 2012). This information can be used as a baseline and as a measure of progress throughout the treatment reporting period. Regardless of how the clinician chooses to analyze language samples, the priority is documenting language production and progress. It is also important to note that language samples can be used as intervention tools for parents. For example, the clinician could provide the parent with a transcript of language produced by their child and ask them to identify language production patterns or errors (e.g., omitting articles or plural –s). For a list of Brown's (1973) grammatical morphemes in order of acquisition, visit: https://www.asha.org/Practice-Portal/Clinical-Topics/Late-Language-Emergence/Grammatical-Morphemes-in-Order-of-Acquisition/.

CAREGIVER COACHING

Research has well established that caregivers play a crucial role in literacy, communication, and academic development of children (Bradshaw, Koegel & Koegel, 2017; Committee on Early Childhood Pedagogy, 2000; DesJardin et al., 2017; Entwisle & Alexander, 1999; Kaiser & Roberts, 2013; Kemp & Turnbull, 2014; Wright & Kaiser, 2017). It is critical that interventionists make caregivers active participants and partners in the evaluation, development of the plan of care, and the therapy provision process. Baumrind, Larzelere, and Owens (2010) reported an authoritarian parenting style during the preschool years consistently lead to adolescents who were maladjusted. Discussing parenting styles and strategies to facilitate communication development may be needed as part of the intervention plan. It may also be appropriate to refer the parent(s) for counseling or parent training. See Table 8.2 *Parent Coaching Strategies*

for a list of ways to help parents become the primary facilitators of language development for their child. An additional resource for learning more about parenting styles and recommendations is the Center for Effective Parenting (https://parenting-ed.org).

Important factors to consider when providing intervention with children or when coaching caregivers is the impact of cultural differences and personal bias. Cultural differences can impact how children develop language and also what interventionists should consider to be disordered or delayed. Interventionists should thoroughly review cultural information presented on case history forms and reported by families. Do not be afraid to ask families questions in an effort to better understand potential cultural differences or preferences. Knowledge of cultural differences may also dictate how therapy lesson plans are designed as well. For example, a child from a family that is Jewish would find importance in learning language about Hanukkah, but likely would not benefit from therapy activities with a Christmas holiday theme.

Cultural bias in standardized testing is well-established in the literature (Hart & Risley, 1995; Lahey, 1990, 1992; Terrell & Terrell, 1983). Researchers are consistently working on developing speech and language assessments that accurately reflect delays and account for cultural differences. This is why it is now recommended that clinicians assess children in their primary language and secondary language before diagnosing a language disorder. If a child is proficient in his/her primary language (e.g., Spanish), but delayed in his/her secondary language (e.g., English), a language disorder is not an appropriate diagnosis. In this case, the child is learning English and would benefit from *English as a Second Language* (ESL) educational activities, but would not be appropriate to see on the caseload of a speech–language pathologist.

Table 8.2   Parent Coaching Strategies

(1) Develop rapport with the child's parent by having consistent, open communication. It is recommended that this communication take place face-to-face; however, if this is not possible, consider keeping a therapy journal or sending short video clips of therapy tasks and objectives to the parent via a secure electronic means.
(2) Provide parents with practical, functional information.
(3) Encourage parents to be partners in the development of therapy goals, objectives, and tasks.
(4) Provide parents with a demonstration of a task, then assist them in leading the task. Finally, let them lead the task so they gain confidence and are competent in leading the task in additional functional contexts with the child.
(5) Provide consistent feedback of expectations for carry over at home. Encourage families to keep a therapy journal, notebook, or binder to track progress and communicate goals with everyone on the intervention team. This could come in written form or through electronic means (e.g., video clip).
(6) Highlight positive parental behaviors and actions.

Compiled from a variety of sources.

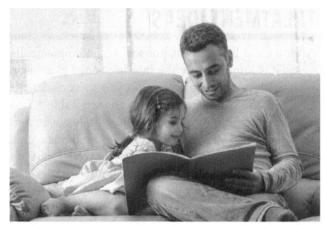

ilkercelik/Shutterstock.com

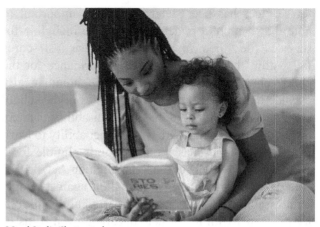

LStockStudio/Shutterstock.com

An interventionist must also consider his or her personal culture and journey. Individuals are shaped by a number of factors (e.g., culture, socioeconomic status, religion, community, etc.) and these must be taken in to account when working as a professional. *Cultural competence*, or the ability to provide services that meet the needs of individuals regardless cultural differences, is an imperative skill for emerging and seasoned professional to develop. One of the first steps in developing cultural competence is to identify the cultural identify of oneself. This often involves self-reflection and contemplation of how one's cultural identity can impact assessment and intervention procedures. According to the American Speech Language Hearing Association (ASHA, 2018), cultural competence in assessment and intervention is important to:

- respond to demographic changes in the United States;
- eliminate long-standing disparities in the health status of people based on racial, ethnic, and cultural backgrounds;
- improve the quality of services and health outcomes; and
- meet legislative, regulatory, and accreditation mandates. (Para. 6)

As mentioned previously, ASHA provides resources such as the Cultural Competence Checklist to help interventionists identify personal biases and reflect on how this cold impact service delivery.

INTRODUCTION TO IEPs

As mentioned in Chapter 6, Public Law 94-142 the Education of All Handicapped Children Act was passed which eventually led to the Individuals with Disabilities Education Improvement Act of 2004, (PL 108-446). This legislation established the need for *free and appropriate*

education (FAPE). This also stipulates that educators develop and annually update the child's *individualized family service plan* (IFSP) from birth through 2 years, 11 months of age and an *individualized education program* (IEP) for 3 through 21 years of age. The focus of this chapter is on children 3–5 years of age which is covered under Part B of IDEA, therefore, the IEP will be further discussed. It is important to note that the IEP developed during the early childhood or preschool years will follow the child to elementary school if services remain to be warranted. For brief examples and explanations of IEPs as well as IEP teams and implantation of IEPs, please view the following websites:

→ www.ed.gov—Search: IEP Guide
→ www.asha.org/SLP/schools/IEPs/
→ www.understood.org—Search: Anatomy of an IEP or IFSP

The child's SLP is typically involved in the evaluation of his/her speech and language skills as well as development of *measurable* goals on the IEP if eligibility

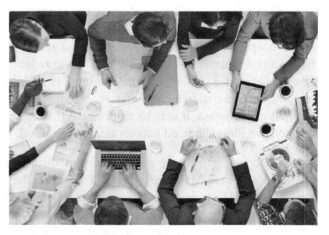

Rawpixel.com/Shutterstock.com

for services has been determined. It is important to note that if a child is determined to be ineligible for services (i.e., their speech and language test scores fall within the average range of performance for the child's chronological age), this does *not* automatically exclude that child from support services in the school setting. If the child has a diagnosed disability that can be documented to interfere with his/her ability to learn in the educational classroom, he/she is eligible for a *504 plan*. Section 504 of the Rehabilitation Act of 1973 (PL- 93-112) prohibits discrimination against people with disabilities. This means that if a child's disability interferes with his or her education (even if his or her speech and language scores are within the average range of performance), he or she is eligible to receive specific accommodations (methods or tools to ensure the child receives FAPE) in his or her educational setting (this could include classroom, playground, etc.). For an explanation of the differences between IEPs and 504 plans, please visit (https://www.understood.org/en/school-learning/special-services/504-plan/the-difference-between-ieps-and-504-plans). 504 Plans do not require schools to modify procedures; however, they do require that educators make sure education is *accessible*.

When IDEA was reauthorized in 2004, one of the major changes was that educators now had the option of using the *response to intervention* (RTI) model to determine if and how a student might respond to intervention services based on research-based intervention. This model was developed over time (Heller, Holtzman, & Messick, 1982; Fuchs & Fuchs, 1998, 2007; Vaughn & Fuchs, 2003). Over a period of time, if the child does not respond well to RTI, that could be an indicator that the child would benefit from special education services, and an IEP. RTI is traditionally explained and conceptualized as a three tier triangle and is often used in early elementary grades. See Figure 8.1, Conceptual framework for RTI. The concept is that most students will respond and learn in a general education setting, while others may learn best in focused group educational settings. If a child has completed a trial in a group education setting and is not making progress, it may be determined that a trial of intensive individualized intervention is warranted.

It is important for future communication disorders professionals to be familiar with RTI because they are primary players in the intervention component of this model. They may be called upon to serve as an observer for a student in tier 1, a consultant for a student in tier two, and the primary interventionist for a student in tier 3 for example.

TREATMENT IDEAS

After a child has been diagnosed with a language disorder, it is important for the interventionist to consider what is developmentally appropriate to consider and target on the child's treatment plan. See Table 8.1 for a review of communication and play milestones for a child three to 5 years of age. Keep in mind that a child with a chronological age of 4 may have the developmental age of 2. After the initial diagnosis and development of the treatment plan, the interventionist must then decide how to target skills directly in therapy session.

It is one thing to know a child needs to be able to expressively describe a familiar object's function. It is a different skill entirely when you are the clinician in a therapy room or classroom with a frustrated four year old whom you now need to get to participate for what may initially seem to be a fairly easy task (i.e., "tell me how we use this" while handing the child a toothbrush) multiple times. Interventionists are tasked with following detailed treatment plans, gathering data, and documenting progress all the while motivating a child to consistently participate in therapy activities.

Keep in mind, if the interventionist is not enjoying his/her time, the child/family likely isn't enjoying their time either. If a child isn't making progress on an objective, it is important the interventionist consider that it may be the method of teaching rather than the child's ability. Developing the ability to be reflective after therapy sessions is a difficult skill. What went well? What could have gone better? Could this task be presented in a way that is more motivating for the child? These are sometimes hard questions, but these are also questions that shape young clinicians into quality service providers.

GOALS AND OBJECTIVES

For additional information on how to generate long- and short-term goals, please refer to chapter one. Sample goals and objectives for early intervention follow. It is important to note there are a variety of ways to write goals and objectives. The list provided below is not a comprehensive list and should not be treated as such.

SAMPLE LONG-TERM GOALS

1. Child will improve receptive language skills to be commensurate with same-aged peers.

2. Child will improve expressive language skills to be commensurate with same-aged peers.

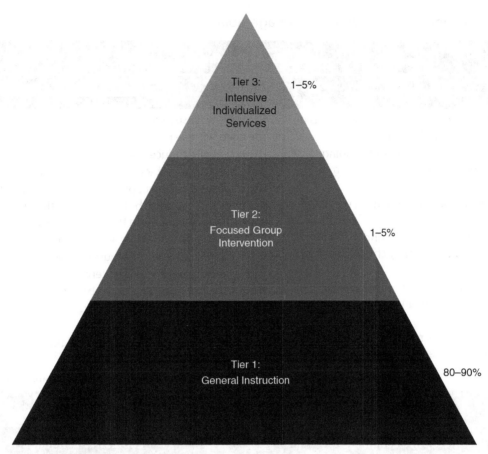

Figure 8.1 Conceptual Framework for RTI

© Kendall Hunt Publishing Company

3. Child will improve receptive language skills to enhance communication.
4. Child will improve expressive language skills to enhance communication.

SAMPLE *DO* AND *CONDITION* STATEMENTS FOR SHORT-TERM OBJECTIVES

For the objectives below to be complete, a *criterion* statement for mastery would need to be added. For example, if a clinician chose to use the same objective, "The child will vocalize in response to speech" the clinician would also need to add a *condition* and *do* statement. See the example provided below.

During semi-structured play activities, = Condition Statement

the child will vocalize in response to speech = Do Statement

5 times during a single session for 3 consecutive sessions. = Criterion Statement

The final draft of the short-term objective would be:

During semi-structured play activities, the child will vocalize in response to speech 5 times during a single session for three consecutive sessions.

For additional information on the development of criterion statements, please see Chapter 1, *Professional Development*. Table 8.3 provides sample language goals for early childhood language intervention. Take note that goals are divided based on *chronological age* and this may not match a child's *developmental age*. Treatment plans (also referred to as Plan of Care (POC) documents should reflect a baseline of the child's developmental age and goals to help bridge the gap between the child's developmental age and chronological age if applicable. Bridging the developmental and chronological age gap may not be possible in all cases. If achieving developmental skills commensurate with chronological age is not judged to be realistic in the reporting period, goals should be developed to help the child improve language skills.

Table 8.3 Sample Early Childhood Language Goals

36–42 Months	
Receptive Language	**Expressive Language**
• The child will match sets/categories of items or pictures (e.g., animals, food clothing). • The child will demonstrate understanding of prepositions by pointing/choosing from pictures. • The child will follow two sequential, unrelated commands. • The child will demonstrate an understanding of first opposites by pointing/choosing in pictures. • Given items/objects/pictures, the child will demonstrate an understanding of comparatives and superlatives. • The child will demonstrate an understanding of basic language concepts: size, color, shape.	• The child will use plural –s, –es. • The child will use possessive 's. • The child will produce first opposites. • The child will use subject pronouns (e.g., we, she, they). • The child will use object pronouns (e.g., her, him, them). • The child will use adverbs for place and time (e.g., behind, in back/front of, between, in the middle of, during). • The child will use copula be + negation (e.g., isn't). • The child will use present progressive verbs. • The child will use regular past tense verbs. • The child will use 3rd person verbs (e.g., sings.) • The child will use days of the week. • The child will ask "When" questions. • The child will take 4–5 conversational turns. • The child will request permission. • The child will provide 2 descriptors of desired object/picture.
43–48 months	
Receptive Language	**Expressive Language**
• This child will demonstrate an understanding of singular vs. plural nouns in sets of items/objects/pictures. • The child will completes 3-part stories in pictures. • The child will answer final word analogies. • The child will identify objects missing from scene. • The child will demonstrate an understanding of time concepts (e.g., day/morning/ afternoon/night). • The child will demonstrate an understanding of quantity concepts (e.g., some, all, numbers 1 through 3).	• The child will use "most, least". • The child will use reflexive pronouns (e.g. myself, himself, and herself). • The child will use possessive pronouns (e.g., its, her, his). • The child will ask "What, Which, Were" questions. • The child will tell 2 events in correct order.
49–60 months	
Receptive Language	**Expressive Language**
• The child will demonstrate an understanding of the function of body parts by pointing (e.g., "Show me what we use to see.") • The child will identify some indefinite pronouns (e.g., both, few, many). • The child will demonstrate an understanding of contractions. • This child will consistently identify the difference between real and fantasy in stories. • The child will demonstrate an understanding of: first, next, last. • The child will demonstrate an understanding of idioms and basic riddles.	• This child will recall 5 related items from a story. • The child will repeat 5 numbers, letters, or words. • The child will appropriately answer "What if…" questions. • The child will use comparatives and superlatives. • The child will use past/present/future tense verbs. • The child will use verb-noun derivation (e.g., teacher, baker, and speaker). • The child will use irregular past-tense verbs. • The child will use politeness markers (e.g., please, thank you).

REFERENCES

American Speech Language Hearing Association (ASHA). (2002). *Cultural competence checklist: Personal reflection.* Retrieved from https://www.asha.org/uploadedFiles/Cultural-Competence-Checklist-Personal-Reflection.pdf

American Speech Language Hearing Association (ASHA). (2010). *Cultural competence checklist: Service delivery.* Retrieved from http://www.asha.org/uploadedfiles/practice/multicultural/servicedelivery.pdf

American Speech Language Hearing Association (ASHA). (2018). *Cultural competence* Retrieved from https://www.asha.org/PRPSpecificTopic.aspx?folderid=8589938.30&section=References

Anderson, L. M., Shinn, C., Fullilove, M. T., Scrimshaw, S. C., Fielding, J. E., Normand, J., Carande-Kulis, V. G., & Task Force on Community Preventive Services. (2003). The effectiveness of early childhood development programs: A systematic review. *American Journal of Preventive Medicine, 24*(3), 32–46.

Barnett, W. S. (1995). Long-term effects of early childhood programs on cognitive and school outcomes. *The Future of Children, 8.*3), 25–50.

Baumrind, D., Larzelere, R. E., & Owens, E. B. (2010). Effects of preschool parents' power assertive patterns and practices on adolescent development. *Parenting: Science and practice, 10*(3), 157–201.

Bradshaw, J., Koegel, L. K., & Koegel, R. L. (2017). Improving functional language and social motivation with a parent-mediated intervention for toddlers with autism spectrum disorder. *Journal of Autism and Developmental Disorders, 47*(8), 2443–2458.

Brown, R. (1973). *A first language: The early stages.* Cambridge, MA: Harvard University Press.

Bowen, C. (2011). *Structural analysis of a language sample.* Retrieved from http://www.speech-language-therapy.com/.

Committee on Early Childhood Pedagogy (2000). Executive summary. In B. Bowman, M. S. Donovan, & M. S. Burns (Eds.), *Eager to learn: educating our preschoolers* (pp. 1-22). Washington, DC: National Academy Press.

DesJardin, J. L., Stika, C. J., Eisenberg, L. S., Johnson, K. C., Ganguly, D. M. H., Henning, S. C., & Colson, B. G. (2017). A longitudinal investigation of the home literacy environment and shared book reading in young children with hearing loss. *Ear and Hearing, 38*(4), 441–454.

Entwisle, D. R., & Alexander, K. L. (1999). Early schooling and social stratification. In R. C. Pianta, S. Rimm-Kaufamn, & M. Cox (Eds.), *The transition to kindergarten* (pp. 13-38). Baltimore, MD: Brookes Publishing.

Fenson, L., Marchman, V. A., Thal, D., Dale, P. S., Reznick, J. S., & Bates, E. (2006). MacArthur-Bates Communicative Development Inventories: User's Guide and Technical Manual. 2. Baltimore, MD: Brookes Publishing.

Fuchs, L. S., & Fuchs, D. (1998). Treatment validity: A unifying concept for reconceptualizing the identification of learning disabilities. *Learning Disabilities Research & Practice, 13*(4), 204–219.

Fuchs, L. S., & Fuchs, D. (2007). A model for implementing responsiveness to intervention. *Teaching Exceptional Children, 39*(5), 14–20.

Hart, B., & Risley, T. R. (1995). *Meaningful differences in the everyday experiences of young American children.* Baltimore, MD: Brookes Publishing.

Hajizadeh, N., Stevens, E. R., Applegate, M., Huang, K. Y., Kamboukos, D., Braithwaite, R. S., & Brotman, L. M. (2017). Potential return on investment of a family-centered early childhood intervention: A cost-effectiveness analysis. *BMC Public Health* (17), 796. doi.org/10.1186/s12889-017-4805-7

Halfon, N., & Hochstein, M. (2002). Life course health development: An integrated framework for developing health, policy, and research. *The Milbank Quarterly, 80*(3), 433–479.

Heller, K., Holtzman, W., & Messick, S. (1982). *Placing children in special education: A strategy for equity.* Washington, DC: National Academy of Science Press

Kaiser, A. P., & Roberts, M. Y. (2013). Parents as communication partners: An evidence-based strategy for improving parent support for language and communication in everyday settings. *Perspectives on Language Learning and Education, 20*(3), 96–111.

Kemp, P., & Turnbull, A. P. (2014). Coaching with parents in early intervention: An interdisciplinary research synthesis. *Infants & Young Children, 27*(4), 308.324.

Lahey, M. (1990). Who shall be called language disordered? Some reflections and one perspective. *Journal of Speech and Hearing Disorders, 55*, 612–620.

Lahey, M. (1992). Linguistic and cultural diversity: Further problems for determining who shall be called language disordered. *Journal of Speech and Hearing Research, 35*, 638–639.

Lazar, I., & Darlington, R. (1982). Lasting effects of early education: A report from the Consortium for Longitudinal Studies. *Monographs of the Society for Research in Child Development, 47*(2–3), 1–151.

Miller, J. F., Freiberg, C., Holland, M. B., & Reeves, M. A. (1992). Implementing computerized language sample analysis in the public school. *Topics in Language Disorders, 12*(2), 69–82.

Owens, R. (2004). *Language disorders* (4th ed.). Boston, MA: Allyn & Bacon.

Paul, R., & Norbury, C. (2012). *Language disorders from infancy through adolescence: Listening, speaking, reading, writing, and communicating.* New York, NY: Elsevier Health Sciences.

Price, L. H., Hendricks, S., & Cook, C. (2010). Incorporating computer-aided language sample analysis into clinical practice. *Language, Speech, and Hearing Services in Schools, 41*(2), 206–222.

Rolnick, A. J., & Grunewald, R. (2003). Early childhood development: Economic development with a high public return. *The Region, 17*(4), 6–12.

Schweinhart, L. L., Weikart, D. P., & Larner, M. B. (1986). Consequences of three preschool curriculum models through age 15. *Early Childhood Research Quarterly, 1*(1), 15–45.

Sklerov, A. J. (1974). The effect of preschool experience on the cognitive style of reflectivity-impulsivity of disadvantaged children. *Graduate Research in Urban Education & Related Disciplines, 7*(2), 77–91

Terrell, S., & Terrell, F. (1983). Distinguishing linguistic differences from disorders: The past, present and future of non-biased testing. *Topics in Language Disorders, 3*, 1–7.

Vaughn, S., & Fuchs, L. S. (2003). Redefining learning disabilities as inadequate response to instruction: The promise and the potential problems. *Learning Disabilities Research & Practice, 18*(3), 137–146.

Wetherby, A. M., & Prizant, B. M. (2002). *Communication and symbolic behavior scales: Developmental profile.* Baltimore, MD: Paul H Brookes Publishing.

Wright, C. A., & Kaiser, A. P. (2017). Teaching parents enhanced milieu teaching with words and signs using the teach-model-coach-review model. *Topics in Early Childhood Special Education, 36*(4), 192–204.

Zigler, E., Abelson, W. D., Trickett, P. K., & Seitz, V. (1982). Is an intervention program necessary in order to improve economically disadvantaged children's IQ scores?. *Child Development, 53*(2), 340–348.

PRACTICE

The purpose of this section is to provide emerging clinicians an opportunity to practice utilizing the information provided in the aforementioned chapter. Case scenarios provided are meant to facilitate discussion between emerging clinicians and educators to provide a foundation for competent clinical practice. There is often more than one way to answer the case scenario questions provided in this section. Long-term goals are meant to be over-arching goals for therapy during the current reporting period. Short-term objectives should correlate with long-term goals and are to be utilized as steps to achieve the long-term goal. Emerging clinicians need to be mindful that short-term objectives should be clearly stated, measurable, and time driven. Tasks should be developmentally appropriate for the child (which may not necessarily correlate with the child's chronological age).

Case Scenario 8-1 Worksheet

NAME: _____   DATE: _____

Isabella is a 4-year-old little girl who recently moved to your school district from Mexico. She was evaluated in both Spanish and English and was diagnosed with a language disorder. Her parents and family are bilingual and they report she is exposed to English and Spanish equally in the home. You have been tasked with providing Isabella language therapy services in English and are collaborating with another SLP who is providing therapy services in Spanish. In English, the evaluation reported receptive language skills within the average range of performance for her chronological age. A severe delay in expressive language (*Strengths: familiar with gender vocabulary, consistently produces 2-word phrases, identifies her name, and identifies body parts and familiar clothing. Weaknesses: no use of negatives (e.g., not, no), inconsistent production of familiar question forms, no production of 4–5 word sentences, no identification of colors or shapes, and significantly struggles with problem-solving and providing descriptions of objects and object use*) was reported. There are currently no concerns with feeding and swallowing and Isabella has age-appropriate play skills. Hearing and vision were also determined to be within normal limits at this time.

1. What might you and your colleague who is co-treating Isabella need to discuss as you develop her treatment plan and subsequent therapy session plans?

   _____

   _____

   _____

2. What is an appropriate LONG-TERM GOAL?

   _____

3. What are <u>three</u> appropriate SHORT-TERM OBJECTIVES? (Hint: Short-term objectives should correlate with the long-term goal listed above.)

   A.

   _____

   _____

   B.

   _____

   _____

C.

_____

_____

4. List the TASK you would use to target the short-term objectives listed above. The task for 3A should pair with the short-term objective listed for 2A. Please list MATERIALS you plan to utilize.

A.

_____

_____

B.

_____

_____

C.

_____

_____

5. How would you introduce and explain the purpose of each short-term objective and task in the therapy session to the parent/caregiver?

A.

_____

_____

B.

_____

_____

C.

_____

_____

Case Scenario 8-2 Worksheet

NAME: _____ DATE: _____

Gavin is a 3-year-old little boy with a diagnosis of a severe mixed (both receptive and expressive) language delay. His family reported they have no concerns with other developmental milestones at this time. His most recent evaluation noted possible concerns with play skills and limited joint attention. Gavin's parents reported he is often frustrated and tantrums a minimum of 10 times each day. Gavin's father is reported to most often be working during the day and his mother is reported to be his primary caregiver. His mother reported often feeling exhausted at the end of each day. Gavin was reported to have the following strengths in receptive language: inconsistently follows simple commands with gestural cues and able to attend to a game or book for one minute. Gavin was reported to have the following strengths in receptive language: *identifying a variety of body parts, consistently recognizing new words, understanding action phrases, and identifying familiar clothing items.* The following weaknesses were reported for receptive language: *understanding personal pronouns, understanding subject pronouns, understanding object function, and understanding size differences.* Gavin was reported to have the following strengths in expressive language*: consistently imitates 2-word phrases, inconsistently produces 1–2 word phrases, asking for "help" using one word, and use of a variety of nouns.* The following weaknesses were reported for expressive language: *production of plural –s, using negation, using subject pronouns, recalling familiar nursery rhymes, and producing 2–3 word phrases.* There are currently no concerns with feeding, swallowing, or play skills. Hearing and vision were also determined to be within normal limits at this time.

1. What referrals might be appropriate?

   _____

   _____

   _____

2. What is an appropriate LONG-TERM GOAL?

   _____

3. What are <u>three</u> appropriate SHORT-TERM OBJECTIVES? (Hint: Short-term objectives should correlate with the long-term goal listed above. So, if you listed a *receptive* long-term goal, the short-term objectives listed below should target *receptive* language development.)

   A.

   _____

   _____

   B.

   _____

   _____

C.

_____

_____

4. List the TASK you would use to target the short-term objectives listed above. The task for 3A should pair with the short-term objective listed for 2A. Please list MATERIALS you plan to utilize.

A.

_____

_____

B.

_____

_____

C.

_____

_____

5. How would you introduce and explain the purpose of each short-term objective and task in the therapy session to the parent/caregiver?

A.

_____

_____

B.

_____

_____

C.

_____

_____

Case Scenario 8-3 Worksheet

NAME: _____   DATE: _____

Lona is a 5-year-old little girl whose recent evaluation indicated a moderate delay in expressive language skills. All other milestones with the exception of communication were reported to have been met within the expected time frames. She has been attending preschool for two years and was initially referred for an evaluation by her primary care physician who felt Lona was not "talking as much as she should." Hearing and vision screenings fell within normal limits at this time. Lona was reported to have the following strengths in expressive language: *producing subject pronouns, use of regular verbs, inconsistent use of conjunctions, appropriately responds to "how" and "when" questions, and stays on topic during conversations turns.* Lona was reported to have the following weaknesses in expressive language: *inconsistent use of possessive pronouns, use of irregular past-tense verbs, use of comparatives and superlatives, use of politeness markers (e.g., please, thank you), and use of irregular plural nouns.* No other concerns with development were reported or documented in the evaluation report.

1. What is an appropriate LONG-TERM GOAL?

   _____

2. What are three appropriate SHORT-TERM OBJECTIVES? (Hint: Short-term objectives should correlate with the long-term goal listed above.)

   A.

   _____

   _____

   B.

   _____

   _____

   C.

   _____

   _____

3. List the TASK you would use to target the short-term objectives listed above. The task for 3A should pair with the short-term objective listed for 2A. Please list MATERIALS you plan to utilize.

   A.

   _____

   _____

   B.

   _____

   _____

   C.

   _____

   _____

4. How would you introduce and explain the purpose of each short-term objective and task in the therapy session to the parent/caregiver?

   A.

   _____

   _____

   B.

   _____

   _____

   C.

   _____

   _____

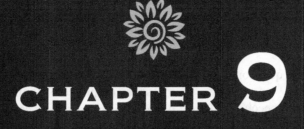

CHAPTER 9

Introduction to Literacy Development and Intervention

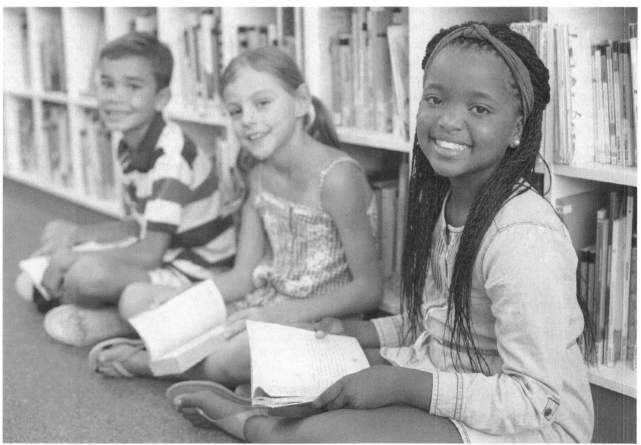

wavebreakmedia / Shutterstock.com

"Literacy is a bridge from misery to hope."

—Kofi Anan

This chapter is aimed to answer these questions:

1. What is the connection between speech and language and literacy?

2. What parts of speech and language are essential for learning to read?

3. What parts of literacy are addressed through speech therapy?

4. Case Studies and Essential Vocabulary

INTRODUCTION

Speech predates literacy by thousands of years. Only in the recent centuries has literacy come to the forefront of humans' consciousness. This is in part thanks to the printing press developed by Johannes Gutenberg in 1439. Until this time, humans told oral accounts of history, stories and expressed thoughts and ideas. This relied on people's ability to speak. Speech is putting language together to express complete thoughts and ideas and verbally expressing these to an audience. The English alphabet has changed over the years based on the invaders in the times of Old English, or Anglo-Saxons. The English alphabet is a phonics-based system, which is symbols based on phonemes or sounds. The combinations of

symbols which follow the rules of spelling to dictate a message comprised of sounds people have previously heard. This processes is called encoding.

The human brain is hardwired to learn and use speech and language (Giraud et al., 2007; Poeppel, 2003; Schroeder, Lakatos, Kajikawa, Partan, & Puce, 2008). The neurological networks within the mind are designed to process language on the left side of the brain, in Wernicke's and Broca's areas. The lexicons (vocabulary) and phonemes (sounds) of language are processed via incoming auditory signals. These signals contain significant amounts of information. The intonation, rate, and fluency of spoken language are processed as part of the message containing meaning.

Literacy, or words on a page, work much the same way as spoken language. A reader decodes the letters into understood words. This forms a mental picture (comprehension) of the message being transmitted. Punctuation marks delineate meaning to help complete the picture in the reader's mind. For a fluent reader, this process happens in milliseconds. However, unlike speech, the visual cortex is involved in reading (Demb, Boynton, & Heeger, 1997). The visual cortex is required to automatically read the symbols that represents the phonemes and to send these visual

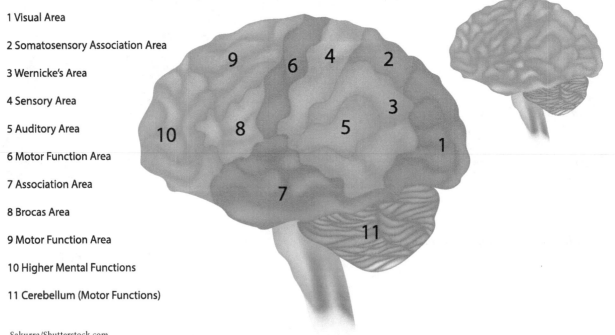

Anatomy and Functional Areas of the Brain

1 Visual Area

2 Somatosensory Association Area

3 Wernicke's Area

4 Sensory Area

5 Auditory Area

6 Motor Function Area

7 Association Area

8 Brocas Area

9 Motor Function Area

10 Higher Mental Functions

11 Cerebellum (Motor Functions)

Sakurra/Shutterstock.com

representations to the language processing center to build recognizable words.

The process of developing a picture from words read from a page to form a connection to a concept involves language. In Wernicke's area, the read word forms are matched to a previously heard or known auditory representation (in most cases). This is why early speech and language development is so critical. Children need exposure to speech, vocabulary and concepts in order to acquire a base of knowledge in which to build upon. If visual representations have no previously heard auditory template, more cognitive processes are required to use context clues and inference to build that representation of knowledge into a person's personal lexicon.

It is essential to develop speech and language skills prior to the introduction of literacy. Literacy skills are not necessary to develop speech and language; however, one cannot build literacy skills without language (Catts, Fey, Shang, & Tomblin, 1999; Dickinson, McCabe, Anastasopoulous, Peisner-Feinberg, & Poe, 2003). Therefore, let us take a closer look at the essential skills of speech and language to necessary to build a solid foundation for literacy.

SPEECH AND LANGUAGE MILESTONES IMPORTANT FOR LITERACY DEVELOPMENT

Before birth, children are hard-wired to learn speech and language. Babies process speech sounds in utero as their parents speak to them (Granier-Deferre, Ribeiro, Jacquet, & Bassereau, 2011). After birth, babies start to process speech sounds and develop their own language through crying. Happy cries, sad cries, mad cries, cries for hunger and tiredness are all ways babies differentiate meanings through verbal expression.

Around 6 months of age, babies begin to put together the phonemes heard to verbally match the world around them. These word forms come out as babble and word play. As babies gain the desired response, these word forms shape into basic words such as, mama and dada. Thus begins the growth of the personal vocabulary, or lexicon of a child. This lexicon grows as the child is exposed to more objects or people, and develops a symbolic representation in the form of speech.

At 1 year of age, babies start to put words together to form strings of words or phrases. Children model the speech heard to develop a sense of syntax, or an order to the words said. Morphological rules also develop through experience, modeling and feedback from the people surrounding the child. If you have ever heard the expression, the apple doesn't fall far from the tree, it all starts at the linguistic level. These strings of words take shape into sentences and stories as a child grows and continues to develop linguistic confidence and experiences. For additional information on language developmental milestones, refer to chapter 4.

Not only does linguistic confidence grow, but phonological processing develops as well. Articulation becomes clearer to match the speech sounds heard in a child's surrounding environment. The initial sounds are shaped into simple words. The words grow in increasing syllable length to match the phonological complexity. As the child is exposed to more concepts, the phonological and syllabic complexity develops to match what is being heard. Multisyllabic words develop sequencing and morphology so a child can distinguish plurals from singular, as well as past, present and future tense. All of these concepts develop at the same time. It's like gears of a machine all working together to develop cognition and the representation of thoughts in a symbolic manner, language. For additional information on speech sound acquisition, refer to Chapter 4.

LITERACY DEVELOPMENT

Pre-literacy skills such as vocabulary development, print knowledge, and phonological sensitivity can start as early as 3 years of age (McCardle, Scarborough, & Catts, 2001; Spira, Bracken, & Fischel, 2005; Storch & Whitehurst, 2003). Pre-literacy skills such as book orientation, tracking print from left to right, and "reading" or describing pictures to make a story with a sequence are developed before a child ever enters an elementary classroom. Children pick up on these skills as books are read and stories explained to them. Comprehension is built upon the pictures that accompany the words from the story.

Formal literacy knowledge grows from the pre-literacy skills. Letter recognition and sequencing are typically introduced in pre-school. Its starts with something familiar, children's names. For example, Andrea starts with the letter A. Finding the letter A in an alphabet is typically one of the first alphabetic knowledge skills taught. The alphabet song is sung and alphabetic

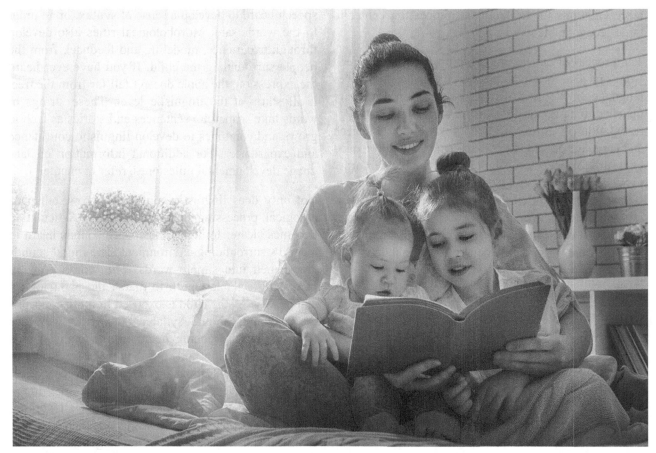

Yuganov Konstantin/Shutterstock.com

sequencing begins. However, environmental print serves a valuable purpose at this point. Children begin to associate the golden arches that make the letter M with McDonalds and fast food. The letter M in the form of golden arches is a symbolic representation of the restaurant. Children begin the print associations with recognizing environmental print to a physical concept at this point.

Print awareness is not just recognizing letters and sounds, but directionality as well. Kids need to start recognizing that the English language is read from left to right and top to bottom. Visual tracking and eye gaze become important at this stage. Children develop the visual cortex in the brain to recognize the symbols as letters with meaning. Visual tracking develops along with print orientation. This is when the child holds a book upright and reads from front to back. All of these skills are expected of children prior to entering elementary school and are to be viewed as potential objectives for SLPs and SLP-As who are working with preschool-age children with delays in language. Readers are encouraged to visit: https://www.theliteracybug.com/ stages-of-literacy/ for additional discussion of stages of literacy development as well as charts for the stages of reading development created by renowned literacy researcher, Dr. Jeannne Chall.

THE 5 PILLARS OF READING

The early elementary years for literacy development are critical. In 1997, Congress asked the Director of the National Institute of Child Health and Human Development (NICHD) to create a panel of experts in the area of reading development. The National Reading Panel (NRP) was soon established and charged with creating a framework for teaching reading skills. The NRP developed the five pillars of reading: phonemic awareness, phonics, fluency, vocabulary and comprehension, which build upon each other and are taught to children starting around the age of 4 (NRP, 2000). The skills of each pillar develop intertwined with each other, much like language development. If any single skill is weak, literacy as a whole will be a struggle.

Phonemic Awareness is the word play that develops the auditory acuity within words. Rhyming is the first skill learned. This word play amongst different words is crucial to hear the similarities and differences of a multitude of words. Segmenting into syllables, isolation of sounds and blending of sounds into words are three very distinct and complex phonemic awareness skills that are essential to build new words. Manipulation and ellison of sounds within the word to make new words are complex skills. The analysis and recognition of word parts to make new words helps to build that visual lexicon. All of these skills build the auditory skills of hearing the distinct components that make up words. These analysis skills then are applied to new words for decoding and reading.

Phonics is the individual skill of isolating letters or graphemes (vowel teams, digraphs, combinations, trigraphs) and matching them to a specific sound. The analytical skills developed during phonological awareness are applied when breaking down words into the significant parts. The parts are identified and matched to a phoneme or sound. The sounds are blended together to make a word. That word has meaning attached to it to build a bigger mental picture. Morphology fits into this skill as well. *Morphology* is the letter or letters added to a base word to change its form or use. Examples would be the plural -s added to the base word cat. One cat is great, but many cats would be problematic.

What happens when the words don't follow the rules or patterns that have been learned? That is when children need to learn instant words. These words have been called a variety of names over the years, sight words, rainbow words, Fry words (https://www.k12reader.com/subject/vocabulary/fry-words/) or Dolch words (http://www.dolchword.net/). For the purpose of this text, they will be called instant words. These are words that children need to know instantly upon coming across them. They do not necessarily follow a pattern or have meaning, yet are necessary for making a syntactic and morphologically correct sentence.

Fluency combines all three previously discussed skills into a single process. *Reading fluency* is different than speaking fluency. Stuttering (a.k.a. speaking disfluency) is a completely different process involving the auditory feedback loop and motoric movements. *Reading fluency* is the instant recognition of words, analysis of word parts to build into a word and attaching meaning to the word. This process happens in a matter of milliseconds through neurological connections within the brain. Auditory and visual processing combine to form new thoughts within the brain. If any part is slow, the processing is slow. This affects fluency, which can make reading a labor intensive chore for some people. The rapid recognition of letters, matched to a sound, built into a word, words combined into thoughts to form a mental picture are the essential building blocks of reading fluency.

The mental picture built through reading cannot be completed without previous word knowledge. This knowledge comes from exposure to words built into a personal lexicon. Everyone's lexicon is different due to personal experiences and exposure. Home and school environments add to this from a variety of factors. Factors such as socioeconomic status, school experience, exposure to new environments and vacations add to the knowledge base an individual holds. The vocabulary from a country life is full of concepts involving animals, crops and agricultural terms. City life involves traffic, buildings, occupations and terms that involve urbanite living.

VOCABULARY

In Beck, McKowen, and Kucan's book (2013), *Bringing Words to Life*, vocabulary is broken down into three tiers. **Tier one** vocabulary is general, everyday terms. Vocabulary at this level are concepts discussed in daily life. Most of the words originated from Old English, from the Anglo-Saxon people. This language contains nouns and verbs, articles and adjectives that are common most people. **Tier two** vocabulary involves academic terms that are used in school. As children continue through school they become fluent with these terms such as exam, evaluation, grades and semesters. By the end of formal schooling, these terms are synonymous with school. **Tier three** vocabulary is subject specific. In the field of speech pathology there are very specific terms used to discuss concepts between other professionals. This professional jargon contains words like dysphagia, lexicon, syntax, pragmatics to name a few. Vocabulary growth occurs when individuals are exposed to a variety of subjects. This knowledge is built upon the basic foundation of tier one vocabulary. This is depicted in Figure 6.1 in chapter 6 with the breakdown of vocabulary into tiers, much like a pyramid.

Words paint a complex picture through comprehension. *Comprehension* is using the known vocabulary to develop a mental image inside one's brain. This image is developed through working memory and permanently stored in long-term memory, or processed to be forgotten. *Cognition* is the process of making decisions on which images are worth remembering and which are worth forgetting in terms of how individuals relate and interact with the images in their environment. Comprehension is the permanent understanding of concepts and thoughts to use for future progressing in answering questions and making statements.

Comprehension also involves higher-level thinking processes such as inference, prediction and using context clues to develop a bigger picture of the situation or thought (Oakhill, 1982, 1984). If the bigger picture is missing information, cognition and comprehension will fill in the blanks. Sometimes this filling of the gaps may be erroneous, while at other times, the picture may be used to reach conclusions. Inductive and deductive thinking processes depend upon a strong comprehension of the events and processing of information to gain the proper perspective on a situation.

WRITING IS RELATED

Reading is a print-based activity, encompassing the transmission of messages in a permanent form. In order to have a message to read, one must be able to write. Written language can be transmitted through a variety of alphabets: phonetic, characters, or hieroglyphics to name a few.

Writing; however, is a more complex process than reading and is considered expressive language. One must know the correlation between sounds and symbols, the rules for combining the symbols to make whole words, and then combine words to make sentences. Sentences express complete thoughts, which are encoded into symbols or words on paper. This (written) expressive language activates the parts of the brain used for expressive (spoken) language, Wernicke's and Broca's areas, frontal cortex, as well as the motor strip and down to the fingertips for writing or typing. The visual cortex is also active during the writing process to monitor and give feedback about the printed message (Cohen et al., 2000; Bolger et al., 2005; Baker et al., 2007).

In order to complete a written message, thoughts must be formed and put into words. The words are encoded into letters and word patterns. Over 80% of the English word spellings are predictable if the spelling rules are known (Pinker, 1994). Not only are the rules of spelling necessary for writing, but the six syllable types need to

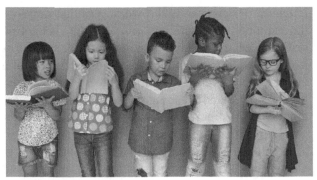

Rawpixel.com/Shutterstock.com

be understood and applied. Of course, all the previous reading concepts are incorporated in this process (phonological awareness, decoding, fluency, vocabulary, and comprehension). This is why writing and spelling typically lag behind reading in the timeline of developmental skill acquisition. Readers are encouraged to visit: https://dyslexiaida.org/scarboroughs-reading-rope-a-groundbreaking-infographic/ and see Figure 9.1 for additional discussion as well as a visual depiction of how reading skills are interwoven into various other language constructs through "The Reading Rope" figure created by Dr. Hollis Scarborough.

The connections between spoken and written language are well established in that (a) spoken language provides the foundation for the development of reading and writing; (b) spoken and written language have a reciprocal relationship, such that each builds on the other to result in general language and literacy competence, starting early and continuing through childhood into adulthood; (c) children with spoken language problems frequently have difficulty learning to read and write, and children with reading and writing problems frequently have difficulty with spoken language; and (d) instruction in spoken language can result in growth in written language, and instruction in written language can result in growth in spoken language (ASHA, 2001).

As with difficulty in learning to listen and speak, difficulty in learning to read and write can involve any of the components of language—phonology, morphology, syntax, semantics, and pragmatics. Problems can occur in the production, comprehension, and awareness of language at the sound, syllable, word, sentence, and discourse levels. Individuals with reading and writing problems also may experience difficulties in using language strategically to communicate, think, and learn. These fundamental connections necessitate that intervention for language disorders target written as well as spoken language (ASHA, 2001).

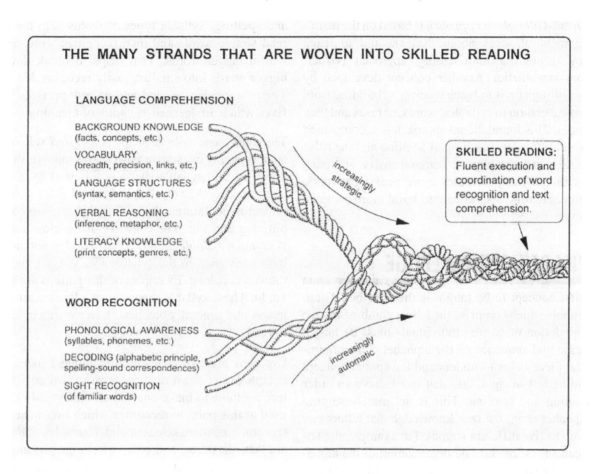

Figure 9.1

Handbook of Early Literacy Research, Volume 1 by Neuman, Susan B.,; Dickinson, David K. Reproduced with permission of Guilford Publications, Incorporated in the format Republish in a book via Copyright Clearance Center.

INTERVENTION

Reading and writing are modern inventions. The human brain has had to develop the cortexes of the brain to build new neurological networks to accommodate this 'new' technology. However, neurology does not always cooperate with technology. Some learners use their whole brain to process a linear technology such as reading. This is when a specialist in language is involved to rewire the neural networks of the brain to process literacy skills in a more timely and efficient manner. The most recent data from the National Assessment of Educational Progress (U.S. Department of Education, National Center for Educational Statistics, 2017) indicated that 32% of fourth graders performed below the basic reading level for their grade. Given that most 4th graders have a chronological age near 9, the aforementioned report is concerning since it has reported that 70% of students who do not learn to read by the age of 9 will not catch up with their peers (Shaywitz, 2003). As shown in the picture below, it is anyone's guess as to who in a group.

Reading and writing are not automatic processes that humans are designed to innately learn. Humans are hard-wired to learn oral language to pass down stories through the generations. Literacy skills must be taught in a systematic, explicit, and comprehensive way. They are not skills that can be obtained through collateral teaching or guessing methods. Humans learned oral language in small increments (babbling, sound play or reduplicated babbling, first words, two word combinations, sentences), learning to read is not such a different process. It is an analytical process that engages several types of cognition.

Many commercial programs are available. These programs each differ in the scope and sequence of material presented. However, the programs share a few commonalities. Each program is based on the concepts developed by Dr. Samuel Orton and Anna Gillingham.

The *Orton-Gillingham approach* is based on the team's development of ideas about dyslexia and to teach literacy through a multisensory approach (visual-auditory-kinesthetic). Another concept developed by Orton-Gillingham is to teach reading by building from phoneme isolation to syllables, words, phrases and then sentences. This foundational approach is accompanied by the simultaneous teaching of spelling and the rules of English orthography. A comprehensive approach to teaching literacy accesses more neural networks; therefore, creating a solid core to build more complex literacy skills.

ALPHABETIC KNOWLEDGE

The first concept to be taught is the alphabet. These 26 symbols which comprise the letters combined make the foundation of words. Individuals must be taught the name and sequence of the alphabet. This organizational piece helps to understand the spatial concept of reading left to right, and that words have an order for reading and spelling. This is not merely singing the alphabet song, but true knowledge that letters can make up to five different sounds. For example, the letter c can say /s/ or /k/. The organization of the alphabet helps teach the analytical skills within words that certain letters before or after a vowel effect how that vowel will sound (short or long). The basis of words consist of at least one vowel. Consonants typically make one sound; therefore, are taught first when learning to read.

PHONOLOGICAL AWARENESS

Phonological awareness begins the necessary skills of sound manipulation to create new words from previously learned words. Rhyming, sound deletion, sound addition, and switching of sounds to create new words also helps to teach word roots, prefixes and suffixes when more complex skills are learned. These phonological awareness skills are taught with alphabetic knowledge and phonemic awareness (sound to symbol correlation). These skills develop individually, while being taught simultaneously.

SYLLABLE TYPES

Once the three previously listed foundational skills have a solid beginning, the next developing skill coincides with learning orthographic patterns for reading and spelling. Syllable types of words help the reader read simple words and then recognize word patterns within bigger words. That helps to break down the bigger words into smaller, easily recognizable words. Then the reader can and add on any prefixes or suffixes which are learned as chunk of meaning.

The most basic syllable shape is a *closed syllable pattern*, typically consonant-vowel-consonant (CVC). The vowel in this syllable shape is followed by a consonant, making the vowel closed in and short. Examples of words containing this syllable shape are cat, beg, pin, dog and fun. The converse of the closed syllable is an *open syllable pattern*. The vowel is not closed in by a consonant in the syllable (VCV, CV); therefore, the vowel is long. Examples of this pattern are he, me, go, hi. These syllable shapes have a limited amount of letters and generally begin as starter words in learning to read.

Digraphs and vowel teams (diphthongs) increase the complexity of word reading because two adjacent letters combine to make one sound. Analytical skills are used at this point to recognize which two adjacent letters combine to make one sound. Examples of *digraphs* are "ch, sh, th, ee, and oo". Vowel digraphs and diphthongs are taught at this point as vowels are combined to make one sound or glide into each other. Rules of when vowel digraphs make particular sounds must also be taught at this point. Rules such as, when the 'a' sound is in the medial position the sound is spelled -ai- and if it is at the final position of a word, the sound is spelled -ay-. More examples are vowel digraphs ea and oe.

Included in this vowel knowledge is another syllable shape, *vowel-consonant-silent e*. This rule goes by many names, "silent e, sneaky e, e makes the vowel say its name" are a few examples of this rule. This orthographic pattern designates the middle vowel before the consonant-letter e will be long, or say its name. Cases in point: cake, five, rope and mule. The pattern of e-consonant-e is always found in two syllable words, like in athlete. This pattern is the next level of complexity in ready one to two syllable words.

As words increase in length, the complexity of the syllable shape also increases. "R" is a consonant that affects many other phonemes due to co-articulation (the effect of one sound upon an adjacent phoneme). The "R" effects the tenseness of the vowel before the r in the medial and final positions of words. Examples include fern, turtle, bird, star, fork and worm. The stress or accent of the syllable affects the final r-controlled vowels. When the accent is on the first syllable, the unaccented second syllable makes the /er/ sound like in doctor and dollar. The finely tuned phonological awareness is extremely important at this point to distinguish between the stress in syllables and the proper vowel sound prior to the r in words.

The sixth syllable shape are *final stable syllables*, consonant-le. These consonant-le patterns can occur with a variety of consonants, "gle, ple, ble, tle, zle, kle" just to name a few. The rules for final stable syllables are that the syllable is always final and unstressed. When the word is broken down into syllables, the first syllable is coded, open, closed, r-controlled, and the second and final stable syllable is bracketed off as a chunk. Examples include: "bubble, dangle, crackle and puzzle." The final stable syllable can be found in longer words such as expandable, but the word can be broken into syllables for easier coding and decoding. Yet, the rules of final stable syllable remain the same.

FLUENCY

Fluency is the culmination of all the previous skills mastered through hours and hours of practice and increasing complexity in texts. Fluency is the mastery of decoding to an automatic level. This only happens through the building and strengthening of neural networks through the cortexes of the brain. Automaticity is reached when the recognition of letters and words matched to the phonemes build to create a mental picture for comprehension within one's head. This process happens in a matter of milliseconds. This can only happen with accurate decoding and a processing rate that allows for the recognition of words into concepts rapidly enough to building a picture within the working memory.

Reading rate is the speed at which words are recognized, decoded and understood in a matter of a minute. The rate at which a person reads varies by the text, the number of familiar and unfamiliar words and complexity of syntax (word order and sentence structure). At www. readingrockets.com, clinicians can view the 2017 Oral Reading Fluency (ORF) data to help set long-term reading fluency goals. Simple, fiction texts tend to be read at a faster rate (think novels and magazine articles). The complexity of the text is simple, written for a 3rd–6th grade reader. Complex, nonfiction text with unfamiliar vocabulary is slower to decode with more complex sentence structures (think textbooks and books with many foreign names). Reading rate will increase with the amount of practice one puts into reading.

The kind of practice necessary to increase reading fluency is to practice an independent reading level. This may seem like the text is too easy, but the speed at which words and letter patterns are recognized will increase the automaticity. Once a person's instructional level of reading increases (reading with some help), then the independent reading level will increase. Reading passages and short stories are examples of items to start with while attempting to increase the reading fluency rate. Re-reading passages will build the familiarity with words and increase rate that will transfer to new passages (Wolf & Katzir-Cohen, 2001).

Another factor that affects reading fluency is accuracy. Reading accuracy is the amount of words read that are correctly decoded and understood. Accuracy affects the message that is intended to portray while reading. Reading accuracy is when words are recognized quickly and correctly. Often this is where people who are dyslexic come into the myth that dyslexia is only when words are read backwards. Truly, for someone who is dyslexic and needs to rewire the neural networks in the brain, the multisensory approach is best. That means visual, auditory, kinesthetic-motor, and tactile (VAKT) for cross-sensory associations between the phonemes and graphemes (Birsh, 2011). Yes, that means more time and energy into reading intervention than someone with a neurotypical brain.

Reading fluency, the measure of accuracy and rate is often used to measure a child's grade level for reading in school. This is not quite the accurate picture to capture a child's true measure of reading ability. Other factors contribute to reading success, such as vocabulary knowledge and comprehension of material. It is not the perfect picture to decode words without being able to gain a mental picture for comprehension. That is considered hyperlexic, and another type of reading disability.

VOCABULARY

Word knowledge is important for any language in all forms, receptive (read) and expressive (oral). Vocabulary is gained through everyday tasks and life experiences (Nelson, 1998). It is gained through the caregivers, friends and family people choose to surround themselves. Socioeconomic status plays a part in vocabulary development due to exposure to a variety of environments and access to books. Interventionists play a crucial role in increasing the exposure to new words and concepts through engaging therapeutic activities.

Exposure to vocabulary concepts requires experiences to build background knowledge. Even a simple trip to the grocery store can be a great opportunity to build vocabulary. Describing the physical attributes of the food, categorizing the types of food, the layout of the store and the process of buying food can be used to build experiential background knowledge for young children. We can expose children to other life experiences through books, videos and role-play activities. When those activities are rich in vocabulary, children learn the words to add to their own personal lexicon.

Personal vocabularies differ based on the individual's exposure to experiences and amount of books read. This is why socioeconomic status related so closely to vocabulary knowledge. Research shows that children from a lower socioeconomic class develop vocabulary at much slower rates that children of higher socioeconomic backgrounds (Arriaga, Fenson, Cronan, & Pethick, 1998; Dollaghan et al., 1999; Morrisset, Barnard, Greenberg, Booth, & Spieker, 1990) and often have limited language enriching experiences when compared to their peers (Hoff, 2003). The less interaction with books means a reduced vocabulary and interaction with print concepts.

COMPREHENSION

Comprehension is the ultimate goal of reading. Reading has no purpose unless a message can be transmitted and comprehended by the receiving party. *Comprehension* is the culmination of decoding the message, applying those decoded words to known vocabulary and background knowledge to remember and use the message

for a variety of purposes. Those purposes can be anything from telling a story to answering a question to generating a novel thought or idea. Comprehension is a multifaceted skill with many moving components and work in sync to create a vivid picture.

Comprehension involves answering the six wh- questions: who, when, where, what, why and how. Who is involved? When did the event/story take place? Where did the event/story take place? What is the problem? Why is it a problem? How did the problem get solved or attempt to be solved? This line of questioning can be applied to fiction and non-fiction texts. The importance of answering these six questions relates to the reader's ability to understand language, process language and apply language to answer questions and make summaries.

The ability to gather information to make inferences and predictions from text requires higher level comprehension skills. These skills involve comprehending the basic text, vocabulary knowledge, as well as incorporating the context clues. Then using background knowledge from previous experiences, the reader will make inferences for the outcome of the problem. The reader can also make predictions once comprehension questions and inferences are completed. For additional resources on literacy development and intervention, see Table 9.1.

Summarizing is a higher level skill necessary for individuals to take large chunks of texts and grasp the main idea and select details. The ability to summarize means a reader truly read and understood the text. The amount of background knowledge and vocabulary has been increased due to the incoming new information. The next time a reader reads about a related topic, previously synthesized text will be used as background information for the new text.

Table 9.1   Literacy Resources

http://www.readingrockets.org/	https://dyslexiaida.org/	https://www.understood.org/en
https://www.readinga-z.com/	https://www.altaread.org/	http://dyslexia.yale.edu/
madebydyslexia.org	dyslexiatraininginstitute.org	headstrongnation.org
http://liguisteducatorexchange.com	etymonline.com	Dyslexiafoundation.org
https://ies.ed.gov/ncee/wwc/		

REFERENCES

American Speech-Language-Hearing Association (ASHA). (2001). *Roles and responsibilities of speech-language pathologists with respect to reading and writing in children and adolescents* [Position Statement]. Retrieved from www.asha.org/policy.

Arriaga, R. J., Fenson, L., Cronan, T., & Pethick, S. J. (1998). Scores on the MacArthur Communicative Development Inventory of children from low- and middle-income families. *Applied Psycholinguistics, 19*, 209–223.

Baker, C. I., Liu, J., Wald, L. L., Kwong, K. K., Benner, T., & Kanwisher, N. (2007). Visual word processing and experiential origins of functional selectivity in human extrastriate cortex. *Proceedings of the National Academy of Sciences, 104*(21), 9087–9092.

Beck, I., McKowen, M., & Kucan, L. (2013) *Bringing words to life: Robust vocabulary instruction* (2nd ed.). New York, NY: Guilford Publications.

Birsh, J. R. (2011). *Multisensory teaching of basic language skills*. Baltimore, MD: Brookes Publishing Company.

Bolger, D. J., Perfetti, C. A., & Schneider, W. (2005). Cross-cultural effect on the brain revisited: Universal structures plus writing system variation. *Human Brain Mapping, 25*(1), 92–104.

Catts, H. W., Fey, M. E., Zhang, X., & Tomblin, J. B. (1999). Language basis of reading and reading disabilities: Evidence from a longitudinal investigation. *Scientific Studies of Reading, 3*(4), 331–361.

Cohen, L., Dehaene, S., Naccache, L., Lehéricy, S., Dehaene-Lambertz, G., Hénaff, M. A., & Michel, F. (2000). The visual word form area: spatial and temporal characterization of an initial stage of reading in normal subjects and posterior split-brain patients. *Brain, 123*(2), 291–307.

Dollaghan, C. A., Campbell, T. F., Paradise, J. L., Feldman, H. M., Janosky, J. E., Pitcairn, D.,. . . Kurs-Lasky, M. (1999). Maternal education and measures of early speech and language. *Journal of Speech, Language, and Hearing Research, 42*, 1432–1443.

Giraud, A. L., Kleinschmidt, A., Poeppel, D., Lund, T. E., Frackowiak, R. S., & Laufs, H. (2007). Endogenous cortical rhythms determine cerebral specialization for speech perception and production. *Neuron, 56*(6), 1127–1134.

Granier-Deferre, C., Ribeiro, A., Jacquet, A. Y., & Bassereau, S. (2011). Near-term fetuses process temporal features of speech. *Developmental Science, 14*(2), 336–352.

Hoff, E. (2003). The specificity of environmental influence: Socioeconomic status affects early vocabulary development via maternal speech. *Child Development, 74*(5), 1368–1378.

Oakhill, J. V. (1982). Constructive processes in skilled and less-skilled comprehenders' memory for sentences. *British Journal of Psychology, 7*, 13–20.

Oakhill, J. V. (1984). Inferential and memory skills in children's comprehension of stories. *British Journal of Educational Psychology, 54*, 31–39.

Pinker, S. (1994). The language instinct: How the mind creates language. New York, NY: William Morrow & Co.

Poeppel, D. (2003). The analysis of speech in different temporal integration windows: cerebral lateralization as 'asymmetric sampling in time'. *Speech Communication, 41*(1), 245–255.

Demb, J. B., Boynton, G. M., & Heeger, D. J. (1997). Brain activity in visual cortex predicts individual differences in reading performance. *Proceedings of the National Academy of Sciences, 94*(24), 13363–13366.

Dickinson, D. K., McCabe, A., Anastasopoulos, L., Peisner-Feinberg, E. S., & Poe, M. D. (2003). The comprehensive language approach to early literacy: The interrelationships among vocabulary, phonological sensitivity, and print knowledge among preschool-aged children. *Journal of Educational Psychology, 95*(3), 465.

McCardle, P., Scarborough, H. S., & Catts, H. W. (2001). Predicting, explaining, and preventing reading difficulties. *Learning Disabilities Research and Practice, 16*, 230–239.

Morrisset, D., Barnard, K., Greenberg, M., Booth, C., & Spieker, S. (1990). Environmental influences on early language development: The context of social risk. *Development and Psychopathology, 2*, 127–149.

National Reading Panel (NRP). (2000). Teaching children to read: An evidence-based assessment of the scientific research literature on reading and its implications. Retrieved from https://www.nichd.nih.gov/sites/default/files/publications/pubs/nrp/Documents/report.pdf

Nelson, K. (1998). *Language in cognitive development: The emergence of the mediated mind*. New York, NY: Cambridge University Press.

Schroeder, C. E., Lakatos, P., Kajikawa, Y., Partan, S., & Puce, A. (2008). Neuronal oscillations and visual amplification of speech. *Trends in cognitive sciences, 12*(3), 106–113.

Shaywitz, S. E. (2003). *Overcoming dyslexia: A new and complete science-based program for reading problems at any level*. New York, NY: Knopf.

Spira, E. G., Bracken, S. S., & Fischel, J. E. (2005). Predicting improvement after first-grade reading difficulties: The effects of oral language, emergent literacy, and behavior skills. *Developmental Psychology, 41*, 225–234.

Storch, S. A., & Whitehurst, G. J. (2003). Oral language and code-related precursors to reading: Evidence from a longitudinal structural model. *Developmental Psychology*, 38, 935–947.

U.S. Department of Education, National Center for Educational Statistics. (2017). *National achievement-level results*. Retrieved from https://www.nationsreportcard.gov/reading_2017/#/nation/achievement?grade=4

Wolf, M., & Katzir-Cohen, T. (2001). Reading fluency and its intervention. *Scientific Studies of Reading, 5*(3), 211–239.

PRACTICE

This purpose of this section is to provide emerging clinicians an opportunity to practice utilizing the information provided in the aforementioned chapter. Case scenarios provided are meant to facilitate discussion between emerging clinicians and educators to provide a foundation for competent clinical practice. There is often more than one way to answer the case scenario questions provided in this section. Long-term goals are meant to be over-arching goals for therapy during the current reporting period. Short-term objectives are to correlate with long-term goals and are to be utilized as steps to achieve the long-term goal. Emerging clinicians need always be mindful that short-term objectives are to be clearly stated, measurable, and time driven. Tasks are to be developmentally appropriate for the child (which may not necessarily correlate with the child's chronological age).

Case Scenario 9-1

NAME: _____   DATE: _____

Hudson is an 8-year, 3-month-old male just finishing the second grade. He has always struggled with reading according to his classroom teachers. He doesn't seem to know his letter sounds and struggles to decode words. Hudson has never repeated a grade in school. He has a history of speech therapy beginning at age four. He has been treated for an articulation disorder, as well as receptive and expressive language disorders. Hudson's articulation disorder has resolved through years of therapy. He continues to receive speech therapy to address his receptive and expressive vocabularies, as well as use of grammar and syntax.

1. What is an appropriate LONG-TERM GOAL to address literacy skills?

   _____

2. What are two appropriate SHORT-TERM OBJECTIVES? (Hint: Short-term objectives should correlate with the long-term goal listed above.)

   A.

   _____

   _____

   B.

   _____

   _____

3. Describe a TASK you would use to target one of the short-term objectives listed above. The task for 3A should pair with one of the short-term objectives listed for 2A.

   A.

   _____

   _____

Case Scenario 9-2

NAME: _____ **DATE:** _____

Madison is a 4-year, 10-month-old female in preschool. She has had a history of speech therapy for articulation, as well as expressive language for the past one and a half years. Madison struggles with rhyming words and remembering letters within the alphabet. Madison has a family history of dyslexia.

1. Would it be appropriate to enroll Madison in speech therapy to address pre-literacy skills?

2. What is an appropriate LONG-TERM GOAL to address literacy skills?

_____

3. What are two appropriate SHORT-TERM OBJECTIVES? (Hint: Short-term objectives should correlate with the long-term goal listed above.)

    A.

    _____

    _____

    B.

    _____

    _____

4. Describe a TASK you would use to target one of the short-term objectives listed above. The task for 4A should pair with one of the short-term objectives listed for 3A.

    A.

    _____

    _____

Case Scenario 9-3

NAME: _____   **DATE:** _____

Shaneice is a 14-year, 2-month-old female who just finished the 9th grade. She has struggled with school all of her life. Her teachers say, "she doesn't try," while Shaneice says she, "can't remember what she read." The Woodcock Test of Reading Mastery was administered which indicated average skills in decoding and word identification. She scored 1.5 to 2 or more standard deviations below average in the areas of word comprehension, listening comprehension and reading comprehension.

1. What is an appropriate LONG-TERM GOAL to address literacy skills?

   _____

2. What are <u>two</u> appropriate SHORT-TERM OBJECTIVES? (Hint: Short-term objectives should correlate with the long-term goal listed above.)

   A.

   _____

   _____

   B.

   _____

   _____

3. Describe a TASK you would use to target one of the short-term objectives listed above. The task for 3A should pair with one of the short-term objectives listed for 2A.

   A.

   _____

   _____

Case Scenario 9-4

NAME: _____   DATE: _____

Markus is a 15-year-old male who just finished the 10th grade. He has struggled with reading all of his school career; however, has never received intervention for reading. He has been given a 504 plan with accommodations for the classroom. Markus was evaluated for dyslexia and was identified as having poor phonological awareness, phonemic awareness and decoding skills.

1. Is Markus an appropriate candidate for speech therapy to address literacy skills?

2. What is an appropriate LONG-TERM GOAL to address literacy skills?

   _____

3. What are <u>two</u> appropriate SHORT-TERM OBJECTIVES? (Hint: Short-term objectives should correlate with the long-term goal listed above.)

   A.

   _____

   _____

   B.

   _____

   _____

4. Describe a TASK you would use to target one of the short-term objectives listed above. The task for 3A should pair with one of the short-term objectives listed for 2A.

   A.

   _____

   _____

CHAPTER 10

Intervention for Language Skills in Schools

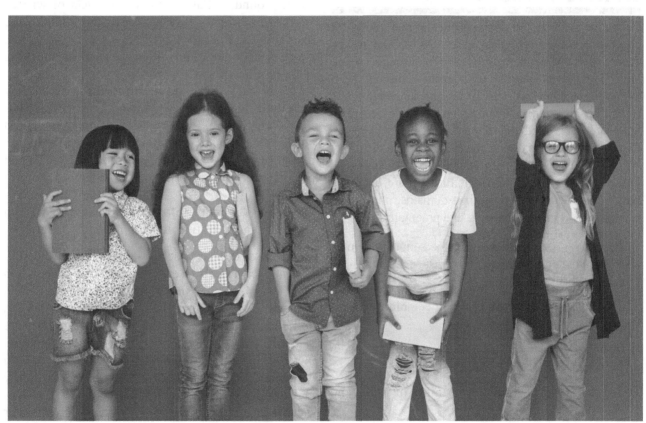

Rawpixel.com / Shutterstock.com

The importance of age-appropriate language in the lives of school-aged children cannot be overstated. Language skills are needed in communicating, and one needs to be able to communicate in order to learn. The better children's communication skills, the better they will do in school. Language skills influence many aspects of school-aged children's lives—academics, the ability to make and maintain friendships with peers, and self-esteem—all affected by one's language abilities. Reading, writing, gesturing, listening, and speaking are all modes of language. Language also overlaps in areas such as cognition, literacy, speech, and perception. Language is the embedded curriculum of school; therefore understanding content-specific language is critical to learning.

WHAT IS LANGUAGE?

Language is an agreed upon set of rules that allows for the expression of thoughts, ideas, wants, and needs. Language may be expressed verbally through speech which is the most common mechanism or through writing, sign, or other gestures. Expressive language refers to one's ability to express thoughts, while receptive language refers to the ability to comprehend language expressed by others. Some children can have difficulty with either expressive or receptive domains of language, or they can have issues with both; furthermore, language may be divided into five distinct domains, phonology, morphology, syntax, semantics, and pragmatics.

Phonology—deals with using the sound system of a language and the rules for how speech sounds are used to form words.

Morphology—deals with rules of combining meaningful units to form words.

Syntax—deals with rules for combining words to form appropriate phrases and sentences.

Semantics—deals with the meanings of words and sentences.

Pragmatics—deals with the appropriate use of language in social contexts. Refer to Chapter 11 for additional information on pragmatic language.

WRITTEN LANGUAGE DISORDERS

Children with written language disorders often have difficulty with the five domains of language listed above. Written language deficits can affect both the comprehension and/or production of language at all levels including: sound, syllable, word, sentence, and discourse. Written language disorders may co-occur along other conditions such of Spoken Language Disorder (SLD), Attention-Deficit Hyperactivity Disorder (ADHD), Autism Spectrum Disorder (ASD), Intellectual Disability (ID), Deaf or Hard-of-Hearing (DHH), or emotional disorders. Characteristics of language disorders are typically recognized before learning disabilities are formally diagnosed (Sun & Wallach, 2014) and due to the intricate relationship among reading, writing, spelling, and language, it is vital to target word recognition, vocabulary, and oral language comprehension in order for children to become strong readers and writers (Tunmer & Chapman, 2012).

At the sound, syllable, and word levels of written language, children may have difficulties with the phonological and morphological structure of words, reading decoding and spelling, and establishing firm associations with printed words. At the sentence and discourse levels, students may display deficits in identifying discourse elements, expressing relationships among ideas using syntax and cohesive devises, reading comprehension, formation of narrative and expository discourse, and social performance. Please refer to https://www.asha.org/Practice-Portal/Clinical-Topics/Written-Language-Disorders/ for more information related to written language and narrative development.

Language is critical to school-aged children and adolescents academic success; however, not all children enter school with the underlying language foundation to access and build upon the school curriculum. When children struggle using language rule systems, they are said to have a language disorder. The goal of speech and language services in schools is to help children with communication impairment do well both academically and socially. It should be noted that literacy development is also critical during the school-age years. For detailed information about literacy development and intervention, see chapter 9. There are a variety of terms used by various researchers in different contexts to label impairments in the use and/or comprehension of language. Box 10.1 is a brief description of each. For additional information, please visit the websites: https://www.asha.org/public/speech/development/communicationdevelopment.htm: https://childdevelopment.com.au/resources/child-development-charts/stages-of-language-development-chart/

Box 10.1 Spoken and Written Language Assessment—School-Age Children and Adolescents

Spoken and written language assessment for school-age children and adolescents is used to evaluate spoken and written language functioning (strengths and weaknesses) in school-age children and adolescents, including identification of impairments, associated activity and participation limitations, and context barriers and facilitators.

Spoken and written language assessment among school-age children and adolescents is conducted according to the *Fundamental Components and Guiding Principles.*

INDIVIDUALS WHO PROVIDE THE SERVICE(S)

Spoken and written language assessments are conducted by appropriately credentialed and trained speech-language pathologists.

Speech-language pathologists may perform these assessments as members of collaborative teams that include the individual, family/caregivers, educators, and other relevant persons.

EXPECTED OUTCOMES

Consistent with the World Health Organization (WHO) framework, assessment is conducted to identify and describe—

- underlying structural/functional strengths and deficits in language and literacy knowledge and skills that affect communication performance;

- effects of spoken and written communication impairments on the individual's activities (capacity and performance in everyday curricular/communication contexts) and participation;

- contextual factors that serve as barriers to or facilitators of successful communication and participation.

Assessment may result in the following:

- Diagnosis of a language disorder involving spoken and written language, or indication that an individual does not have a disorder.

- Clinical description of the spoken and written language disorder.

- Identification of a communication difference, possibly co-occurring with a language disorder.

- Evaluation of the effectiveness of prior intervention and supports.

- Prognosis for change (if a disorder is diagnosed).

- Recommendations for intervention and contextual modifications or other follow-up activities.

- Referral for other assessments or services.

CLINICAL INDICATIONS

Spoken and written language assessment services are provided to school-age children and adolescents as needed, requested, or mandated or when other evidence suggests that individuals may have spoken and written language impairments associated with their body structure/function and/or activities/participation.

Assessment is prompted by referral, by the individual's educational or medical status, or by failing a speech and language screening that is sensitive to cultural and linguistic diversity backgrounds.

CLINICAL PROCESS

Comprehensive assessment is sensitive to cultural and linguistic diversity and addresses components within the WHO's *International Classification of Functioning, Disability and Health* (2001) framework including body structures/functions, activities/participation, and contextual factors.

Assessment may be static (i.e., using procedures designed to describe current levels of functioning within relevant domains) or dynamic (i.e., using

(Continued)

hypothesis testing procedures to identify potentially successful intervention and support procedures) and includes the following:

- Review of auditory, visual, motor, and cognitive status.
- Collection of relevant case history information, including medical and educational status, and teacher, parent, and client/patient perspectives on the problem.
- Administration of standardized assessment tools and/or nonstandardized sampling or observation methods.
- Knowledge and use of language for listening, speaking, reading, writing, and thinking, including—
  ○ phonology and print symbols (orthography) for recognizing and producing intelligible spoken and written words;
  ○ syntactic structures and semantic relationships for understanding and formulating complex spoken and written sentences;
  ○ discourse structures for comprehending and organizing spoken and written texts;
  ○ pragmatic conventions (verbal and nonverbal) for communicating appropriately in varied situations;
  ○ metacognitive and self-regulatory strategies for handling complex language, literacy, and academic demands.
- Examination of how language strengths and weaknesses affect the individual's activities and participation in specific educational, social, and vocational activities identified as problematic by the assessment team.
- Examination of contextual factors that influence the individual's relative success or difficulty in educational, social, and vocational activities.
- Selection of standardized measures for spoken and written language assessment with consideration for documented ecological validity (including relevance to the student's sociocultural experiences, educational curriculum, and/or vocational needs).
- Follow-up services to monitor cognitive-communication status and ensure appropriate intervention and support for children and adolescents with identified spoken and written language disorders.

SETTING, EQUIPMENT SPECIFICATIONS, SAFETY AND HEALTH PRECAUTIONS

Setting: Assessment is conducted in clinical and/or educational environments conducive to eliciting representative samples of the patient's/client's spoken and written language functioning. Selection of settings for assessment is based on the input of others (including the child or adolescent), goals of assessment, and in consideration of the WHO framework. Identifying the influence of contextual factors on functioning (activity and participation) requires the collection of assessment data from multiple language contexts and settings.

Equipment Specifications: Children and adolescents who use AAC devices and techniques are assessed with the devices; those with hearing impairment are assessed using their preferred mode of communication and with optimal amplification.

All equipment and measurement tools are used in accordance with the manufacturer's specifications.

Assessment tools are selected with regard to—

- evidence of adequate reliability and validity, including ecological validity (e.g., curriculum-based assessment may be conducted with components of a student's actual school curriculum and with reference to educational agency standards);
- appropriateness for the cultural and linguistic backgrounds of the individual.

Safety and Health Precautions: All services ensure the safety of the patient/client and clinician and adhere to universal health precautions (e.g., prevention of bodily injury and transmission of infectious disease). Decontamination, cleaning, disinfection, and sterilization of multiple-use equipment before reuse are carried out according to facility-specific infection control policies and services and according to manufacturer's instructions.

DOCUMENTATION

Documentation includes pertinent background information, results and interpretation of assessments and observations, prognosis, and recommendations. Recommendations may include the need for further assessment, follow-up, or referral. When treatment is recommended, information is provided concerning recommended frequency, estimated duration, and type of service (e.g., individual, group, classroom-based, home program).

Documentation addresses the type and severity of the child or adolescent's spoken and written language disorder or difference and associated conditions (e.g., medical diagnoses or special education category).

Documentation may include a portfolio of the child or adolescent's communication samples (e.g., audiotaped or videotaped interactions, transcripts of spoken conversations or print samples read aloud, descriptions of nonverbal interactions or writing processes, written products).

Documentation includes summaries of previous services in accordance with all relevant legal and agency guidelines.

The privacy and security of documentation are maintained in compliance with the regulations of the Health Insurance Portability and Accountability Act (HIPAA), the Family Educational Rights and Privacy Act (FERPA), and other state and federal laws.

Results of the assessment are reported to the individual and family/caregivers, as appropriate. Reports are distributed to the referral source and other professionals when appropriate and with written consent.

ASHA POLICY DOCUMENTS AND SELECTED REFERENCES

American Speech-Language-Hearing Association. (1982). Definitions of language. *Asha, 24*(6), 44.

American Speech-Language-Hearing Association. (1991). Guidelines for speech-language pathologists serving persons with language, sociocommunication, and/or cognitive-communication impairments. *Asha, 33*(Suppl. 5), 21–28.

American Speech-Language-Hearing Association. (1996). Inclusive practices for children and youths with communication disorders. *Asha, 38*(Suppl. 16), 35–44.

American Speech-Language-Hearing Association. (2001). Roles and responsibilities of speech-language pathologists with respect to reading and writing in children and adolescents (position statement, executive summary of guidelines, technical report). *ASHA Supplement, 21,* 17–28.

American Speech-Language-Hearing Association. (2002). Knowledge and skills needed by speech-language pathologists with respect to reading and writing in children and adolescents. *ASHA 2002 Desk Reference, 3,* 455–464.

American Speech-Language-Hearing Association. (2004). Admission/discharge criteria in speech-language pathology. *ASHA Supplement, 24,* 65–70.

World Health Organization. (2001). *International classification of functioning, disability and health.* Geneva, Switzerland: Author.

LANGUAGE DIFFERENCE OR LANGUAGE DISORDER

Specific language disorder (SLD) is an impairment that deals with the mastery of language skills. There are many disorders and syndromes that affect a child's development and use of language (e.g., autism, Down syndrome, and intellectual disability). Children can also experience problems with language independent of known cause. Other related terms used to describe disorders involving language are "speech/language impairment" (sometimes also abbreviated as S/LI), "speech delay," "language delay," "developmental language disorder," and "persistent language impairment."

A *Language Difference* occurs when the child's first language L1 is developing normally while the child's second language L2 is being acquired. *Language Delays* refer to a sequentially normal, but slower pace of language development. A *Language Disorder* is characterized by deficit in in the comprehension and/or production of language. For children who are acquiring English as a second language (ESL) in order for a Language Disorder to be considered, they must have language deficits in both L1 and L2. When evaluating a child for which English is a second language, it is important to consult an ESL teacher to determine the student's competence of L1 and L2.

SPECIFIC LANGUAGE IMPAIRMENT (SLI)

When a child experiences difficulties acquiring language absent any neurological, sensory, intellectual, or emotional disorder, specific language impairment (SLI) may be diagnosed. SLI is typically first identified when children struggle to obtain oral language skills during their preschool years. The underlying cause of SLI is unknown but is not thought to be related to intelligence, i.e., children with SLI may be of average intelligence or even above-average intelligence except for the difficulty they experience with language. Children with SLI are often "late-talkers" who use fewer words when forming sentences and have a limited vocabulary when they do start talking. Children with SLI often experience life-long difficulties with language-based tasks and these issues may change over time. There is a well-established relationship between spoken and written language in those children who experience difficulties with verbal expression, and who may also display similar issues with written language.

LANGUAGE LEARNING DISABILITIES (LLD) AND SPECIFIC LEARNING DISABILITY (SLD)

Specific learning disability (SLD) is one of the 13 diagnostic categories for which children can receive special education services under the Individuals with Disabilities Education Act (IDEA, 2004). Children and adolescents with learning disabilities can have issues with reading, spelling, and writing which are all skills related to language. Math and social skill problems can also occur for children with learning disorders. Dyslexia is a term that is often used to describe problems with reading; however, because students demonstrating issues with reading frequently have language problems as well, SLD is the preferred label. Other terms used to describe SLD include language-based learning disabilities and specific learning disorder.

Data suggest that 80% of students shown to have a learning disability also have a language disorder. Due to the high percentage of those exhibiting language problems, good clinical practice suggests a speech and language assessment be conducted as a part of all diagnostic evaluations for children suspected of having a learning disability. LLD is not part of any official diagnosis under IDEA; rather it is applied to children and adolescents who could fit both the SLI or SLD diagnostic labels. For children diagnosed with SLD and language-based issues, school-based SLPs must consider ways that students' language abilities effect and interact with academic success (Wallach, 2014). One commonality among school-aged children with language learning difficulties is that they struggle daily with the academic language demands of listening, speaking, reading, and writing (Scott, 2014).

Social studies, science, mathematical story problems, and other academic areas all have a discipline-specific vocabulary that can pose challenges for students with comprehensive language learning problems (Ehren, Murza, & Malani, 2012; Faggella-Luby, Graner, Deshler, & Drew, 2012). SLPs must consider how the student's language abilities affect the active engagement of acquiring knowledge, skill, and strategies needed to access and retain not only the curricular content but also in dealing with the social and emotional demands each subsequent academic year brings (Ehren & Ehren, 2001). As Ehren, Hatch, and Ukrainetz (2012) remarked, language and literacy evolve from "learning to read" to "reading to learn" in the later elementary years, and then, the middle school years brings having to "learn to read" at even higher level texts. Frequently, students with language learning issues fall further and further behind affecting not only academic functioning but social performance and self-esteem.

SLPs offer services that assist students in becoming effective communicators, problem-solvers, and decision makers. School-based language services help students be more successful not only in academic aspects of school life but also in improving social aspects through better peer relationships. Specific services such as memory retraining, cognitive reorganization, language enhancement, and efforts to improve abstract thinking, can help children obtain the knowledge, skills, and abilities they will need to lead self-determined lives as adults.

ELIGIBILITY FOR SPEECH-LANGUAGE SERVICES

Speech and language services are a related service provided by the Individuals with Disabilities Education Act (IDEA, 2004) to eligible students. In order to qualify for service a child's school performance must be "adversely affected" by one of the 13 conditions as delineated by the IDEA. See chapter 13 for additional information about disability and Table 13.2 for list and description of the 13 disability categories.

Special education law outlines detailed procedures and criteria for establishing eligibility for special education services. These guidelines were enacted by Congress in the 1975 Public Law 94-142, also known as The Education for All Handicapped Children, which guarantees a free and appropriate education (FAPE) for all children with disabilities. Congress amended,

Table 10.1 Signs of Learning Disabilities

A Child With A Learning Disability May Have Difficulty	Examples
Talking about their own thoughts and ideas.	May seem as if the correct words are on the tip of the child's tongue. May use vague words, such as "thing" or "stuff". May pause to remember words.
Learning new words acquired in the school setting.	Such as words heard in class or seen in books.
Understanding questions and following directions.	
Remembering numbers in an ordered sequence.	Such as numbers in a telephone number or address.
Remembering details.	Such as details in a story plot, or in a teacher's instructions.
Understanding written information.	
Learning words to songs and rhymes.	
Distinguishing left from right.	This contributes to reading and writing difficulties.
Learning the alphabet and numbers.	
Sound-letter correspondence.	This contributes to reading and writing difficulties.
Writing.	May mix up the order of letters in words.
Spelling.	
Math.	May mix up the order of numbers.
Memorizing times tables.	

(Continued)

Table 10.1 Signs of Learning Disabilities (Continued)

A Child With A Learning Disability May Have Difficulty	Examples
Telling time.	
Producing speech sounds.	May have difficulty saying sounds. May not speak clearly. May be difficult to understand.
Language and literacy.	May have difficulty understanding auditory information. May not follow directions or answer questions well. May not say the correct words. May communicate in only short sentences. Language problems may also make reading and writing more difficult.
Social communication.	May have difficulty talking with other children. May not make friends easily. May not understand what others think or how they feel.
Cognitive communication.	May have difficulty with the thinking skills needed to remember, solve problems, and use imagination. May be caused by learning disabilities and/or brain damage.

updated and renamed the law several times since 1975. In 2004 the reauthorized statute, the Individuals with Disabilities Education Improvement Act of 2004 (IDEA, 2004), emphasized reading, early intervention, and research-based instruction provided by highly qualified educators to increase both accountability and improved outcomes for students.

In order to determine if students are eligible to receive special education services it must be determined that a disability exists, that the disability poses an adverse effect on educational performance, and that special services and/or supports are required for progress in the general education curriculum. It is important to understand that eligibility is determined by an interdisciplinary team of professionals that includes the parents and is based on an analysis of data from many sources. The diagnostic reports conducted by SLPs and other professionals are considered by the eligibility committee to determine if services are warranted under IDEA.

RESPONSE TO INTERVENTION AND MULTI-TIER SYSTEM OF SUPPORTS

First introduced with the reauthorization of the Individuals with Disabilities Act (IDEA) in 2004, response-to-intervention is a process to help identify students with SLD. A multilevel prevention system which integrates assessment and intervention is used to maximize student success while reducing problem behaviors. The only category that allows for utilization of response to interventions for identification purposes is specific learning disabilities. SLPs provide valuable input in regards to assessment methods and intervention practices recommended for students with language-based learning disabilities. See chapter 8 for additional information on RTI and Figure 8.1 for a visual depiction of RTI.

A Multi-tier System of Supports (MTSS) is a more comprehensive level of support to ensure that students get the help they need to learn. MTSS may incorporate RTI, but also may include social and emotional supports. It also provides mechanisms for adults to collaborate to help students who not only struggle academically, but also with social and emotional issues.

TRANSITION PLANNING

Transition planning has been mandated for students with disabilities and is an essential function of the IEP team—SLPs are vital to this process. In accordance with IDEA (2004) transition planning must: (a) begin by the time the student with a disability turns 16 years of age; (b) be developed by the IEP team; (c) be individualized, based on strengths, preferences and interests; and (d) provide opportunities for the student to develop skills in preparation for further education, employment, and independent living. The transition plan should address vocation, recreation, independent community living, and the identification of needed supports. It is imperative that the transition team consider

requisite skills for adult living including employment, access to community events and recreation, and adult social relationships.

Effective communication skills are vital to students leading self-determined lives. SLPs are critical to the

---

Box 10.2 Spoken and Written Language Intervention—School-Age Children and Adolescents

Intervention services (including academic instruction) are provided for school-age children and adolescents with spoken and written language.

Intervention is conducted according to the *Fundamental Components and Guiding Principles.*

INDIVIDUALS WHO PROVIDE THE SERVICES

Spoken and written language interventions for school-age children and adolescents are conducted by appropriately credentialed and trained speech-language pathologists, possibly supported by speech-language pathology assistants under appropriate supervision.

Speech-language pathologists may provide these services as members of collaborative teams that include general and special education teachers, the individual, family/caregivers, and other relevant persons.

EXPECTED OUTCOME(S)

Consistent with the World Health Organization (WHO) framework, intervention is designed to—

- capitalize on strengths and address weaknesses related to underlying structures and functions that affect spoken and written language development and use;
- facilitate the individual's social, educational, and vocational activities and participation by assisting the person to acquire new spoken and written language skills and communication strategies (verbal and nonverbal);
- modify contextual factors to reduce barriers and enhance facilitators of successful spoken and written communication and participation and to provide appropriate accommodations and other supports, as well as training in how to use them.

Intervention is expected to result in improved spoken and written language abilities; improved social, academic, and/or vocational functioning and participation; and improved contextual facilitators. Intervention also may result in recommendations for spoken and written language reassessment or follow-up, or in a referral for other services.

CLINICAL INDICATIONS

Spoken and written language interventions for children and adolescents are prompted by referral, mandate sand/or by the results of a spoken and written language assessment. Children and adolescents receive intervention services (including consultation) when their ability to communicate effectively and to participate in social, educational, or vocational activities is impaired because of a spoken and written disorder and when there is a reasonable expectation of benefit to the individual in body structure/function and/or activity/participation. Interventions that enhance activity and participation through modification of contextual factors may be warranted even if the prognosis for improved body structure/function is limited.

Speech-language pathologists also may provide services aimed at enhancing spoken and written language abilities and participation in social, education, and vocational activities, if so requested, when a communication difference is present or when spoken/written language development risks have been identified and service delivery is requested.

CLINICAL PROCESS

Intervention includes collaborative problem solving and providing information and guidance to patients/clients, families/caregivers, teachers, and other significant persons about spoken and written

(Continued)

language development and disorders, the course of intervention, an estimate of intervention duration, and prognosis for improvement.

Intervention goals and objectives are determined from assessment (including input from parents, teachers, the child or adolescent, and other relevant persons); are relevant to the educational curriculum, vocational and social interaction priorities; and are reviewed periodically to determine continued appropriateness.

Depending on assessment results and the age/stage of the child or adolescent, intervention addresses the following:

- Knowledge and use of language for listening, speaking, reading, writing, and thinking, including—
    - phonology and print symbols (orthography) for recognizing and producing intelligible spoken and written words;
    - syntactic structures and semantic relationships for understanding and formulating complex spoken and written sentences;
    - discourse structures for comprehending and organizing spoken and written texts;
    - pragmatic conventions (verbal and nonverbal) for communicating appropriately in varied situations;
    - metacognitive and self-regulatory strategies for handling complex language, literacy, and academic demands.
- Spoken and written language for social, educational, and vocational functions, with an emphasis on participation in specific activities identified as problematic for the individual.
- Contextual factors that influence the individual's relative success or difficulty in those activities.

Progress is measured by comparing changes in speech-language skills to established performance baselines, including curriculum-based language assessments and classroom or workplace observations.

Intervention extends long enough to accomplish stated objectives/predicted outcomes and ends when there is no expectation for further benefit during the current developmental stage.

SETTING, EQUIPMENT SPECIFICATIONS, SAFETY AND HEALTH PRECAUTIONS

Setting: Intervention may be conducted in a variety of settings, including regular or special education classes or in individual/group treatment outside the classroom/workplace setting, selected on the basis of intervention goals and in consideration of the social, academic, and/or vocational activities that are relevant to or desired by the individual.

In any setting, intervention addresses the personal and environmental factors that are barriers to or facilitators of the patient's/client's spoken and written language production. There is a plan to generalize and maintain intervention gains and to increase participation in relevant settings and activities.

Speech-language pathologists serve as members of education teams including special education preferral teams and problem-solving teams (e.g., teacher assistance teams). In addition, speech-language pathologists serve as members of an education team when they are providing speech-language instruction in the context of the academic program.

Equipment Specifications: All equipment is used and maintained in accordance with the manufacturer's specifications. Assistive technology needs (e.g., classroom or personal amplification systems, modified computer access software or hardware, augmentative and alternative communication [AAC] systems) are provided as needed and documented in the intervention plan.

Safety and Health Precautions: All services ensure the safety of the patient/client and clinician and adhere to universal health precautions (e.g., prevention of bodily injury and transmission of infectious disease). Decontamination, cleaning, disinfection, and sterilization of multiple-use equipment before reuse are carried out according to facility-specific infection control policies and services and according to manufacturer's instructions.

DOCUMENTATION

Documentation includes the following:

- Written record of the dates, length, and type of interventions (including consultations) that were provided.

- Consideration of the need for assistive technology (e.g., classroom or personal amplification systems, modified computer access software or hardware, AAC systems) and a plan for monitoring, maintaining, and updating any technological supports.

- Progress toward stated goals (relative to baseline levels and with relevance to the general education curriculum or vocational activities), updated prognosis, and specific recommendations.

- Evaluation of intervention outcomes and effectiveness within the WHO framework of body structures/functions, activities/participation, and contextual factors.

The privacy and security of documentation are maintained in compliance with the regulations of the Health Insurance Portability and Accountability Act (HIPAA), the Federal Educational Rights and Privacy Act (FERPA), and other state and federal laws.

Documentation may be a part of the patient's/client's individualized education program or other collaborative treatment plan.

ASHA POLICY DOCUMENTS AND SELECTED REFERENCES

American Speech-Language-Hearing Association. (1982). Definitions of language. *Asha, 24,* 44.

American Speech-Language-Hearing Association. (1991). A model for collaborative service delivery for students with language-learning disorders in the public schools. *Asha, 33*(Suppl. 5), 44–50.

American Speech-Language-Hearing Association. (1991). Guidelines for speech-language pathologists serving persons with language, sociocommunication, and/or cognitive-communication impairments. *Asha, 33*(Suppl. 5), 21–28.

American Speech-Language-Hearing Association. (1996). Inclusive practices for children and youths with communication disorders. *Asha, 38*(Suppl. 16), 35–44.

American Speech-Language-Hearing Association. (2000). *Guidelines for the roles and responsibilities of the school-based speech-language pathologist.* Rockville, MD: Author.

American Speech-Language-Hearing Association. (2001). Roles and responsibilities of speech-language pathologists with respect to reading and writing in children and adolescents (position statement, executive summary of guidelines, technical report). *ASHA Supplement, 21,* 17–28.

American Speech-Language-Hearing Association. (2002). Knowledge and skills needed by speech-language pathologists with respect to reading and writing in children and adolescents. *ASHA 2002 Desk Reference, 3,* 455–464.

American Speech-Language-Hearing Association. (2003). Appropriate school facilities for students with speech-language-hearing disorders: Technical report. *ASHA Supplement, 23,* 83–86.

American Speech-Language-Hearing Association. (2004). Admission/discharge criteria in speech-language pathology. *ASHA Supplement, 24,* 65–70.

National Joint Committee on Learning Disabilities. (1991). Providing appropriate education for students with learning disabilities in regular education classrooms. *Asha, 33*(Suppl. 5), 15–17.

World Health Organization. (2001). *International classification of functioning, disability and health.* Geneva, Switzerland: Author.

transition process due to their knowledge and expertise in the areas of technology and the communication needs of students with severe disabilities that are required for success in employment settings and in adult life. Speech-language services have the potential to provide students with the strategies needed for self-advocacy, problem-solving, conflict resolution, executive function, social-emotional competence, and independent living skills. The transition from high school to young adulthood is a crucial period for learning these skills (Davis, Koroloff, & Ellison, 2012).

Speech-language services are an essential part of the overarching curriculum for public school students with communication disorders (Powell, 2018). By focusing on communication for success in the academic arena, in addition to social skill supports designed to foster relationships with peers and others, speech-language services provide the foundation for successful transitions from school to adult living.

REFERENCES

ASHA. *Learning Disabilities*. Retrieved from https://www.asha.org/public/speech/disorders/Learning-Disabilities/

Davis, M., Koroloff, N., & Ellison, M. L. (2012). Between adolescence and adulthood: Rehabilitation research to improve services for youth and young adults. *Psychiatric Rehabilitation Journal, 35*, 167–170.

Ehren, B. J., & Ehren, T. C. (2001). New or expanded literacy roles for speech-language pathologists: Making it happen in the schools. In *Seminars in Speech and Language* (Vol. 22, No. 03, pp. 233–244).

Ehren, B. J., Hatch, P., & Ukrainetz, T. (2012). SLPs: At the core of the Common Core State Standards (CCSS). In *Seminar presented at the American Speech-Language-Hearing Association Convention, Atlanta, GA.*

Ehren, B. J., Murza, K. A., & Malani, M. D. (n.d.). *Disciplinary Literacy From a Speech–Language Pathologist's... : Topics in Language Disorders*. Retrieved from https://journals.lww.com/topicsinlanguagedisorders/Fulltext/2012/01000/Disciplinary_Literacy_From_a_Speech_Language.8.aspx

Faggella-Luby, M. N., Graner, P. S., Deshler, D. D., & Drew, S. V. (2012). Building a house on sand. *Topics in Language Disorders, 32*(1), 69–84.

Individuals with Disabilities Education Improvement (IDEA). Act of 2004, Pub. L. 108–466. Secondary Transition CFR 300.1(a); Summary of Performance 34 CFR 300.305(e)(3); Summary of Performance 20 U.S.C. 1414(c)(5)(B)(ii).

Powell, R. K. (2018). Unique contributors to the curriculum: From research to practice for speech-language pathologists in schools. *Language, Speech & Hearing Services in Schools, 49*, 140–147.

Scott, C. M. (2014). One size does not fit all: Improving clinical practice in older children and adolescents with language and learning disorders. *Language, Speech & Hearing Services in Schools, 45*(2), 145–152.

Sun, L., & Wallach, G. P. (2014). Language disorders are learning disabilities: Challenges on the divergent and diverse paths to language learning disability. *Topics in Language Disorders, 34*(1), 25–38.

Tunmer, W. E., & Chapman, J. W. (2012). The simple view of reading redux: Vocabulary knowledge and the independent components hypothesis. *Journal of learning disabilities, 45*(5), 453–466.

Wallach, G. P. (2014). Improving clinical practice: A school-age and school-based perspective. *Language, Speech & Hearing Services in Schools, 45*(2), 127–136.

Chapter 10   Activities

NAME: _____   **DATE:** _____

The following 10 therapy goals are missing vital details. Apply the skills you learned in Chapter 1 to correct these goals and make them *SMART* goals.

SCHOOL-AGED LANGUAGE:

Receptive:

1. By the end of the IEP, the patient will sequence picture cards with 90% accuracy as measured by observation, when given pictures and a verbal prompt.

2. By the end of the IEP, the patient will identify and discriminate sizes of toy vehicles with 80% accuracy as measured by observation, given a closed set of toy vehicles.

3. By the end of the IEP, the patient will follow specific and clear directions with 80% accuracy, as measured by observation, with no repetitions of requested instruction.

4. By the end of the IEP, the patient will identify classroom objects with 90% accuracy, as measured by observation, when given a description and closed set of five objects.

Expressive:

5. By the end of the IEP, the patient will incorporate vocabulary into a two-word phrase with 80% accuracy when given a picture card.

6. By the end of the IEP, the patient will communicate using 4- 5 words per sentence during 80% of utterances.

7. The patient will produce irregular past tense verbs during spontaneous speech with 80% accuracy as measured by observation.

8. By the end of the IEP, the patient will be able to give specific and clear directions with 80% accuracy, as measured by observation.

Literacy:

9. By the end of the IEP, the patient will understand the main idea of stories with 80% accuracy, as measured by observation.

10. By the end of the IEP, the patient will organize a story in correct order from memory with 80% accuracy, as measured by observation, given a closed set of story picture cards.

Report Writing Practice

Use the following case history and diagnostic information along with skills learned in this Chapter and Chapter 1 to write a diagnostic report (See Appendix for a diagnostic report example).

Report Writing Activity: SCHOOL-AGE LANGUAGE

SPEECH/LANGUAGE/HEARING Case History/ CHILD

SPEECH AND HEARING CLINIC

TO THE PARENTS OR GUARDIAN:

You have requested an appointment for an evaluation of your child's speech, language, hearing problem. To plan ahead for this interview, we need certain information. Please complete this form to the best of your ability.

All information will be held confidential.

I. General Information Child's Name: **Emma Lewis** Phone: **863-0126**

Birth Date: **June 7ᵗʰ, 2008**   Age: **7 years**   Sex: **Female**   Grade: **2nd Grade**

Address: **645 Blanchard Street**   City: **Tulsa**   State: **Oklahoma**   Zip: **74101**

School: **Tulsa Middle School**   Teacher: **Mrs. Lopez**   School District: **Tulsa School District**

Father's Name: **James Lewis**   Age: **38**   Address: **645 Blanchard Street**   City: **Tulsa**
State: **Oklahoma**   Zip: **74101**   Occupation: **Realtor**   Business Phone: **785-9006**
Place of Occupation: **American Dream Realty**   Education; number of years completed: **13 yr; high school diploma**

Mother's Name: **Tara Lewis**   Age: **35**   Address: **645 Blanchard Street**   City: **Tulsa**
State: **Oklahoma**   Zip: **74101**   Occupation: **Registered Nurse**   Business Phone: **800-7420**
Place of Occupation: **Tulsa Regional Hospital**   Education; number of years completed: **13 yr; high school diploma 4 yr; higher education**

If mother is employed, who cares for the child?   **Emma's father has a more flexible schedule and is typically with Emma and her younger brother when I can't be with them. On occasion, we do have James' mother, who lives with us, watch the kids when we both can't be home.**

Who will be responsible for payment of charges?   **Medicaid**

Brothers and/or sisters of the child: Name: **Eli Lewis**   Age: **7** School: **Tulsa Primary School** Grade: **Kindergarten**

Relatives or others living in the home: Name: **Barbara Lewis**   Relationship: **Grandmother (James' mother)**

Who referred you to the University of Arkansas Speech and Hearing Clinic?

Name: **Mrs. Hall**   Relationship: **The Speech-Language Pathologist at Emma's school**   Address: **9021 Main Street**   City: **Tulsa**   State: **Oklahoma**   Zip: **74101**

II. Statement of the Problem:

Describe the problem: **Mrs. Lopez, Emma's school teacher, asked the SLP at the school to evaluate her, but having too many students on her case load already, she referred us here for the eval. Emma doesn't seem to have the same language skills as her friends and we've been told by Mrs. Lopez that Emma doesn't talk much at all during class activities.**

When was the problem first noticed?

Emma has always been a little behind on her language, we've just thought that she would catch up on her own.

What has been done about it?

This is the first time we are recognizing that Emma being behind in her language is a problem to be treated.

What is the child's reaction to the problem?

Emma has not expressed to us that her language delay is a problem for her; I'm not sure she even notices it.

III. Pregnancy and Birth History:

During this pregnancy did the mother experience any unusual illness, condition or accident? If so, describe:

No

Were there any complications during the delivery such as caesarean, extremely long labor, or use of instruments?

No complications during Emma's birth

IV. Developmental History:

At what age did the following occur?

Sat alone unsupported: **6 months**   Crawled: **8 months**   Walked alone: **12 months**

Maintained bowel and bladder control while awake: **3 years**   asleep: **4 years**

Does the child seem awkward or uncoordinated?   **No**

V. Medical History:

Does your child have any long-term medical conditions for which they are now being or have been treated?   **No**

Does your child take any medication regularly?   **No**

Has your child had a speech examination prior to this time?   **No**

Where? _____

When?_____

What were the results?

Has your child had a hearing test prior to this time?   **Yes**

Where? **School** When?   **Last year**

What were the results?   **Normal**

Has your child had a neurological examination prior to this time?   **No**

Where? _____

When? _____

What were the results?

Has your child had a psychological examination prior to this time?   **No**

Where? _____

When? _____

What were the results?

Has your child had an eye examination prior to this time?   **Yes**

Where? **School** When?   **Last year**

What were the results?   **Normal**

Has your child had a recent medical examination?   **No**

Where? _____

When? _____

What were the results?

Name of child's pediatrician/physician: **Dr. Rufus Willams**

Address: **746 Get Well Soon Ave.**

City, State, Zip: **Tulsa, Oklahoma 74102**

Phone #: **670-4070**

Check the following illnesses this child has had:

_____ Measles __ **X** _____ Influenza _____ Draining Ears _____ Head Injury

_____ Mumps _____ Meningitis _____ Chronic Colds _____ Heart Disease

_____ Whooping Cough _____ Encephalitis _____ Allergies _____ Kidney Disease

_____ Chicken Pox _____ Epilepsy _____ Sinus Problems _____ High Fever

_____ Scarlet Fever _____ Tonsillitis _____ Excessive Ear Wax

Has this child ever had earaches or ear infections? ___ **X** _____ Yes _____ No. If yes, how often and in which ear(s)? _____ **Emma has only had a few minor ear infections** _____

How was it treated?

_____ **Antibiotics** _____

Has this child ever had a PE tubes, tonsillectomy and/or adenoidectomy? _____ Yes ____ **X** _____ No.

If yes, when _____ Physician _____

Is there a history of hearing loss in the family? _____ Yes ____ **X** _____ No. If yes, indicate which relative and at what age the hearing loss was diagnosed.

_____

_____

_____

Has your child ever worn a hearing aid? _____ Yes ____ **X** _____ No. If yes, what kind of aid and in which ear (s)? _____

_____

_____

VI. Daily Behavior:

Has your child been harder to manage than other children?   **Not really**

Describe any unusual behavior:

Describe your child's interests: **Emma loves anything and everything pink. She just turned 7 in June and we had a unicorn party. She also enjoys painting and expressing herself through arts and crafts.**

VII. Speech and Hearing History:

Does your child talk?   **Yes, some, but she also uses a lot of gestures.** If not, how does your child communicate?

When did your child first use words meaningfully?   **Around 24 months**

When did your child begin to use two-word sentences?   **Around 36 months**

Does your child understand what you say to him/her?   **I think she does. When I ask her to do something, she typically understands me enough to get the task done**

How well is s/he understood by parents?   **Emma doesn't talk much, but because I'm her mother, I can usually make out what she is trying to tell me.**

By others?   **Other friends and family have a difficult time understanding Emma**

Do you think your child hears adequately?   **Yes**

If not, what do you feel is the reason?

Has your child had frequent colds or ear problems?   **Not really**

VIII. Educational History:

Has your child repeated any grades?   **No**   If so, which ones?

With what subjects has your child had particular difficulties?   **Reading and writing**

Has your child ever had special help through the school?   **No**

If so, please describe:

How does your child feel about school? **Emma enjoys going to school for art class and seeing her friends, however, she doesn't like class activities or doing class work.**

After receiving Emma's case history, a date was scheduled for an evaluation. During the evaluation, an OME and hearing test were performed as well as standardized tests. The results of each of those are as follows:

Summary of Findings:

Emma's hearing test revealed that his hearing was within normal limits.

The two Assessment tests that Mrs. Hairston used to evaluate Emma were:

1. Expressive One-Word Picture Vocabulary Test (EOWPVT)

Raw Score	Standard Score	Percentile Rank
42	66	1

2 .Receptive One-Word Picture Vocabulary Test (ROWPVT)

Raw Score	Standard Score	Percentile Rank
79	94	34

3. Clinical Evaluations of Language Fundamentals, Fifth Edition (CELF-5)

Test	Scaled Score
Sentence Comprehension	11
Linguistic Concepts	10
Word Structure	6
Word Classes	9
Following Directions	8
Formulated Sentences	5
Recalling Sentences	5
Understanding Spoken Paragraphs	6
Pragmatics Profile	

Core and Index Scores	Standard Score
Core Language Score	96
Receptive Language Score	96
Expressive Language Score	83

Emma scored a severe score of 66 on the EOWPVT and an average score of 94 on the ROWPVT. She scored within normal limits for receptive language on the CELF-5 but she scored in the mild delay range with a standard score of 83 in the expressive language portion.

Given the case history, and results from the oral-mech, hearing screening and Assessment tests, Mrs. Hairston believes the prognosis for Emma to improve her expressive language is good. Mrs. Hairston recommends that Emma be seen for therapy to work on her expressive language skills once a week for an hour.

CHAPTER 11

Social Communication Disorders

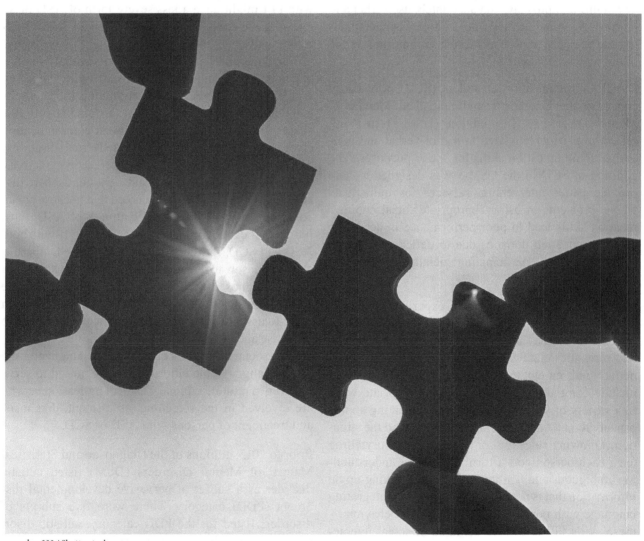

maradon 333 / Shutterstock.com

Language is a social tool that is used to form and maintain emotional relationships with those around us. Language occurs in a social context; this process, referred to as social communication, encompasses our ability to use language rule systems of form (syntax, morphology, and phonology) and semantics (word meanings). Pragmatic language gives our communication attempts function and intent and is an essential aspect of social communication. According to ASHA, social communication comprises "social interaction, social cognition, pragmatics, and language processing" (ASHA). Without it, other language aspects would have no meaning. The effective use of language encompasses much more than correct use of syntax, morphology, phonology, and vocabulary; one must apply these rule systems in the appropriate context. The ability to detect and express subtle nuances conveyed through prosody, and adequately use verbal and nonverbal communication rules, as well as understanding the perspective of others is just as important as the other aspects of language.

Social Communication Disorders (SCD), a category added to the Diagnostic and Statistical Manual of Mental Disorders, fifth edition (DSM-5) in 2013, reflect impairments related to use of verbal and nonverbal communication skills for social purposes. The addition of SCD in the DSM-5 was designed to help provide better intervention services for individuals whose problems in using appropriate social communication skills lead to poor performance in academic and/or occupation domains due to deficits communicating effectively, participating socially, or maintaining social relationships.

Individuals exhibiting SCD can experience life-long and wide-ranging issues that may impede performance in social situation, hinder development of friendships and romantic relationships, and limit success in academic and employment settings. Specific deficits include communicating in socially appropriate ways in a variety of social contexts; communicating appropriately to meet the needs of the listener and the situation, following rules for conversation and storytelling (e.g., each person gets a turn); using and understanding ambiguous and nonliteral language; picking-up on information that is not explicitly stated, and integrating language with nonverbal communicative behaviors—these skills fall under the domains of social interaction, social cognition, and pragmatic language.

Traditionally impairments in social pragmatic aspect of language have been thought to involve individuals with Autism Spectrum Disorder (ASD) solely; however, research has shown that not all children with social language concerns exhibit the complete diagnostic criteria of ASD (Adams, 2012). Historically, pragmatic language impairments (PLI) have been conceptualized as a type of specific language impairment (SLI), but rather than grammatical and lexical development being the primary concern, language function is the primary deficit. Current research has shown that, while children with SLI can also have difficulty with the social aspects of language, these impairments are less severe than those observed in PLI. Research has also shown that social language difficulties observed in individuals with PLI are less severe than in children with ASD, and there may be continuity in the social dimension of impairment between language impairments and ASD. Previously it was suggested that individuals with PLI might have a less severe form of ASD or an intermediate condition between SLI and ASD. PLI has traditionally been defined as deficits in the social use of language and has not included nonverbal communication; SCD, although often used interchangeably with PLI, includes nonverbal communication deficits and will be the preferred term for the remainder of this chapter. SCD can co-occur with other communication disorders in the DSM-5 (e.g., intellectual disability, traumatic brain injury, attention-deficit/hyperactivity disorder, learning disability, and right-hemisphere disability); however, it should be noted that because social communication deficits are a hallmark of ASD, thus, individuals cannot be diagnosed concurrently with both ASD and SCD. If all criteria are met for ASD, there is also no reason to identify SCD as well. SCD should not be diagnosed until the age of 4–5 years because children must demonstrate adequate language skills in order to assess higher-order pragmatic deficits. Due to expertise and understanding of the intricate connection among social communication, spoken language, and written language modalities, SLPs are poised to serve as part of a multidisciplinary team of professionals who are involved in the screening, assessment, diagnosis, and treatment of persons with ASD or SCD.

Prior to 2013, editions of the Diagnostic and Statistical Manual of Mental Disorders (DSM) listed autistic disorder as a subset of pervasive developmental disorders (PDD) category. There were five subsets of disorders listed for the PDD category: autistic disorder, Asperger's disorder, and pervasive developmental disorder, not otherwise specified (PDD-NOS), Rhett syndrome, and childhood disintegrative disorder. ASD was created as a new category, replacing the previous

Table 11.1 Social (Pragmatic) Communication Disorder

Diagnostic Criteria 315.39 (F80.89)
A. Persistent difficulties in the social use of verbal and nonverbal communication as manifested by all of the following:
1. Deficits in using communication for social purposes, such as greeting and sharing information, in a manner that is appropriate for the social context.
2. Impairment of the ability to change communication to match context or the needs of the listener, such as speaking differently in a classroom than on a playground, talking differently to a child than to an adult, and avoiding use of overly formal language.
3. Difficulties following rules for conversation and storytelling, such as taking turns in conversation, rephrasing when misunderstood, and knowing how to use verbal and nonverbal signals to regulate interaction.
4. Difficulties understanding what is not explicitly stated (e.g., making inferences) and nonliteral or ambiguous language (e.g., idioms, humor, metaphors, multiple meanings that depend on the context for interpretation).
B. The deficits result in functional limitations in effective communication, social participation, social relationships, academic achievement, or occupational performance, individually or in combination.
C. The onset of symptoms is in the early developmental period (but deficits may not become fully manifest until social communication demands exceed limited capacities).
D. The symptoms are not attributable to another medical or neurological condition or to low abilities in the domains of word structure and grammar, and are not better explained by autism spectrum disorder, intellectual disability (intellectual developmental disorder), global developmental delay, or another mental disorder.

PDD one. Prior diagnostic frameworks outlined a triad of impairments to identify ASD; the DSM-5, however, focuses on two symptom dimensions: social communication deficits and restricted and repetitive interests and behaviors. According to the DSM-5, ASD is characterized by impairments in social communication and social reciprocity and by the presence of restricted interests and repetitive behaviors. It is the presence of restricted interests and repetitive behaviors that primarily differentiates ASD from SCD.

DEVELOPMENT OF SOCIAL SKILLS

Emotional Intelligence (EQ)

The best predictor of life and career success is said to be determined by Emotional Intelligence, the ability to understand oneself and others, relate to people, and adapt and cope with changing situations and surroundings. We have an innate desire to be social, and this need manifests itself in our quest for acceptance in all areas of human interactions. Emotional Intelligence is said to be a better predictor of success than IQ which is thought to contribute only 20–25% to life goals, and is a weak predictor of overall wealth and happiness. EQ is three times better at predicting vocational success than does the social class to which one is born and luck. Other areas for which EQ is a strong predictor include: academic retention, the ability to cope with severe medical issues, aggressive behaviors in the workplace, suicide attempts, employment retention, and incarceration (Baron-Cohen).

Although the development of EQ is thought to be controlled by genetics, social and emotional skills must be taught in order to ameliorate the effects. Early expression of emotion by parents increases the development of EQ, while abuse is a significant hindrance. Social situations from real experiences provide the foundation for development because many social language skills are obtained through exposure to situations that are observed or overheard (i.e., incidental learning); however, children's social lives are decreasing as screen addiction is on the rise. Also, children have less time spent with adults who foster development of social skills, such as parents, grandparents, and aunts and uncles (Grayson, 2002).

Domains of EQ and specific skills include:

- Intrapersonal
  - Emotional self-awareness
  - Assertiveness
  - Self-regard
  - Self-actualization
  - Independence
- Interpersonal
  - Empathy
  - Interpersonal relationships
  - Social responsibility
- Adaptability
  - Problem-solving
  - Reality testing
  - Flexibility
- Stress Management
  - Stress tolerance
  - Impulse control
- General Mood
  - Happiness
  - Optimism

Theory of Mind

People who lack a well-developed Theory of Mind (ToM) have difficulties understanding the beliefs of others. ToM refers to the ability to predict and explain human behavior in terms of mental states such as intention, emotions, desires, and beliefs, and states of knowledge and ignorance. Starting around the ages of 3–5 years, children demonstrating typical development start to make links between the behaviors of others and their beliefs, desires and intentions. Specifically, deficits in ToM affect a person's ability to pick-up on deception, understand metaphorical language, follow the use of humor, and reason from a moral standpoint. Children who establish ToM early or have a strong sense of ToM are often more popular among their peers, and enjoy more life success in general.

Two stages of ToM development (Baron-Cohen, 1989)

1st Order ToM

- The understanding that people have different thoughts
- Children start to acquire this skill by age 4
- This skill is well-developed by age 5

2nd Order ToM

- The understanding that people have thoughts about other people
- This skill is not well developed until age 6

Early ToM Development

9 months of age

- Children begin to demonstrate intentionality
- Children begin to follow gaze and use gestures such as pointing

18 months of age

- Children begin to engage in behaviors to satisfy an adult's desire

24 months of age

- Children begin to communicate desires

3 years of age

- Children begin to make references to desires and beliefs as is evidenced by use of terms such as "think," and "know."
- Children begin to distinguish mental from physical entities (e.g., children understand that an actual kitty must be fed and not the thought of a kitty must be fed).

4 years of age

- Children become interested in and engages in deception
- Children begin to acquire 1st order ToM

5–6 years of age

- Children develop false-belief understanding (See Sally-Anne test explanation below).
- Children acquire 2nd order ToM

7–8 years of age

- Children begin to justify beliefs
- Children can attribute a variety of interpretations
- Children enjoy the humor of lexical ambiguity (e.g., "Time flies like an arror. Fruit flies like a banana).
- Children begin to negotiate dual-word meanings.

Poor ToM affects social interaction in a number of ways. For example, individuals with poor ToM may not,

- realize that they don't fit in when interacting socially
- correctly perceive social situations
- read social cues correctly, or may miss them entirely
- understand that some comments can offend or embarrass others
- pick up on facial expressions, body language, or tone of voice
- understand that our behavior affects how others think or feel about us
- adjust behavior to accommodate a particular social situation
- infer mental states of others including the mental states of story characters

By 4 years of age a child can pick out words that tell what goes on in the mind (Baron-Cohen, 1992):

Think	Know	Jump	Dream	Pretend
Eat	Hope	Wish	Move	Imagine

Sally-Anne Test

In this scenario, children with a well-defined 2nd order ToM will respond that Sally will look for her marble in the basket, because that is the last place that Sally knew the marble to be placed; however, children being tested (and Anne) know something that Sally doesn't know—the marble has been moved to the box. The majority (85%) of typically developing 5 year olds 'pass' the test by answering correctly, whereas the majority of 5 years old with ASD (80%) answer incorrectly by answering or pointing to the box. See Figure 11.1.

Executive Function

Executing functions are the neurologically-based processes that allow for self-management and self-regulation, making the achievement of goals—from preparing a meal to graduating from college—realities. Executive Function (EF) abilities are unique to humans. Dawson and Guare (2004) described these skills as necessary for overriding immediate rewards in favor of achieving longer-term goals. For example, as I am writing these words, it is an absolutely beautiful Fall Saturday. Fall is my favorite time of year. Typically on a lovely Fall Saturday, I would be visiting our local farmers' market, drinking a latte, and visiting with my fellow farmers' market goers. Instead of engaging in my favorite activity during my favorite time of the year, I am in my office writing. Because of my excellent EF capabilities, I can override immediate rewards—visiting the farmers' market—in favor of accomplishing a longer term goal—finishing this text. You are probably demonstrating your EF skills, as well. Would you rather be binge-watching your favorite program while sharing a bowl of popcorn with a friend, or would you rather be reading this text? I thought so. It is due to EF abilities that we can plan and accomplish goals.

Executive Function skills are mediated by the prefrontal cortext. This portion of the brain is the last to develop fully and is what makes us human and separates us from other species. Your personality and the very essence of who you are as a person are controlled by this portion of the brain. The sub-cortex is the part of our brain that drives such basic functions as hunger and thirst, sleeping and waking patterns, sex drive and bio-rhythms. If the sub-cortex is in control, our behavior may be characterized by intense emotions, impulsive reactions, rigid and repetitive responses, and lack of self-reflection and perspective-taking.

There are many components that make-up EF, which has often been referred to as the "CEO" of the brain. The foundation for EF is laid early in life and develops in a continuous rather than stage-wise fashion all through school reaching full development in the early 20s. Maturation without rich life-experiences will not result in well-developed EF. Everyday life experience provide the platform for honing EF in youths.

Experiences are paramount to the development of EF. Because executive control skills predict academic success more effectively than tests of academic achievement or cognitive ability, fostering these vital functions throughout childhood and into early adulthood is crucial. Facilitation of EF should focus on providing learning experiences with clearly defined expectations for different circumstances and environments. Rather than merely attempting to manage problem behaviors of children and youths through this vital developmental stage proactive teaching is required because EF is

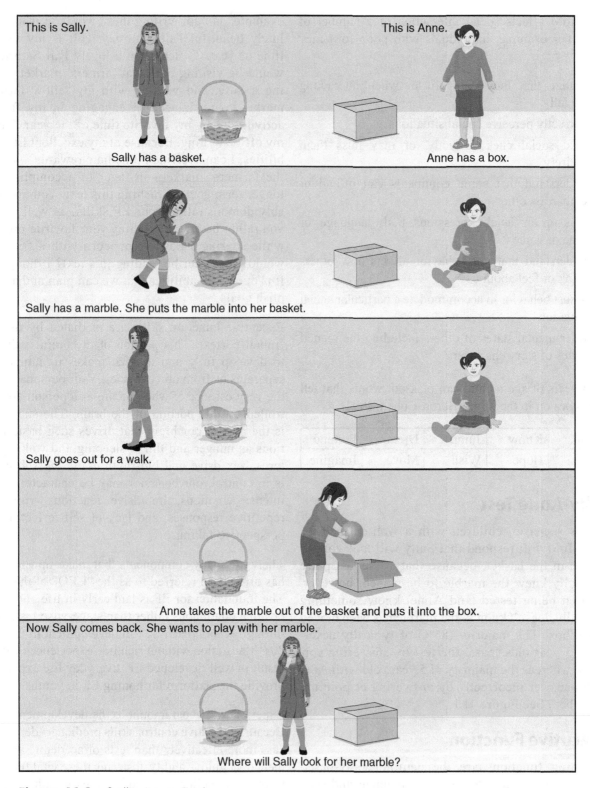

Figure 11.1 Sally-Anne Test

© Kendall Hunt Publishing Company

also essential for the development of ToM. One effective strategy is for adults to relate verbally when planning and executing our own goals when in the presence of youths. For example, a parent might list the steps needed to complete the preparation of a meal, or even a task such as doing the laundry. Also, talking through

Table 11.2 Social Communication Benchmarks

Consider cultural and linguistic factors that may influence appropriateness and/or relevance of benchmarks.

SOCIAL COMMUNICATION BENCHMARKS

Consider cultural and linguistic factors that may influence appropriateness and/or relevance of benchmarks.

AGE	BENCHMARK
Birth to 12 months	prefers looking at human face and eyes; prefers listening to human voice; looks for source of voice; differentiates between tones of voice (angry, friendly); smiles back at caregiver; follows caregiver's gaze; participates in vocal turn-taking with caregiver; vocalizes to get attention; demonstrates joint attention skills (sharing attention); uses gestures to make requests and direct attention; plays simple interactive games such as peek-a-boo
12 – 18 months	brings objects to show caregivers; requests by pointing and vocalizing; solicits attention vocally; practices vocal inflection; says "bye" and other ritualized words; protests by shaking head, saying "no"; supplements gestures with verbal language; aware of social value of speech; responds to the speech of others with eye contact; demonstrates sympathy, empathy, and sharing nonverbally
18 – 24 months	uses single words to express intention; uses single and paired words to command, indicate possession, express problems and gain attention; uses *I, me, you, my* and *mine*; participates in verbal turn-taking with limited number of turns; demonstrates simple topic control; interrupts at syntactic junctures or in response to prosodic cues
24 – 36 months	engages in short dialogues; verbally introduces and changes topic; expresses emotion; begins to use language in imaginative way; relates own experiences; begins to provide descriptive details to enhance listener understanding; uses attention-getting words; clarifies and asks for clarification; introduces and changes topics; uses some politeness terms or markers; begins to demonstrate some adaptation of speech to different listeners
3 – 4 years	engages in longer dialogues; anticipates next turn at talking; terminates conversation; appropriately role-plays; uses fillers—such as *yeah* and *okay*— to acknowledge a partner's message; begins code-switching and uses simpler language when talking to very young children; uses more elliptical responses; requests permission; begins using language for fantasies, jokes, teasing; makes conversational repairs when not understood and corrects others, uses primitive narratives—events follow from central core/use of inferences in stories
4 – 5 years	uses indirect requests; correctly uses deictic terms (e.g., *this, that, here, there*); uses twice as many effective utterances as 3-year-olds to discuss emotions and feelings; uses narrative development characterized by unfocused chains—stories have sequence of events but no central character or theme; develops basic understanding of Theory of Mind (ToM); shifts topics rapidly
School-Age Years	demonstrates increased understanding of ToM (e.g., reads body language, facial expressions, and prosodic characteristics of language to predict behavior; takes perspective of another and modifies language use accordingly); provides assistance and demonstrates altruism; uses narrative development characterized by causally sequenced events using "story grammar"; demonstrates improved conversational skills (e.g., topic maintenance, repair, and increased number of turns); extends topic of conversation; demonstrates refined social conventions; uses language for varied functions including persuading and advancing opinion
Adulthood	uses verbal and nonverbal language competently and flexibly; navigates multiple registers flexibly and fluidly; demonstrates refined understanding and use of nonverbal behavior; develops close friendships and romantic relationships

Table based on information from Gard, Gilman, & Gorman (1993) and Russell (2007).

Table 11.3   Components of Social Communication

SOCIAL INTERACTION	• Speech style and context • Cultural influences • Gender communication differences • Language interference (influence of one language on another) • Code switching • Rules for linguistic politeness	• Social reasoning • Peer-related social competence • Social tasks (e.g., accessing peer groups, cooperative play) • Conflict resolution • Power relationships (e.g., dominance/deference)

SOCIAL COGNITION	• Theory of Mind (ToM) (ability to connect emotional states to self and others; understanding that others have knowledge, desires, and emotions that may differ from one's own); ability to take the perspective of another and modify language use accordingly
	
	• Emotional competence
	
	  ○ emotional regulation
	
	  ○ emotional understanding
	
	  ○ emotional expression, (e.g., effectively regulating one's emotional state and behavior while focusing attention on salient aspects of the environment and engaging in social interaction)
		• Executive functioning (e.g., organization, planning, attention, problem solving, self-monitor future, goal-directed, behavior)
		
		• Joint attention - (e.g., social orienting, establishing shared attention, monitoring emotional states, and considering another's intentions)
		
		• Inference
		
		• Presupposition

PRAGMATICS — **VERBAL COMMUNICATION**	• Speech acts (e.g., requests, responses, comments, directives, demands, promises, and other communication functions)
	• Communicative intentions (communicative acts)
	• Perlocutionary/illocutionary/locutionary acts
	• Prosody
	• Grice maxims of conversation (quantity, quality, relevance, manner)
		• Discourse
		
		  ○ Style—Conversation, narration, expository, procedural
		
		  ○ Interaction/transaction
		
		  ○ Cohesion/coherence
		
		  ○ Responsiveness/assertiveness
		
		  ○ Topic maintenance/introduction/responsiveness/shift
		
		  ○ Social reciprocity (e.g., initiating and responding to bids for interaction, taking turns)
		
		  ○ Communication breakdown and repair
		
		  ○ Deictic forms
		
		  ○ Contingency/adjacency
		
		  ○ Co-construction of meaning
		
		  ○ Event knowledge
		
		  ○ Scripts

NONVERBAL COMMUNICATION	• Body language (posture and positioning) • Gesture • Facial expression • Eye contact	• Gaze (gaze shifts) • Proxemics • Deictic gestures • Challenging behavior as communication
LANGUAGE PROCESSING (EXPRESSIVE AND RECEPTIVE)	• Spoken and written language comprehension • Spoken and written language expression • Morphology (word forms)	• Syntax (word order) • Semantics—general and discipline-specific vocabulary (e.g., science, math, social studies) • Phonological skills for spelling and reading decoding

This table was generated using the following resources: Grice, 1975; Nelson, 1978; and Timler, Olswang, & Coggins, 2005.

having to delay a fun activity in order to accomplish a goal, such as, "I would really love to go to the ballgame, but then I would not get my shopping done for my trip next week" are effective strategies.

Problems with EF abilities can be seen in adulthood as well and may arise secondary to aphasia, traumatic brain injury, right-hemisphere damage, Alzheimer's disease, and other neurodegenerative disorders (Cummings, 2007). Intervention for adult populations should focus on enhancing conversational skills, navigating social situations, and facilitating full participation in daily activities. Frazier (2018) suggested that involving the family in the components of intervention is critical for the adult who has sustained injury leading to deficits in EF.

Behaviors suggesting poor executive function abilities:

Loses/breaks everything

Yells out answers in class/difficulty sitting in seat

Talks to you when you are on the phone

Messy room, desk, locker

Coat & Shoes dumped on the hallway floor

Forgets water bottle, permission slip, etc.

Takes things without asking

Uses the last of something & does not tell

Does not read directions

Starts building project on kitchen table at 6 pm

Leaves front door open, light on, etc.

Needs to use the restroom 5 minutes into a long car trip

Table 11.2 lists social communication benchmarks and is a good reference for expectations of certain social behaviors, however, keep in mind that social communication skills may vary and are depended on personal, familial, and cultural expectations (e.g., in some cultures, making direct eye-contact may be seen as an aggressive act).

Table 11.3 lists components of social performance.

COMPREHENSIVE ASSESSMENT

ASHA recommends an age-appropriate, culturally sensitive, and functional comprehensive assessment which includes collaboration among families, caregivers, classroom teachers, SLPs, special educators, psychologists, and other professionals across multiple partners, topics and settings. Assessment is warranted to diagnose SCD, to describe the characteristics and severity of the disorder, to make appropriate referrals to other services providers as needed, and to make recommendations for intervention and support services. Also, the communication expertise of SLPs is invaluable in the differential diagnosis of social communication disorder and ASD. Because SCD is pervasive in scope and far-reaching in its effects on performance across multiple domains, school-aged children are eligible for speech-language pathology services regardless of their performance on standardized tests measuring cognitive skills or language abilities. Because it is common for SCD to occur alongside other diagnoses, the SLP must be aware of overlapping symptomology in order to evaluate factors related to social communication. Unfortunately, reliable and culturally valid assessment measures with which to make a differential diagnosis are lacking. This does not mean, however, that we as SLPs are unable to assess social communication skills and provide diagnostic data needed to construct appropriate intervention plans. Accurate diagnosis is vital to designing effective intervention and possible through use of formal and informal measures. Rating scales and communication checklists, completed either by the individual, teacher, or parent, have become increasingly popular because it is difficult to extrapolate social skill in everyday contexts from pragmatic performance in a clinical setting. The following are recommendations outline areas to be addressed during social communication skill assessment (Norbury, 2014; Bishop, 1998; Roth & Spekman, 1984)

- Verbal and non-verbal modes of communication—this may include speech, signs, natural gestures, pictures, writing, and any augmentative and alternative communication (AAC) systems.

- Comprehension and interpretation of verbal and nonverbal communication—this includes gestures, body language, facial expression, and prosody.

- Initiation of spontaneous communication and conversation—this includes the ability to follow the rules that guide the maintenance and termination of conversation.

- Turn-taking abilities—this includes skills across various setting and communication partners.

- Comprehension of verbal and non-verbal discourse—this includes discourse used in social, academic, vocational, and community settings.

- Comprehension of figurative language and inference making—this includes idioms, ambiguous language and drawing conclusions when information is not overtly stated.

- Attribution of mental and emotional states of self and others—this includes theory of mind (TOM) which is discussed below.

- Communication abilities in a variety of settings that are reciprocal and lead to the development of friendships and other rewarding interpersonal relationships—this includes relationships in academic, extracurricular, vocational, and recreational settings.

No evaluation of any type of communication disorder would be complete without assessment of communication skills and communication-related domains, co-occurring disorders and health conditions, functional communication skills and participation in social activities, description of both barriers to and facilitator of successful social performance, as well as, a description of the impact the communication disorder has on the person's ability to lead a self-determined life.

TREATMENT OF SOCIAL COMMUNICATION DEFICITS

As with any intervention plan, treatment approaches for social communication deficits should involve family and educators and be individualized to meet the specific needs of each child. School-aged children will require help with making friends, navigating school life and other settings, and participating in extracurricular activities. It is helpful to begin therapy with a one-on-one instructional approach to teach new skills and practice those skills in a protected environment before moving on to more natural and functional communication settings and different communication partners. Teacher-mediated interventions and peer-mediated interventions are often used in school settings, as well, as arranging the environment to maximum best performance (Timler, 2008).

SLPs work closely with other service providers such as classroom teachers, special educators, psychologists, and vocational counselors to help maximize strengths and address weaknesses connected to primary functions affecting social communication in hopes of building independence in everyday social contexts. Some strategies for fostering social competency includes teaching skills and strategies that will increase the individual's participation in social interactions and adjusting contextual dynamics that may be barriers to both successful communication and participation in social situations and identifying and enhancing factors that facilitate improved social performance.

REFERENCES

Adams, C., Lockton, E., Freed, J., Gaile, J., Earl, G., McBean, K., . . . Law, J. (2012, March 27). *The Social Communication Intervention Project: A randomized controlled trial of the effectiveness of speech and language therapy for school-age children who have pragmatic and social communication problems with or without autism spectrum disorder.* Retrieved from http://onlinelibrary.wiley.com/doi/10.1111/j.1460-6984.2011.00146.x/abstract

Bishop, D. V. (1998). Development of the Children's Communication Checklist (CCC): A method for assessing qualitative aspects of communicative impairment in children. *The Journal of Child Psychology and Psychiatry and Allied Disciplines, 39*(6), 879–891.

Cummings, L. (2007, May). Pragmatics and adult language disorders. In *Seminars in Speech and Language* (Vol. 28, No. 02, pp. 093-095). Copyright © 2007 by Thieme Medical Publishers, Inc., 333 Seventh Avenue, New York, NY 10001, USA.

Grayson, R. (2002). Emotional Intelligence: Understanding, Applying, and Measuring.

Guare, R., & Dawson, P. (2004). Executive skills in children and teens: parents, teachers and clinicians can help. *Brown University Child & Adolescent Behavior Letter, 20*(8), 1–7.

Frazier, K. F. (2018). Executive function and social skill support after traumatic brain injury. *Journal of Life Care Planning. 16*(1), 47–51.

Roth, F. P., & Spekman, N. J. (1984). Assessing the pragmatic abilities of children: Part 1. Organizational framework and assessment parameters. *Journal of speech and Hearing Disorders, 49*(1), 2–11.

Norbury, C. F. (2014). Practitioner review: Social (pragmatic) communication disorder conceptualization, evidence and clinical implications. *Journal of Child Psychology and Psychiatry, 55*(3), 204–216.

Timler, G. (2008, November 01). *Social communication: A framework for assessment and intervention.* Retrieved from https://leader.pubs.asha.org/article.aspx?articleid=2288092

Chapter 11   Activities

NAME: _____   DATE: _____

The following 10 therapy goals are missing vital details. Apply the skills you learned in Chapter 1 to correct these goals.

SOCIAL LANGUAGE:

1. By the end of the IEP, the patient will use appropriate nonverbal communication skills when engaging in activities with age equivalent peers, with 4/5 opportunities as measured through observation.

2. By the end of the IEP, the patient will greet peers and adults, during appropriate times, with 80% accuracy given 4/5 opportunities as measured by observation.

3. By the end of the IEP, the patient will understand positive and negative behaviors with 80% accuracy when given a picture and description of a positive or negative behavior.

4. By the end of the IEP, the patient will request needs and wants appropriately using the phrase "May I have ___ please?" during structured tasks, as measured by observation.

5. By the end of the IEP, the patient will take turns appropriately with 80% accuracy, as measured by observation, given 2 prompting cues or less.

6. By the end of the IEP, the patient will use appropriate tone of voice and volume with 90% accuracy, as measured by observation, given a structured role-playing task.

7. By the end of the IEP, the patient will infer the feelings and emotions of others with 80% accuracy, as measured by observation, given limited cues.

8. By the end of the IEP, the patient will initiate interactions with other students in at least one activity throughout the day, within the classroom setting, out of five consecutive data collection days (one whole week of school).

9. Over 5 consecutive sessions, the patient will keep his or her hands and feet to himself or herself when interacting with peers with 80% accuracy, as measured by observation, given verbal and gestural cues.

10. By the end of the IEP, the patient will follow expected classroom rules and behaviors within the classroom setting with 80% accuracy, as measured by observation, given limited verbal or gestural cues.

Report Writing Practice

Use the following case history and diagnostic information along with skills learned in this Chapter and Chapter 1 to write a diagnostic report (See Appendix for a diagnostic report example).

Report Writing Activity: SOCIAL LANGUAGE

SPEECH/LANGUAGE/HEARING Case History/ CHILD

SPEECH AND HEARING CLINIC

TO THE PARENTS OR GUARDIAN:

You have requested an appointment for an evaluation of your child's speech, language, hearing problem. To plan ahead for this interview, we need certain information. Please complete this form to the best of your ability.

All information will be held confidential.

I. <u>General Information</u>

Child's Name**: Henry Thompson**

Phone: **745-6201**

Birth Date: **March 25th, 2004**   Age: **14 years**   Sex: **Male**   Grade: **8th grade**

Address: **421 McAllister Drive**   City: **Charolette**   State: **North Carolina**   Zip: **28202**

School: **Charolette Middle School**   Teacher: **Mrs. Stacy**   School District: **Charolette School District**

Father's Name: **Charles Thompson**   Age: **42**   Address: **421 McAllister Drive**   City: **Charolette** State: **North Carolina**   Zip: **28202**   Occupation: **Pharmacist**   Business Phone: **950-3277** Place of Occupation: **Side Effects Pharmacy**   Education; number of years completed: **13 yr; high school diploma   8 yr; higher education**

Mother's Name: **Carol Thompson**   Age: **39**   Address: **421 McAllister Drive**   City: **Charolette** State: **North Carolina**   Zip: **28202**   Occupation: **5th Grade Math Teacher**   Business Phone: **236-2531**   Place of Occupation: **Charolette Elementary School**   Education; number of years completed: **13 yr; high school diploma 4 yr; higher education**

If mother is employed, who cares for the child?   **Being a teacher, I have the same schedule as Henry, so I typically watch him when he is not in school.**

Who will be responsible for payment of charges?   **Private Insurance**

Brothers and/or sisters of the child:

Name: **Elizabeth Thompson**   Age: **10**   School: **Charolette Middle School**   Grade: **5th grade**

Name: **Catherine Thompson**   Age: **7**   School: **Charolette Primary School**   Grade: **2nd grade**

Relatives or others living in the home: Name: **N/A**   Relationship: **N/A**

Who referred you to the University of Arkansas Speech and Hearing Clinic?

Name: **Mrs. Stacy**   Relationship: **Henry's school teacher**   Address: **6503 School Street** City: **Charolette**   State: **North Carolina**   Zip: **28202**

II. Statement of the Problem:

Describe the problem:

We've been told by Mrs. Stacy that Henry doesn't work well with others and gets frustrated easily when forced to do group work in school. At home, Henry often isolates himself in his room and doesn't bother interacting with the rest of the family. Sometimes getting Henry to leave his room and participate with the rest of the family can lead to a fight. In public, I've noticed that Henry doesn't engage in conversation or greet others appropriately.

When was the problem first noticed?

Henry has been this way since I can remember. At first we thought Henry was just shy and introverted, but years have gone by and things haven't changed and he hasn't evolved out of those 'shy' habits.

What has been done about it?

We have just now become aware of Henry's condition; nothing has been done about his 'behavior' in the past

What is the child's reaction to the problem?

I don't believe Henry knows that he isn't acting appropriately at school or in public.

III. Pregnancy and Birth History:

During this pregnancy did the mother experience any unusual illness, condition or accident? If so, describe:

No

Were there any complications during the delivery such as caesarean, extremely long labor, or use of instruments?

I did have to have a c-section with Henry.

IV. Developmental History:

At what age did the following occur?

Sat alone unsupported: **9 months**   Crawled: **11 months**   Walked alone: **13 months**

Maintained bowel and bladder control while awake: **4 years** asleep: **5 years**

Does the child seem awkward or uncoordinated? **No**

V. Medical History:

Does your child have any long-term medical conditions for which they are now being or have been treated? **No**

Does your child take any medication regularly? **No**

Has your child had a speech examination prior to this time? **No**

Where? _____

When?_____

What were the results?

Has your child had a hearing test prior to this time? **Yes**

Where? **School** When? **Last year**

What were the results? **Normal**

Has your child had a neurological examination prior to this time? **No**

Where? _____
When?_____

What were the results?

Has your child had a psychological examination prior to this time? **No**

Where?_____
When?_____

What were the results?

Has your child had an eye examination prior to this time? **Yes**

Where? **School** When? **Last year**

What were the results? **Normal**

Has your child had a recent medical examination? **No**

Where? _____
When?_____

What were the results?

Name of child's pediatrician/physician: **Dr. Ted Hide**

        Address: **411 Main Stree**

        City, State, Zip: **Charolette, North Carolina 28202**

        Phone #: **980-7200**

Check the following illnesses this child has had:

_____ Measles _____ Influenza _____ Draining Ears _____ Head Injury

_____ Mumps _____ Meningitis _____ Chronic Colds _____ Heart Disease

_____ Whooping Cough _____ Encephalitis __ **X** __ Allergies _____ Kidney Disease

_____ Chicken Pox _____ Epilepsy __ **X** __ Sinus Problems _____ High Fever

_____ Scarlet Fever _____ Tonsillitis _____ Excessive Ear Wax

Has this child ever had earaches or ear infections? __ **X** __ Yes _____ No. If yes, how often and in which ear(s)? ___ **Henry had one or two ear infections when he was younger** _____

How was it treated? _____ **Antibiotics** _____

Has this child ever had a PE tubes, tonsillectomy and/or adenoidectomy? ___ Yes ___ **X** ___ No.

If yes, when _____ Physician _____

Is there a history of hearing loss in the family? ___ Yes ___ **X** ___ No   If yes, indicate which relative and at what age the hearing loss was diagnosed.

_____

_____

_____

Has your child ever worn a hearing aid? ___ Yes ___ **X** ___ No   If yes, what kind of aid and in which ear (s)?
_____

_____

_____

VI. <u>Daily Behavior:</u>

Has your child been harder to manage than other children? **Sometimes. His younger sisters are definitely easier to manage than him most of the time.**

Describe any unusual behavior: **For him to actually do as I ask, the first time, is a rare occasion. Following directions is difficult for him it seems. I just thought it was because he was a teenager and a boy.**

Describe your child's interests:

Henry loves creating and building detailed objects out of Legos, especially Star Wars ships and figurines.

VII. <u>Speech and Hearing History:</u>

Does your child talk? **Yes, but it's limited** If not, how does your child communicate?

When did your child first use words meaningfully? **Around 14 months**

When did your child begin to use two-word sentences? **Around 24 months**

Does your child understand what you say to him/her? **I'm pretty sure he does**

How well is s/he understood by parents? **When Henry talks, we can understand him well**

By others? **When Henry talks, others seem to be able to understand him pretty well**

Do you think your child hears adequately? **Yes**

If not, what do you feel is the reason?

Has your child had frequent colds or ear problems? **Not really**

VIII. Educational History:

Has your child repeated any grades? **No** If so, which ones?

With what subjects has your child had particular difficulties? **There isn't one specific subject he has difficulty in**

Has your child ever had special help through the school? **Sometimes his teachers have to get with him one-on-one to explain the task more clearly, but nothing like special education.**

If so, please describe:

How does your child feel about school? **Henry doesn't particularly enjoy going to school, he would rather stay home and build with Legos by himself. He has told us that he doesn't have many friends at school, which could be part of the reason it has been difficult to get him up and out of the door in the morning.**

Diagnostic Information:

After receiving Henry's case history, a date was scheduled for an evaluation. During the evaluation, an OME and hearing test were performed as well as two standardized tests. The results of each of those are as follows:

Summary of Findings:

Henry's hearing screening suggested that his hearing was within normal limits, bilaterally.

The two Assessment tests that Mrs. Patterson used to evaluate Henry were:

1. Test of Pragmatic Language (TOPL-2)

Raw Score	Pragmatic Language Usage Index	Percentile Rank	Descriptive Rating
9	70	2	Severe

The Test of Pragmatic Language, Second Edition (TOPL-2) assesses the use of language skills and the ability to react in social settings by problem solving, predicting, and analyzing. Henry scored a severe score of 70 on the TOPL-2 and ranks in the 2nd percentile for his age group.

2. Social Language Development Test, Adolescent

The Social Language Development Test assesses social language skills in adolescents ages 12-17:1. This tests assesses perspective taking, making inferences, problem solving, interpreting social language, and understanding idioms, irony and sarcasm. The standard scores are based on a mean of 100 with a standard deviation of 15.

	Making Inferences	Interpreting Social Language	Problem Solving	Social Interaction	Interpreting Ironic Statements	Total Test
Raw Score	4	4	4	4	4	4
Percentile Rank	11	3	1	<1	5	<60
Standard Score	81	71	65	<60	76	<60

Henry scored a severe score of 70 on the TOPL-2 and a severe score of <60 on the Social Language Development Test.

Given the case history, and results from the oral-mech, hearing screening and standardized tests, Mrs. Patterson believes the prognosis for Henry to make improvement in his social skills is good. Mrs. Patterson recommends that Henry comes in for speech therapy to work on his pragmatic social skills once a week for an hour.

CHAPTER 12

Intervention for Stuttering

Ashlen Thomason, Ph.D., CCC-SLP

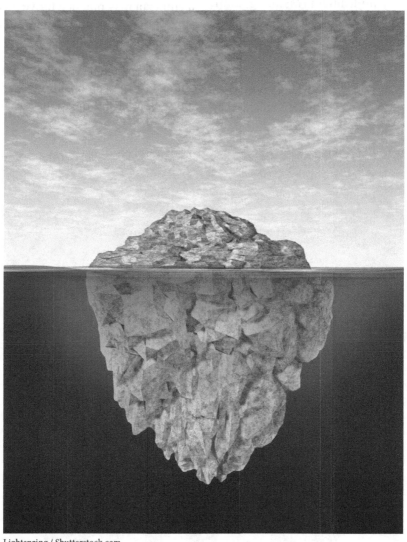

Lightspring / Shutterstock.com

THERE'S A CLIENT WHO STUTTERS ON MY CASELOAD. NOW WHAT?

Taking on a client who stutters may seem daunting for a new clinician. Unfortunately, treating a client who stutters might even seem intimidating for a seasoned speech–language pathologist (which may explain the worried look on your supervisor's face). Stuttering is an area in which speech–language pathologists traditionally report feeling ill-equipped to treat and university program directors report having low confidence in the training they provide their students (Matkin, Ringle, & Snope, 1983; Curlee, 1985; Sommers & Caruso, 1995). One reason that many licensed clinicians may feel underprepared is because coursework in fluency disorders was not a required part of university curricula until the early millennium (Manning, 2001; Yaruss & Quesal, 2002). In a 1988 survey of school based speech–language pathologists, on half had taken a course in stuttering, and 5% reported that the course work emphasized treatment (Mallard, Gardner, & Downey, 1988). Nearly a decade later, only 54% of bachelors level and 65% of graduate students had taken a course that was entirely or partially devoted to stuttering; approximately half of those surveyed indicated that they felt inadequate when attempting to treat people who stutter (Kelly et al., 1997). Having both speech and affective components that should be addressed, the overt and covert nature of stuttering treatment can deter many clinicians. Van Riper (1982) called stuttering "..more than a riddle. It is at least a complicated, multidimensional jigsaw puzzle with many pieces still missing. Unlike many other disorders in the Big Nine for which treatment is aimed at remediating the disorder, stuttering treatment goals are generally targeting compensatory strategies and management of affective components. Not being able to "fix" the client's problem can discourage many clinicians. Additionally, stuttering has a prevalence of 1% (Andrews & Harris, 1964; Mansson, 2000). Therefore, a clinician may practice for years before treating a person who stutters and applying his or her knowledge from graduate school.

Take a deep breath (but please don't ask your client who stutters to do deep breathing exercises), and move past any potential intimidation you are feeling. Stuttering

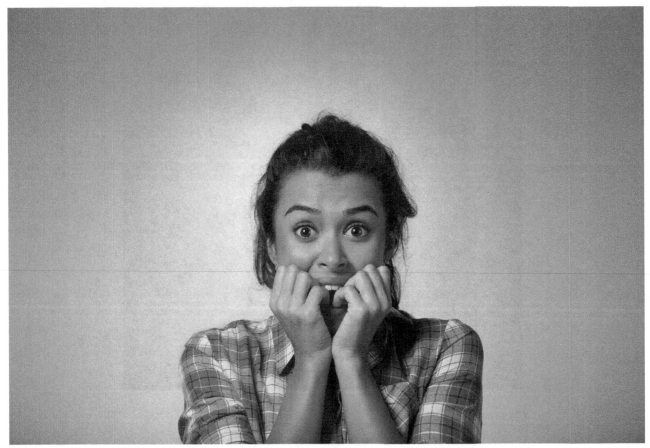

WAYHOME studio/Shutterstock.com

treatment strategies can easily be learned. This chapter will provide you with information about defining stuttering, stuttering etiology, distinguishing stuttering from other fluency disorders, prognostic indicators that can predict if a child will have life-long stuttering or stuttering that goes away on its own, optimal timing for assessing and treating stuttering in early childhood, when therapy is appropriate for clients whose stuttering has persisted, the basics of fluency shaping and stuttering modification, data collection, and goal writing.

WHAT IS STUTTERING?

Stuttering is easy to recognize when you see it, but it is a tricky disorder to define. Having a one-dimensional definition of stuttering can lead to one-dimensional therapy. Stuttering is a multifactorial disorder, so it is paramount for clinicians to understand that stuttering is more than just surface speech characteristics. According to the World Health Organization (1977), stuttering is defined as "a disorder of the rhythm of speech in which the individual knows precisely what he wishes to say, but at the time is unable to say it because of an involuntary, repetitive prolongation or cessation of sound" (p. 202). While this definition captures the involuntary nature of stuttering and the fact that disfluencies are not indicative of a word-finding problem, it only addresses overt stuttering characteristics. Van Riper, known as the 'Father of Speech Pathology,' said that "Stuttering occurs when the forward flow of speech is interrupted by a motorically disrupted sound, syllable, or word, or the speaker's reactions thereto" (Van Riper, 1971). Van Riper's definition captures the component involving the speaker's reaction to the disruptions of a stuttering event. A more complete definition captures both the involuntary nature of stuttering, the speech characteristics that are visible to outside listeners, and the speaker's feelings and avoidance of various speech tasks as a result of the stuttering. Stuttering, is a speech disorder characterized by the involuntary disruption of the flow of speech, manifesting in repetitions of single-syllable whole-words, sounds or syllables in words, prolonging of sounds, and/or interruption of sounds, sometimes accompanied by secondary characteristics, and the speaker's avoidance of particular sounds, words, or speaking tasks.

Fluency disorders cover a variety of speech conditions involving the disruption to the flow of speech. Generally in the field of speech pathology, when we use the term "fluency," we are referring to stuttering,

more formally known in research as "persistent developmental stuttering" (PDS) (Yairi & Ambrose, 2005). This chapter is not dedicated to other disorders of fluency such as cluttering, a language-based fluency disorder characterized disorganized language, rapid rate, irregular prosody, and excessive use of "other disfluencies" (ODs)—multisyllabic whole-word repetitions, phrase repetitions, abandoned utterances, and interjections; neurogenic stuttering, a type of stuttering that occurs following a neurological injury or progression of neurological disease, typically characterized by rapid whole-word and part word repetitions, usually with a higher percentage syllables stuttered than occurring in even severe persistent developmental stuttering; psychogenic stuttering, sudden onset stuttering that is often transient occurring suddenly after a trauma or co-occurring with a psychological disorder (Yairi & Seery, 2015; Bloodstein & Bernstein Ratner, 2008).

True stuttering events are often referred to in research as stuttering-like disfluencies (SLDs). The four SLDs are single-syllable whole word repetitions (e.g., "I-I-I-I-I want to go outside."), part-word repetitions (e.g., "I w-w-w-want to go outside."), prolongations (I waaaaaaaaaaaant to go outside."), and blocks (I want t------to go outside."). These SLDs always occur within a single syllable (Manning, 2001; Bloodstein & Bernstein Ratner, 2008; Yairi & Seery, 2015). Secondary characteristics are tic-like movements, pitch rise of the voice, or increasing intensity of the voice that occur only during stuttering events. Some common secondary characteristics are rapid blinking, head-nodding, facial grimacing, and articulatory posturing.

As mentioned above, there are other facets to stuttering that cannot be viewed on the surface. After years of experiencing peoples' reactions to their stuttering, people who stutter can develop fear and of many different sounds, words, and speaking tasks and an overall negative communication attitude (Manning, 2001; Caruso, Chodzko-Zajko, Bidinger, & Sommers, 1994; Blomgren, 2010). This affective impact of stuttering should be assessed and incorporated into a holistic treatment plan.

WHAT CAUSES STUTTERING?

The short answer: we don't know. The more accurate short answer: we don't know exactly what causes stuttering, but we have mounting evidence that stuttering is a neurological condition with a significant genetic component (Kidd, 1980; Ambrose, Yairi, & Cox, 1993;

Ambrose, 2004). Copious neuroimaging studies have revealed many aberrant neurological findings in people who stutter, some of which include: regional cerebral bloodflow to the right temporal lobe rather than the left during moments of fluent speech and normal bloodflow to the left perisylvian region during moments of disfluency (Fox et al., 1996; Braun et al., 1997); three times higher dopamine uptake across the striatum during speech (Giraud et al., 2008); abnormally symmetric planum temporale with large right-sided volume (Foundas, Bollich, Corey, Hurley, & Heilman, 2001); cortical disconnection immediately below the laryngeal and tongue representation in the left sensorimotor cortex (Sommer et al., 2002); and many more. The majority of these neuroimaging studies have been conducted in adults who stutter, previously making it difficult for researchers to determine if the abnormal neurological findings have been present since the onset of stuttering in childhood or of these differences are a manifestation of years of stuttering. Recent neuroimaging studies of children who stutter reveal that many of the neuroanatomical and neurophysiological findings of adults with persistent stuttering are present from childhood, including decreased white matter integrity in the superior longitudinal fasciculus underlying the ventral sensorimotor cortex (rolandic operculum); differences in white matter integrity in an area that contains thalamocortical and corticonuclear tracts connecting cortical brain regions with deep subcortical areas and cranial nerves that directly control speech musculature (Chang, Erickson, Ambrose, Hasegawa-Johnson, & Ludlow, 2008); caudates with reduced volume on the right side and leftward asymmetry (Foundas, Cindass, Mock, & Corey, 2013); atypical development of basal ganglia networks, namely, unnaturally thin white-matter in neural networks that support temporal motor control for speech production in the auditory motor and basal ganglia-thalmocortical networks (Chang & Zhu, 2013); cortical thickness of grey matter comprising the left pars opercularis of people who stutter was abnormally thick in childhood and failed to thin normally with age (Beal et al., 2015).

HOW DO I KNOW IF THIS CHILD WHO STUTTERS NEEDS THERAPY?

It has been well-established in literature that approximately 74% of children who stutter will undergo spontaneous recovery, while 26% will have stuttering that persists through the lifespan (Bryngelson, 1938;

Sheehan & Martyn, 1970; Yairi & Ambrose, 1999b, 2005). Longitudinal studies of preschoolers who stutter have analyzed the key prognostic indicators differentiating between those children whose stuttering persists versus those who recover (Andrews & Harris, 1964; Panelli, McFarlane, & Shipley, 1978; Yairi & Ambrose, 1992a; Kloth, Kraaimaat, Janssen, & Brutten, 1999; Rommel, Hage, Kalehne, & Johannsen, 2000; Mansson, 2000; Yairi & Ambrose, 2005; Throneburg & Yairi, 2003).

The strongest predictive factor for stuttering persistence or recovery among preschoolers who stutter is family history (Ambrose et al., 1993) Children who have relatives who have stuttered for more than 4-years are likely to have their stuttering persist into adulthood without therapy. Children who have relatives whose stuttering underwent natural remission or children with no family history of stuttering are more likely to undergo natural recovery. In children who have a first order relative (parent or sibling) of the same gender who stuttered, the child has a 65% chance of following that family member's course of persistence or recovery.

The second strongest predictor of stuttering persistence or recovery is gender. Males tend to persist in stuttering, while girls tend to recover naturally. Only one in five adults who stutter is female (Yairi & Ambrose, 1992; Yairi, Ambrose, Paden, & Throneberg, 1996).

The third largest predictive factor for stuttering persistence or recovery among preschoolers who stutter is the course of stuttering across the first 6 months following onset (Yairi et al.,1996). In all children, those who persist or recover, there is typically a worsening of stuttering severity at the 2-month mark after stuttering onset. From there, children who recover naturally tend to have a marked lessening in stuttering severity by the 7-month mark post onset. Children who tend to persist in their stuttering typically have steady or increasing stuttering severity compared to their severity at onset.

The next strongest predictive factors for stuttering persistence or recovery are the presence of certain stuttering characteristics at month seven following onset. Interestingly, stuttering severity near onset is not a predictive factor for persistence or recovery; many children who start off stuttering severely recover and many children who start off with mild stuttering persist and vice versa (Yairiet al., 1996). At 7 months following onset, if a child has single-syllable whole word repetitions or part-word repetition of three or more units, prolongations, blocks, or secondary movements, those characteristics are prognostic indicators for stuttering persistence (Yairiet al., 1996) Children who tend to naturally recover do not usually have aberrant phonations (blocks and prolongations), secondary movements, or repetitions beyond three units at month 7 following onset.

There are multiple indicators with less predictive value that help predict stuttering remission or persistence, including age at stuttering onset, co-occurring speech or language delays, and length of time since onset (Yairi et al., 1996). The average age of stuttering onset is between 25 and 36 months of age (Yairi & Ambrose, 1999a). Children who tend to recover naturally from stuttering are usually less than 3 years 6 months of age at stuttering onset, while children who persist usually have stuttering onset after 3 years 6 months of age. The presence of concomitant speech or language delays, such as weaknesses in speech intelligibility, syntax, grammar, or receptive language skills is a risk factor for persistence (Watkins & Yairi, 1997; Watkins, Yairi, & Ambrose, 1999b). Children who tend to persist also have stuttering that is showing no signs of recovery around a year status post onset (Yairiet al., 1996).

Given these research findings, children who have just started stuttering should ideally be tested when they are at least 7 months following stuttering onset, as all prognostic indicators cannot be determined before that point. This assessment should include formal stuttering test with a speech analysis, such as the *Stuttering Severity Instrument 4th-Edition* (Riley, 2009). Beyond the typical domains of frequency (percentage of syllables stuttered), duration (average length of the three longest stuttering events), and physical concomitants (ratings of secondary movements), a risk analysis should be completed using evidence-based prognostic indicators for natural remission and persistence into adulthood (Yairi et al., 1996). Children with greater than two risk factors for persistence who are within 3 years of stuttering onset (but at least 7 months from onset) should be enrolled in direct speech therapy.

Unfortunately, a major finding in the same longitudinal research studies is that a child's chance of stuttering recovery, even with therapy, drops to <5% after he or she has been stuttering for 3 years following onset; stuttering is considered persistent if the child has stuttered for 4 years after onset (Yairi & Ambrose, 1999b; Yairi, Ambrose, & Niermann 1993). Thus, the critical window for stuttering treatment aimed at complete recovery from stuttering in childhood should take place before a child has been stuttering for 3 years.

WHAT ARE TREATMENT OPTIONS FOR PEOPLE WHO STUTTER?

For young children who have been stuttering for less than 3 years since onset, therapy is aiming at complete remission—though early childhood therapy is never a guarantee that the client will not have persistent stuttering. To facilitate recovery, a clinician can help the child to be fluent in two ways: *indirect therapy* or *direct therapy*.

In *indirect therapy*, the goal is to reduce the child's stuttering frequency without instructing the child to change his or her speech in any way (Bloodstein & Bernstein Ratner, 2008; Millard & Cook, 2010; Yaruss & Bernstein Ratner, 2010). The clinician models and teaches caregivers to create a fluency-facilitating environment that will cause the child to stutter less often. Indirect therapy is only employed with young preschoolers and is not appropriate for older children who stutter.

The speech–language pathologist might alternatively choose *direct therapy*, addressing a young child's stuttering by teaching the child to speak in a manner which makes the child more fluent with a method (discussed below) called fluency shaping (Bloodstein & Bernstein Ratner, 2008; O'Brian, Onslow, Cream & Packman, 2003; Yairi & Seery, 2015). Direct teaching of fluency shaping may also be appropriate for young preschoolers who stutter who can understand some basic terminology (slow, stretched, gentle, etc.) and can follow the clinician's direct model. The goal of direct therapy with a young preschooler is to reduce a child's stuttering frequency by getting them to use fluency shaping as much as possible.

Fluency shaping is a method of causing clients who stutter to be essentially fluent by speaking in a different manner (Bloodstein & Bernstein Ratner, 2008, O'Brian et al., 2003; Yairi & Seery, 2015). The three main components of fluency shaping are continuous voicing, slowed rate, and easy onset. The use of prolonged, drone speech to create continuous voicing is the component of fluency shaping that induces fluency by causing the speaker to use alternate premotor control that theoretically bypasses aberrant basal ganglia functioning (Alm, 2004; Neumann et al., 2005). The goal of fluency shaping is to eliminate stuttering and cause the client to be essentially 100% fluent while these techniques are employed. Fluency shaping can be used by people who stutter of all ages.

Stuttering modification is another direct therapy method to address stuttering (Van Riper, 1971; Blomgren, 2010; Yairi & Seery, 2015). The overall goal of stuttering modification is to change moments of stuttering such that they are as short and relaxed as possible so that the flow of speech is maximized. With stuttering modification, clients will stutter with the same frequency that they stuttered before; the reduction in severity comes from the shorter duration of stuttering events and lack of tension. With stuttering modification, non-stuttered words are said with natural prosody and rhythm—only stuttered words are altered. Concepts of stuttering modification are generally too complex for proper execution in young children; thus, fluency shaping is the only direct therapy options for young children who stutter.

Indirect Preschool Stuttering Treatment

As mentioned above, children are not specifically directed to speak in a different manner in indirect treatment. Rather, caregivers change the child's environment to be fluency-facilitating in an attempt to target decreased stuttering. With indirect treatment caregivers slow down their speaking rate, slow down the pace of play activities, reduce the language complexity that they use while speaking with their child, stick to a single topic at a time that is simple for the child to discuss during discourse, and space out questions and prompts for the child to comment (Yairi & Seery, 2015; Millard & Cook, 2010; Yaruss & Bernstein Ratner, 2010; Bloodstein & Bernstein Ratner, 2008). Caregivers must be involved in order to successfully implement indirect stuttering treatment in a young child, a caveat that may preclude this type of treatment from being carried out in regular sessions through a school-based provider. When carried out successfully, clinician's monitor the client's fluency in 1 month intervals throughout the course of treatment and attain caregiver report on how much the client is stuttering at home. Clinicians have sessions with the children and caregivers in which they instruct and model indirect stuttering therapy strategies while the caregivers watch, then facilitate the techniques. Play-based client-directed activities are recommended for indirect therapy methods. For indirect therapy, clinicians should meet with caregivers for direct sessions as often as necessary to ensure that they can carry out indirect strategies in the home environment. For some families, that means may warrant multiple direct sessions, weekly phone calls to monitor progress, and once monthly sessions for ongoing assessment of stuttering.

Fluency Shaping

The three main components of fluency shaping are continuous voicing, slowed rate, and easy onset. The use of prolonged, drone speech to create continuous voicing is the component of fluency shaping that induces fluency (Bloodstein & Bernstein Ratner, 2008, O'Brian et al., 2003; Yairi & Seery, 2015). For continuous voicing, one speaks across a single breath unit with essentially continuous airflow across the glottis with vowels prolonged and negligible spaces between words, as if "sing-talking." Continuous voicing induces fluency in a similar matter to singing, correcting the aberrant over activation of the basal ganglia by using alternative premotor support from the pre-motor cortex (Alm, 2004; Goldberg, 1985, Giraud et al., 2008). Continuous voicing is a vital part of fluency shaping and cannot be left out of a fluency shaping approach. Continuous voicing can be taught using modeling (e.g., exhibiting proper continuous voicing, showing the child contrasting between continuous voicing and regular prosody or choppy speech, etc.), direct instruction (e.g., "use your sing-talking," "keep your voice motor on"), and/or tactile cueing (e.g., running a finger across a table, placing the fingers on the throat to feel continuous voicing, etc.)

Slowed rate is a component of fluency shaping; however, using a slowed rate of speech alone is not effective use of fluency shaping (Yairi & Seery, 2015). Clinicians should work to find an optimal rate of speech that facilitates fluency but is fast enough to sound natural. Slowed rate should always be used concurrently with continuous voicing.

Easy onset is a technique used in fluency shaping to start utterances or resume utterances after pauses (Bloodstein & Bernstein Ratner, 2008, O'Brian et al., 2003; Yairi & Seery, 2015). Though continuous voicing is the primary agent in fluency-shaping, many people who stutter cannot get out the first sound in an utterance to begin continuous voicing. Easy onset allows people who stutter to begin utterances with less likelihood of stuttering. Easy onset is employed by letting air through the glottis as if making a quiet /h/ sound and blending that /h/ with the first sound in an utterance. The typical locus of stuttering is at the beginning of an utterances (Manning, 2001; Bloodstein & Bernstein Ratner, 2008; Yairi & Seery, 2015) so easy onset is typically an important element to fluency shaping. However, for some people who stutter, continuous voicing without easy onset can be effective enough for inducing fluency that it is not needed for fluency shaping. Easy onset can be taught with modeling, direct instruction (e.g., "let out your /h/ sound," "use an easy beginning," etc.) and tactile cueing (e.g., holding the hand in front of the mouth to feel the air coming out). Be aware that many young children mistakenly exhibit an inspiratory /h/ sound while learning easy onset and need immediate correction before the pattern becomes a habit.

For children who stutter, fluency shaping should be taught in a hierarchy that gradually taxes a child's language. The goal is to get children to use slow rate, easy onset, and continuous voicing in conversational exchanges and narratives. For many children, that means starting with instruction at the single-word level, moving through two-word utterances, carrier phrases, rote sentences, and isolated self-created sentences (e.g., "Tell me something about a _____"), before reaching conversational speech and story-telling.

One method for generalization of fluency shaping is using constant verbal contingencies (Yairi & Seery, 2015). This type of therapy involves the clinician and caregivers constantly modeling and providing children with feedback about fluency shaping. Clinicians (then later caregivers) respond to every one of a child's utterances with feedback about his or her use of techniques. If a child attempts to use techniques appropriately, the clinician or caregivers provide positive verbal feedback (e.g., "I heard your voice motor on," "that was the new way," "Awesome slow, gentle speech," etc.). When the child speaks without techniques, speaks particularly fast, or has a stuttering event, approximately 75% of the time, the clinician or caregiver will recast what the child just said using fluency-shaping. The other 25% of the time that the client does not use techniques, the clinician or caregiver will ask the child to try saying the utterance again while using techniques (e.g., "That was bumpy. Can you say it the new way?"). A clinician should use his or her judgement regarding how often and for how many sessions the caregivers need to attend sessions before being able to carry out generalization methods accurately at home.

For adults who stutter, fluency shaping should be mastered in a hierarchy of functional speaking tasks that

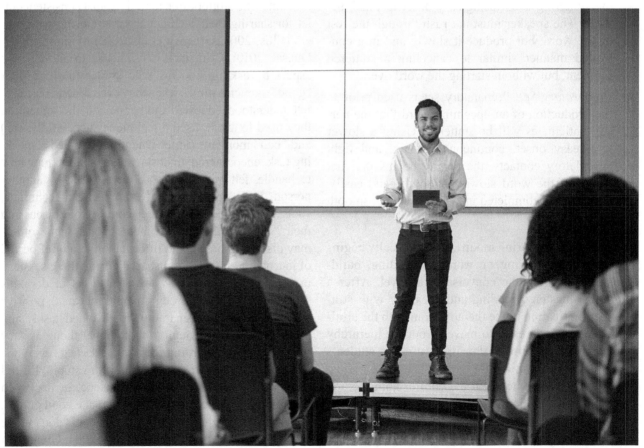

Monkey Business Images/Shutterstock.com

gradually tax their limbic system reactions (Caruso et al., 1994; Blomgren, 2010). To ensure that the client has mastery of skills for generalization—not just speaking to the clinician in the comfortable therapy environment—it is paramount to target speaking tasks that the client faces each day as part of social, academic, or work-related participation.

Stuttering Modification

Traditional stuttering modification approaches employ three techniques: cancellations (a.k.a. post blocks) after a stuttering event, slides (a.k.a. pull-outs or in-blocks) during a stuttering event, and preparatory set (a.k.a. pre-block) before an anticipated stuttering event (Van Riper, 1971; Yairi & Seery, 2015). Below are more detailed descriptions of each:

- *Cancellation*: After a stuttering event has occurred, the person stops the disfluency, releasing tension, and then produces the word again in an easier manner that is slower and controlled with easy onset.

- *Slide (a.k.a. "pull-out")*: The individual must catch themselves in a moment of stuttering and then produce a slide by easing themselves out of the stuttering event using easy onset to finish the word. The speaker must not rush through the rest of the word, but produce it slowly and in a controlled manner similar to canceling a stuttered moment, but without starting the word over.

- *Preparatory Set*: Preparatory set is used prior to the production of an upcoming word that the person anticipates will be stuttered. Using a slower rate, easy onset, continuous voicing, and light articulatory contacts, the person begins the first sound of the word slowly, smoothly, and easily. The word is completed in a slow, relaxed, smooth manner.

Instruction of stuttering modification typically begins with pseudo stuttering on words in reading, building up to skills at the conversational level. After a client has mastered reading and speaking with stuttering modification in the therapy room with the clinician, he or she is ready to move through a hierarchy of functional speaking tasks. To ensure that students have mastery of skills for generalization (not just speaking to the clinician in the comfortable therapy environment), it is paramount to target speaking tasks that maximizes the social and academic participation of students outside of therapy (Yairi & Seery, 2015; Caruso et al., 1994).

HOW DO I ADDRESS AFFECTIVE ASPECTS OF STUTTERING?

Children who stutter generally gain awareness about their stuttering when they are 5-years of age (Yairi & Ambrose, 2005). Clinicians can use a combination of affective scale results, student self-report, caregiver report, and teacher report, to gather information about the client's baseline level of knowledge about stuttering and compensatory strategies, participation level, and communication attitude. From this baseline information, clinicians should develop objectives to address these domains of the affective aspects of stuttering. Holistic treatment of stuttering should aim to ensure that students who stutter are knowledgeable regarding stuttering, have a high level of recall and understanding about speech techniques they are learning, have a positive communication attitude, and participate in all social and academic aspects of their school day. Addressing affective aspects empowers students who stutter to become their own advocates, reduces feelings of guilt and shame, and maximizes participation (Gregory, Campbell, Gregory, & Hill, 2003; Miller & Rollnick, 1991; Wolpe, 1969).

Students who stutter often benefit from a consistent outlet for sharing their feelings about stuttering with others (Ellis, 2004; Gregory et al., 2003; Manning, 2001; Quesal, 2010). Clinicians may choose to address this aspect by asking students who stutter to share their "good" moments (times when they overcame an obstacle, felt understood, educated another person, did something they used to avoid, used a technique successfully, etc.) and "bad" moments (times when they avoided a speaking task, encountered an obstacle they didn't know how to handle, felt misunderstood, were teased by another person, were not successful with using a technique, etc.). Some students may feel comfortable discussing their "good" and "bad" moments aloud, while others may disclose more candid information in a brief period of journaling. Information shared during these sessions may help the clinician to see what tasks or domains should be addressed through mental rehearsal, positive self-talk, teaching preparation for avoided tasks, and talking a student through any irrational thoughts they may experience regarding speaking tasks (e.g., everyone will laugh, my classmates will think I'm stupid, I'll fail the class, etc.) by discussing the evidence against such thoughts (e.g., you have friends, you make good grades, not everyone laughed last time, most people don't judge others who are struggling, etc.) (Ellis, 2004; Gregory et al., 2003; Manning, 2001; Quesal, 2010).

HOW DO I KEEP DATA?

Data on a child's fluency level during session activities is not serving the overall goal, which is getting the client to show mastery of skills up through the conversational level and consistent use of the techniques across all environments. Clinicians may find that collecting data based on if the client did or did not use techniques, per utterance, yielding a percentage of accuracy, may be an easy, clean way of tracking a client's mastery of techniques.

Two primary types of data should be gathered from pre-persistent clients who stutter: (1) Data on the child's mastery of skill with techniques during everyday therapy activities, and (2) Data taken around once monthly regarding the client's stuttering severity—monitoring for recovery. In pre-persistent children, it is important to intermittently track their conversational speech without being cued to use techniques, to determine if they are reaching recovery. A straightforward way to collecting that data is by recording a brief open-ended sample of the client's conversational speech and getting a percentage of syllables stuttered, just as one would do for the Frequency subtest of the *SSI-4* (Riley, 2009). Clinicians may find it beneficial to take this data during the first 10 minutes of sessions once monthly.

As with all speech production related goals, clinicians must ensure that affective-based goals have a quantitative aspect to measure progress (Gregory et al., 2003; Manning, 2001; Quesal, 2010). Measuring progress with affective aspects is traditionally carried out in two ways. One way to quantify progress with affective aspects of stuttering is to compare a student's affective scale scores before and after periods of treatment (e.g., Given repeated lessons regarding stuttering, mental rehearsal before previously avoided speaking tasks, and outlet discussion regarding "good" moments and "bad" moments of stuttering, the student's affective scale total overall score will reduce from the severe range to the moderate range after two semesters of weekly therapy). Another way to quantify progress with affective aspects of stuttering is performance on recall tasks. This technique for goal quantification typically only works for knowledge goals (e.g., Given repeated lessons on the three fluency shaping techniques, the client will recall slow rate, easy onset, and continuous phonation, with 100% accuracy at the beginning of every therapy session).

When taking data, clinicians should be mindful of false fluency. False fluency is a term used to describe how school-age children, teens, and adults who stutter may exhibit significantly more fluent speech when speaking during a one-on-one task in an environment and with a listener with whom he or she is comfortable. This level of fluency is considered "false," because the same person would have significantly more stuttering because with regular limbic system reactions compounding stuttering events. Clinicians should be mindful of false fluency during assessments, keeping in mind that sampling may need to take place with functional speaking tasks rather than one-on-one conversation. Clinicians should also be aware of the potential for False Fluency in therapy: is the client fluent because he or she is using fluency shaping or is the client just comfortable talking to me and is not attempting any strategies?

WHAT ABOUT STUDENTS WHO DO NOT WANT THERAPY?

A student with persistent stuttering may also choose dismissal, even without mastery of compensatory fluency shaping or stuttering modification strategies. If a school-age child or teen who stutters states explicitly that he or she does not want to be enrolled in therapy, consideration should be made for dismissal from direct intervention. If that child is fully participating in class based on the report of multiple teachers—is okay with openly stuttering while participating in all aspects of academic tasks—and does not want therapy, the students should not be enrolled in direct treatment. If the child is avoiding functional speaking tasks for school (e.g., taking 0% grades for class presentations, will not raise his or her hand to ask questions, refuses reading aloud, etc.) and does not want to be enrolled in therapy, a team discussion should take place with the child regarding his or her enrollment in therapy based on the reported speaking avoidance. A discussion among the client, caregivers, speech–language pathologist, teachers, and special education administrators should take place to determine if classroom modifications should be considered in lieu of direct speech therapy.

What Else Should I do to Help My School-Age Client Who Stutters Succeed in School?

Each student's educational team should discuss ways to make the student's academic and social environments at school as accommodating to the client's persistent stuttering as is possible and reasonable. The following are some potential classroom accommodations that the team may find beneficial for school-age and teen students with persistent stuttering:

- Advanced notice for practicing oral presentations like book reports or speeches

- Giving presentations in front of the SLP, then the teacher, then the teacher and a few friends, before finally giving it in front of the class

- Sending the student home with a copy of passage that the teachers plans to have he/she read out loud in class the night before to allow practice time

- Avoiding scenarios with timed pressure to speak such as game show type review games in which students are racing to see who can call out an answer first

- Allowing the student to finish his or her dysfluent sentences without being interrupted by others or having the sentence finished for them

- Facilitating an environment of respect with a no-tolerance policy for bullying or teasing

- Allowing the client, potentially as a part of a therapy goal, to give a brief presentation to educate his/her fellow students about stuttering to further their acceptance of his disfluencies and his/her comfort with stuttering in front of her peers

WHAT ARE SOME SUGGESTED GOALS FOR MY CLIENT WHO STUTTERS?

Preschool: Direct Fluency Shaping Therapy

- **Preschool (Fluency Shaping, working up to conversational level)**
  - Given direct instruction and modeling of easy onset, slowed rate, and continuous voicing, the patient will use fluency shaping for producing:
    - single words with ##% accuracy
    - two-word utterances with ##% accuracy
    - carrier phrases with ##% accuracy
    - rote utterances with ##% accuracy
    - self-created sentences with ##% accuracy
    - conversational exchanges with ##% accuracy
    - narratives with ##% accuracy

- **Preschool (Fluency Shaping, conditioning after mastering conversational and narrative level in therapy)**
  - Given direct modeling of fluency shaping accompanied by verbal praise for all utterances using fluency-shaping, clinician and/or caregiver recasting of fast of 75% of dysfluent utterances, and clinician and/or caregiver verbal prompts for the patient to restate fast or dysfluent utterances with fluency shaping, the patient will produce conversational speech with fluency-shaping in ##% of utterances.

School-Age/Adult: Direct Fluency Shaping

- **Persistent (Early Fluency Shaping Teaching Activities)**
  - Given direct instruction and modeling of easy onset, slowed rate, and continuous voicing, the patient will use fluency shaping for producing:
    - single words with ##% accuracy
    - two-word utterances with ##% accuracy
    - carrier phrases with ##% accuracy
    - rote utterances with ##% accuracy
    - self-created sentences with ##% accuracy
    - conversational exchanges with ##% accuracy
    - narratives with ##% accuracy

- **Persistent (School-Age and Teens, Fluency Shaping Functional Activities)**
  - Given direct instruction and modeling of easy onset, slowed rate, and continuous voicing, the patient will use fluency shaping for:
    - conversational exchanges with the clinician with ##% accuracy
    - reading aloud in front of the clinician with ##% accuracy
    - phone call with the clinician with ##% accuracy
    - answering job (or scholarship) interview questions with the clinician with ##% accuracy
    - ordering food (cafeteria or restaurant) with ##% accuracy
    - reading aloud in front of a small peer group with ##% accuracy
    - giving a 1–2 minute presentation in front of a small peer group with ##% accuracy

○ talking on the phone with an unfamiliar listener for a semi-scripted conversational exchange with ##% accuracy

○ reading aloud in front of a large group of peers with ##% accuracy

○ giving a full class (or work) presentation in front of a small peer group with ##% accuracy

○ answering job (or scholarship) interview questions with an unfamiliar listener with ##% accuracy

School-Age/Adult: Stuttering Modification

● **School-Age, Teens, and Adults (Stuttering Modification, Teaching Activities)**

○ Given instruction and modeling of a tension and release activity, the patient will demonstrate release of tension on pseudo-stuttering events of pre-selected words in a reading passage with ##% accuracy.

○ Given instruction and modeling of cancellations, the patient will demonstrate cancellations with pseudo-stuttering events of pre-selected words in a reading passage with ##% accuracy.

○ Given instruction and modeling of slides (pull-outs), the patient will demonstrate slides with pseudo-stuttering events of pre-selected words in a reading passage with ##% accuracy.

○ Given instruction and modeling of preparatory set, the patient will demonstrate fluent speech with easy onset, slowed rate, and continuous voicing through pre-selected words in a reading passage with ##% accuracy.

● **School-Age, Teens, and Adults (Stuttering Modification, Functional Activities)**

■ Given instruction and modeling of stuttering modification techniques, the patient will modify all pseudo-stuttering events and real stuttering events with cancellations, slides, or preparatory during:

○ conversational exchanges with the clinician with ##% accuracy

○ reading aloud in front of the clinician with ##% accuracy

○ phone call with the clinician with ##% accuracy

○ answering job (or scholarship) interview questions with the clinician with ##% accuracy

○ ordering food (cafeteria or restaurant) with ##% accuracy

○ reading aloud in front of a small peer group with ##% accuracy

○ giving a 1–2 minute presentation in front of a small peer group with ##% accuracy

○ talking on the phone with an unfamiliar listener for a semi-scripted conversational exchange with ##% accuracy

○ reading aloud in front of a large group of peers with ##% accuracy

○ giving a full class (or work) presentation in front of a small peer group with ##% accuracy

○ answering job (or scholarship) interview questions with an unfamiliar listener with ##% accuracy

Affective Components: Knowledge-Based Objectives

● Given repeated lessons, the student will recall the following information with 100% accuracy across at least three therapy sessions by the end of the semester:

○ the three fluency shaping techniques (slow rate, easy onset, continuous phonation)

○ the three stuttering modification techniques (cancellations, slides, preparatory set)

○ descriptions/definitions of each of the three fluency shaping techniques

○ descriptions/definitions of each of the three stuttering modifications

○ three famous people who stutter

○ three fluency-inducing conditions (singing, choral reading, metronome effect, whispering, acting, speaking in an accent, speaking to a baby or pet, delayed auditory feedback, etc.)

○ prevalence of stuttering (1%)

○ define the Adaptation Effect

○ describe how the Adaptation Effect can be used to prepare for reading aloud or giving a presentation

○ contemporary etiology theories (neurological differences and genetics)

○ what makes stuttering worse (limbic system reactions)

- define cycling
- discuss/disclose their current level of stuttering in their present cycle
- describe how to prepare for reading aloud in front of others
- describe how to prepare for giving a presentation

REFERENCES

Alm, P. (2004). Stuttering and the basal ganglia circuits: A critical review of possible relations. *Journal of Communication Disorders, 37,* 325–369.

Ambrose, N. (2004). Theoretical perspectives on the cause of stuttering. *Contemporary Issues in Communication Science and Disorders, 31,* 80–91.

Ambrose, N., Yairi, E., & Cox, N. (1993). Genetic aspects of early childhood stuttering. *Journal of Communication Disorders, 35,* 63–82.

Andrews, G., & Harris, M. (1964). *The syndrome of stuttering. Clinics in developmental medicine, No. 17.* London: William Heineman Medical Books Ltd.

Beal, D., Lerch, J., Cameron, B., Henderson, R., Gracco, V., & De Nil, L. (2015). The trajectory of gray matter development in Broca's area is abnormal in people who stutter. *Frontiers of Human Neuroscience, 9,* 1–9.

Blomgren, M. (2010). Stuttering treatment for adults: An update on contemporary approaches. *Seminars in Speech and Language, 31*(4), 272–282.

Bloodstein, O., & Bernstein Ratner, N. (2008). *A handbook on stuttering* (6th ed.). New York, NY: Cengage.

Braun, A. Varga, M. Stager, S., Schulz, G., Selvie, S., Maisog, J., Carsn, R., & Ludlow, C. (1997). Altered patterns of cerebral activity during speech and language production in developmental stuttering. *Brain, 120,* 761–784.

Bryngelson, B. (1938). Prognosis of stuttering. *Journal of Speech Disorders, 3,* 121–123.

Caruso, A., Chodzko-Zajko, W. J., Bidinger, D. A., & Sommers, R. K. (1994). Adults who stutter: Responses to cognitive stress. *Journal of Speech and Hearing Research, 37,* 746–754.

Chang, S., & Zhu, D. (2013). Neural network connectivity differences in children who stutter. *Brain, 136,* 3709–3726.

Chang, S., Erickson, K., Ambrose, N., Hasegawa-Johnson, M., & Ludlow, C. (2008). Brain anatomy differences in childhood stuttering. *Neuroimage, 39,* 1333–1344.

Curlee, R. (1985). Training students to work with stutterers. In Boberg, E. (Ed.), *Stuttering: Part one. Seminars in speech and language* (pp. 131–144). New York, NY: Thieme-Stratton.

Ellis, A. (2004). *Rational emotive behavior therapy: It works for me—It can work for you.* Amherst, NY: Prometheus Books.

Foundas, A., Bollich, A., Corey, D., Hurley, M., & Heilman, K. (2001). Anomalous anatomy of speech-language areas in adults with persistent developmental stuttering. *Neurology, 57,* 207–215.

Foundas, A., Cindass, R., Mock, J., & Corey, D. (2013). Atypical caudate anatomy in children who stutter. *Perceptual & Motor Skills: Physical Development & Measurement, 116,* 528–543.

Fox, P, Ingham, R., Ingham, J., Hirsch, T., Hunter-Downs, J., Martin, C., Jerabek, P., Glass, T., & Lancaster, J. (1996). A PET study of the neural systems of stuttering. *Nature, 382,* 158–162.

Giraud, A., Neumann, K., Bachoud-Levi, A., von Gudenberg, A., Euler, A., Lanfermann, H., & Preibisch, C. (2008). Severity of dysfluency correlates with basal ganglia activity in persistent developmental stuttering. *Brain and Language, 104,* 190–199.

Goldberg, G. (1985). Supplementary motor area structure and function: Review and hypothesis. *Behavioral Brain Science, 8,* 567–616.

Goldberg, G. (1991). Microgenetic theory and the dual premotor systems hypothesis. *Cognitive Microgenesis,* 32–52. doi:10.1007/978-1-4612-3056-4_2.

Kelly E., Martin, J., Baker, K., Rivera, N., Bishop, J., Krizike, C., Stettler, D., & Stealy, J. (1997). Academic and clinical preparation and practices of school speech-language pathologists with people who stutter. *Language, Speech, and Hearing Services in Schools, 26,* 195–212.

Kidd, K. (1980). Genetic models of stuttering. *Journal of Fluency Disorders, 5,* 187–201.

Kloth, S., Kraaimaat, F., Janssen, P., & Brutten, G. (1999). Persistence and remission of incipient stuttering among high-risk children. *Journal of Fluency Disorders, 24,* 253–265.

Mallard, A., Gardner, L., & Downey, C. (1988). Clinical training in stuttering for school clinicians. *Journal of Fluency Disorders, 13*(4), 253–259.

Manning, W. (2001). *Clinical decision making in fluency disorders.* New York, NY: Delmar.

Mansson, H. (2000). Childhood stuttering: Incidence and development. *Journal of Fluency Disorders, 25,* 47–57.

Matkin, N., Ringle, R., & Snope, T. (1983). Master report of surveys discrepancies. In Rees, N. & Snope, T. (Eds.), *Proceedings of the Conference on Undergraduate, Graduate and Continuing Education. ASHA Reports, 13.* Rockville, MD: American Speech-Language Hearing Association.

Millard, S., & Cook, F. (2010). Working with young children who stutter: Raising our game. *Seminars in Speech and Language, 31*(4), 283–285.

Miller, W., & Rollnick, S. (1991). *Motivational interviewing: Preparing people to change addictive behavior.* New York, NY: Guilford Press.

Neumann, K., Preibisch, C., Euler, H., von Gudenberg, A., Lafermann, H., Gall, V., & Giraud, A. (2005). Cortical plasticity associated with stuttering therapy. *Journal of Fluency Disorders, 30*, 23–39.

O'Brian, S., Onslow, M., Cream, A., & Packman, A. (2003). The Camperdown Program: Outcomes of a new prolonged-speech treatment model. *Journal of Speech, Language, and Hearing Research, 46*, 933–946.

Panelli, C., McFarlane, S., & Shipley, K. (1978). Implications of evaluating and intervening with incipient stutterers. *Journal of Fluency Disorders, 3*, 41–50.

Quesal, R. (2010). Empathy: Perhaps the most important E in EBP. *Seminars in Speech and Language, 31*(4), 217–226.

Riley, G. (2009). *Stuttering severity instrument for children and adults* (4th ed.). Austin, TX: Pro-Ed.

Rommel, D., Hage, A., Kalehne, P., & Johannsen, H. (2000). Developmental maintenance and recovery of childhood stuttering: Prospective longitudinal data 3 years after first contact. In *Proceedings of the Fifth Oxford Disfluency Conference* (pp. 168–182).

Sheehan, J., & Martyn, M. (1970). Spontaneous recovery from Stuttering. *Journal of Speech and Hearing Research, 13*, 279–289.

Sommers, R., & Caruso, A. (1995). Inservice training in speech-language pathology: Are we meeting the needs for fluency training? *American Journal of Speech–language Pathology, 4*, 22–28.

Throneburg, R. & Yairi, E. (2003). Secondary characteristics of children whose stuttering persisted and recovered. *ASHA Leader, 8*(15), 150.

Van Riper, C. (1971). *The nature of stuttering.* Elglewood Cliffs, NJ: Prentice-Hall.

Van Riper, C. (1982). *The nature of stuttering* (2nd ed.). Elglewood Cliffs, NJ: Prentice-Hall.

Watkins, R., & Yairi, E. (1997). Language production abilities of children who persisted and recovered from stuttering. *Journal of Speech, Language, and Hearing Research, 40*, 385–399.

Watkins, R., Yairi, E., & Ambrose, N. (1999). Early childhood stuttering III: Initial status of expressive language abilities. *Journal of Speech-Language and Hearing Research, 42*(5), 1125–1135.

Wolpe, J. (1969). *The practice of behavior therapy.* New York, NY: Pergamon Press.

World Health Organization. (1977). *Manual of the international statistical classification of diseases, injuries, and causes of death* (Volume 1). Geneva: World Health Organization.

Yairi, E., & Ambrose, N. (1992). A longitudinal study of stuttering in children: A preliminary report. *Journal of Speech and Hearing Research, 35*, 755–760.

Yairi, E., & Ambrose, N. (1999a). Early childhood stuttering. I: Persistency and recovery rates. *Journal of Speech, Language, and Hearing Research, 42*, 1097–1112.

Yairi, E., & Ambrose, N. (1999b). Spontaneous recovery and clinical trials research in early childhood stuttering: A response to Onslow and Packman. *Journal of Speech, Language, and Hearing Research, 42*, 402–410.

Yairi, E., & Ambrose, A. (2005). *Early childhood stuttering for clinicians by clinicians.* Austin, TX: PRO-ED.

Yairi, E., & Seery, C. (2015). *Stuttering: Foundations and clinical applications* (2nd ed.). Boston, MA: Pearson.

Yairi, E., Ambrose, N., & Niermann, R. (1993). The early months of stuttering: A developmental study. *Journal of Speech and Hearing Research, 36*, 521–528.

Yairi, E., Ambrose, N., Paden, E., & Throneberg, R. N. (1996). Predictive factors of persistence and recovery. Pathways of childhood stuttering. *Journal of Communication Disorders, 29*, 51–77.

Yaruss, J., & Quesal, R. (2002). Academic and clinical education in fluency disorders: An update. *Journal of Fluency Disorders, 27*(1), 43–62.

Case Scenario 12-1 Worksheet

NAME: _____ DATE: _____

Caleb is a 4-year 2-month old boy who has been stuttering for 1 year. He has a family history of stuttering with his maternal uncle who continues to stutter into adulthood. Caleb exhibits moderate-range stuttering as compared to other preschoolers, characterized by part-word repetitions of up to 4 units, prolongations, and a few fleeting blocks. During some repetitions, you note that he tilts his head back. An analysis of a cell phone video from Caleb's stuttering at onset also reveals moderate-range stuttering. The father reported that Caleb does not appear to be aware of his stuttering or frustrated during moments of disfluency. Caleb's father also reports cycles of periods of time when Caleb has essentially fluent speech for a few days. While testing other domains of his communication, you find that Caleb has normal receptive and expressive language skills and a mild phonological delay.

1. Perform a risk analysis, listing out prognostic indicators for natural remission and persistence of his stuttering into adulthood.

Natural Remission	Persistence

Based on this analysis would you recommend that Caleb receive treatment?

_____

2. What is an appropriate LONG-TERM OBJECTIVE for Caleb?

_____

_____

3. What are <u>three</u> appropriate SHORT-TERM OBJECTIVES for Caleb if the clinician is choosing to use a fluency-shaping approach?

A.

_____

_____

B.

_____

_____

C.

_____

_____

4. List activities you might use to target the short-term objectives listed above. The task for 4A should pair with the short-term objective listed for 3A. Please list materials you might use.

A.

_____

_____

B.

_____

_____

C.

_____

_____

Case Scenario 12-2 Worksheet

NAME: _____   **DATE:** _____

Jacob is a 15-year-old high school sophomore who has stuttered since he was 4 years of age. Testing reveals that Jacob has mild-range stuttering compared to other school-aged children characterized by blocks, prolongations, and single-syllable whole-word repetitions of up to 2 units; his stuttering events are occasionally accompanied by rapid blinking. Other evaluation results include an affective scale score of moderately impacted communication attitude, normal language scores, and normal articulation skills relative to his age. Jacob's parents report that he has been in speech therapy since he was 5 years old; however, he does not employ the fluency-shaping strategies that he has learned through treatment. The parents also indicate that Jacob will not order his own food in a restaurant, insists on texting rather than talking on the phone to avoid making phone calls, and refused to join the science quiz-bowl team despite his teacher's nomination. The parents relayed that his teachers indicate that Jacob does not raise his hand to answer questions in class and is taking zero scores when it is time to give an oral presentation in front of his classmates. The parents report that Jacob says that he really does not want therapy any more since it cannot fix his stuttering, and he does not want to "talk like a robot" as he was taught in speech therapy.

1. What is a therapy approach for addressing the speech component of Jacob's stuttering without having him continue fluency shaping?

   _____

2. What is an appropriate LONG-TERM OBJECTIVE for Jacob's affective component?

   _____

   _____

3. What is an appropriate LONG-TERM OBJECTIVE for Jacob's speech component?

   _____

   _____

4. What are <u>three</u> appropriate SHORT-TERM OBJECTIVES for addressing speech strategies with Jacob for functional communication tasks for which the parents and teachers raise specific concerns?

A.

_____

_____

B.

_____

_____

C.

_____

_____

5. Write an example of an appropriate SHORT-TERM OBJECTIVE for increasing Jacob's knowledge regarding stuttering?

_____

_____

Case Scenario 12-3 Worksheet

NAME: _____ **DATE:** _____

Tara is a 10-year-old girl who has a history of stuttering since 3 years of age and mild intellectual disability. During your testing session you find that Tara exhibits severe stuttering characterized by blocks of up to 5 seconds in length, prolongations, part-word repetitions, and whole-word repetitions of up to 7 units in length, with many disfluencies accompanied by eye-closing and articulatory posturing. Tara's teachers and parents report that she isolates herself from most people aside from a few close friends, walking around with headphones in her ears between classes and never raising her hand in class to ask or answer questions. Her affective scale results were of compromised validity due to her lack of literacy and receptive vocabulary abilities for words like "often," "rarely," "never," "difficulty," etc.

1. What is an appropriate LONG-TERM GOAL for Tara's affective component?

   _____

2. What is an appropriate LONG-TERM GOAL for Tara's stuttering component?

   _____

3. What are <u>three</u> appropriate SHORT-TERM OBJECTIVES?

   A.

   _____

   _____

   B.

   _____

   _____

   C.

   _____

   _____

4. List the TASK you would use to target the short-term objectives listed above. The task for 3A should pair with the short-term objective listed for 2A. Please list MATERIALS you plan to use.

A.

_____

_____

B.

_____

_____

C.

_____

_____

CHAPTER 13

Introduction to Disability and Transition Services

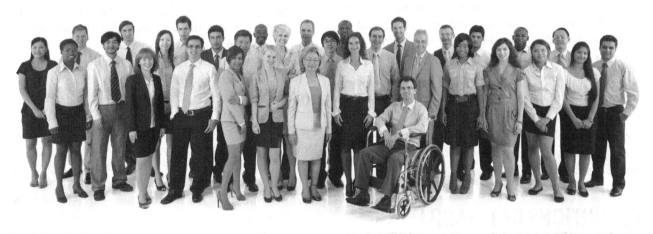

Rawpixel.com/Shutterstock.com

"Disability is a matter of perception. If you can do just one thing well, you're needed by someone."

—Martina Navratilova

OVERVIEW

According to the Pew Research Center (Bialik, 2017), in 2015, there were nearly 40 million Americans with a disability, which represented 12.6% of the population. The purpose of this chapter to provide an introduction and overview of the concepts of disability, chronic illness, relevant disability legislation, and relevant disability services. This chapter will use, and it is recommended that everyone use, person-first language. The use of this type of language stresses the importance of the person before the disability. For example, you would say, "a person who is blind" or "a person with a visual impairment," rather than saying "a blind person." Or it would be more appropriate to say, "a person with a disability" rather than "a disabled person." "Person-first language may appear to be more cumbersome, but it serves the purpose of emphasizing that individual is a person first and the disability is secondary" (Smart, 2009a, p. 95). There is one caveat to person-first language.

> However, individuals who are deaf, especially those in the Deaf Culture, prefer to be referred to as 'a Deaf person' . . . This insistence on putting the word 'Deaf' before the word 'person' is based on the Deaf's identity as a culture, as a group not unified by a disability, but rather unified by shared experiences and a common language. (Smart, 2009a, p. 95).

There are individuals with disabilities who do not use or like person-first language. When working with people with disabilities, it is best to start with person-first language and allow the individual to tell you the language that he/she prefers.

DEFINITIONS OF DISABILITY

> There are hundreds of different disabilities. Some are congenital; most come later in life. Some are progressive, like muscular dystrophy, cystic fibrosis, and some forms of vision or hearing loss. Others, like seizure conditions, are episodic. Multiple sclerosis is episodic and progressive. Some conditions are static, like loss of limb. Still others, like cancer and occasionally paralysis, can even go away. Some disabilities are "hidden," like epilepsy or diabetes. Disability law also applies to people with perceived disabilities such as obesity or stuttering, which are not disabling but create prejudice and discrimination (Shapiro, 1994, p. 5).

There are different definitions of the term disability, and these definitions are typically either a medical definition or a legal definition. According to the Americans with Disabilities Act National Network, a person with a disability is "a person who has a physical or mental impairment that substantially limits one or more major life activities" (2018, para 2). This is a legal definition of disability and comes directly from the Americans with Disabilities Act, which will be discussed in greater detail later in this chapter. The World Health Organization (WHO) provides the following definition of disability:

> Disabilities is an umbrella term, covering impairments, activity limitations, and participation restrictions. An impairment is a problem in body function or structure; an activity limitation is a difficulty encountered by an individual in executing a task or action; while a participation restriction is a problem experienced by an individual in involvement in life situations (WHO, 2018, para 1).

CATEGORIES OF DISABILITIES

There are four broad categories of disabilities: physical, intellectual, cognitive, and psychiatric. "Physical disabilities include mobility impairments; neurologic impairments such as cerebral palsy and seizure disorders; traumatic brain injuries; musculoskeletal conditions, such as muscular dystrophy and arthritis; sensory loss; and health disorders" (Smart, 2009a, p. 23). Individuals with visual impairments, hearing impairments, and chronic illness are included in this category. The American Association of Intellectual and Developmental Disabilities (AAIDD) defines an intellectual disability as one "characterized by significant limitations both in intellectual functioning (reasoning, learning, problem solving) and in adaptive behavior, which covers a range of everyday social and practical skills (AAIDD, 2018, para 1). Examples of intellectual disabilities include Down Syndrome, Autism Spectrum Disorders, and Fragile X Syndrome. "Cognitive disabilities impair perception, memory, information processing, reasoning, sensory discrimination (auditory and visual), and attention" (Smart, 2009a, p. 30). Examples of cognitive disabilities include learning disabilities, traumatic brain injury, and attention deficit hyperactivity disorder (ADHD). Psychiatric disabilities impact mental health. Examples of psychiatric disabilities include depression, bipolar disorder, anxiety disorders, and schizophrenia. See **Table 13.1**, Broad Disability Categories, below for examples of disabilities and the categories in to which they fit.

Table 13.1 Broad Disability Categories

Disability Category	Examples
Physical	Mobility impairments Seizure disorders Traumatic brain injury Musculoskeletal disorders
Intellectual	Down Syndrome Autism Spectrum Disorders Fragile X Syndrome
Cognitive	Learning disabilities ADHD
Psychiatric	Depression Bipolar disorder Anxiety disorders Schizophrenia

Under the Individuals with Disabilities Education Act (IDEA), there are 13 categories of disabilities. These are applicable to individuals with disabilities in the school system, ages 3–21. The categories of disability are: autism, deaf-blindness, deafness, emotional disturbance, hearing impairment, intellectual disability, multiple disabilities, orthopedic impairment, other health impairment, specific learning disability, speech or language impairment, traumatic brain injury, and visual impairment. See **Table 13.2**, IDEA 13 Diagnostic Categories.

For professionals in communication disorders, it is important to be familiar with the 13 categories of disability under IDEA because many services may be provided in schools within the K-12 system. Communication disorders professionals may be integral members of the individualized education plan (IEP) team involved in serving students with a variety of disabilities. The next

Table 13.2 IDEA 13 Diagnostic Categories

Condition	Description
Specific learning disability (SLD)	The conditions covered by the umbrella term "SLD" may affect a child's ability to read, write, listen, speak, reason, or do math.
Other health impairment	The conditions covered by the umbrella term "other health impairment" limit a child's strength, energy, or alertness. One example is an attention issue such as <u>ADHD</u>. Limited strength, vitality, or alertness, including heightened alertness to stimuli in the environment are also examples.
Autism spectrum disorder (ASD)	ASD is a developmental disability, which encompasses a wide range of symptoms and skills, but mainly affects a child's communication and social skills. ASD may also impact behavior.
Emotional disturbance	Children covered by the umbrella term "emotional disturbance" may have a number of mental disorders. Some examples of these include anxiety disorder, schizophrenia, bipolar disorder, obsessive-compulsive disorder, and depression. Some of these issues may also be covered under "other health impairment." The child may exhibit one or more of the following characteristics: • Inability to learn not explained by other factors • Inability to build or maintain interpersonal relationships • Inappropriate feelings given normal circumstances • General pervasive unhappy or depressed mood • Tendency to develop physical symptoms or fears accompanying school or personal problems
Speech or language impairment	The umbrella term "speech or language impairment" covers a wide range of communication problems. Some examples of these include stuttering, impaired articulation, language impairment, or voice impairment.
Visual impairment, including blindness	The umbrella term "visual impairment" includes any vision problem, such as partial sight and blindness, which cannot be corrected with eyewear. Vision problems that can be corrected with eyewear do not qualify.
Deafness	Children with a diagnosis of deafness have a severe hearing impairment which prevents them from processing language through hearing.

(Continued)

Table 13.2 IDEA 13 Diagnostic Categories (Continued)

Condition	Description
Hearing impairment	The term "hearing impairment" refers to a hearing loss not covered by the definition of deafness. This type of loss can fluctuate or change over time. Having a hearing impairment is not the same thing as having an auditory processing disorder.
Deaf-blindness	Children diagnosed with deaf-blindness have both hearing and visual impairments. Their communication needs are so great that they are beyond what programs for the deaf or blind can meet.
Orthopedic impairment	The umbrella term "orthopedic impairment" covers any impairment to a child's body, no matter what the cause.
Intellectual disability	Children diagnosed with an intellectual disability have below-average intellectual ability. These children may also exhibit poor communication, self-care, and social skills. One example of an intellectual disability is Down syndrome. Significantly subaverage general intellectual functioning, co-occurring deficits in adaptive behavior that appear during the developmental period.
Traumatic brain injury	The term "traumatic brain injury" encompasses any injury to the brain caused by an accident or physical force. Impairments may be in one or more areas: • Cognition • Language • Memory • Attention • Reasoning • Abstract thinking • Judgment • Problem solving • Sensory, perceptual, and motor abilities • Psychosocial behavior • Physical functions • Information processing • Speech
Multiple disabilities	Children with multiple disabilities have more than one condition covered by IDEA. Having multiple issues creates greater educational needs than can be met in a program for any one condition.

National Dissemination Center for Children with Disabilities, 2012, p 2–4 and a variety of additional sources.

section will cover four broad models of disability that can be useful for understanding disability when working both inside and outside of the school system.

MODELS OF DISABILITY

Models of disability provide different ways to conceptualize disability. There are five models of disability: the biomedical model, the environmental model, the functional model, the sociopolitical model, and the biopsychosocial model (see **Table 13.3**, Models of Disability). Each model has strengths and weaknesses. The biomedical model is the oldest and most

understood model of disability. "Disability is thought to be pathology, disorder, dysfunction, or deformity that is located within the individual . . . disability can be classified, quantified, measured, and standardized" (Smart, 2009b, p. 4). In this model, the problem lies within the individual and treatment is concerned with changing the individual. In the functional model of disability, "disability is defined as a three-way interaction between the individual, the disability, and the function of the individual" (Smart, 2009b, p. 6). Interventions are designed to adapt the function of the individual.

The basis of the environmental model is that the individual's social and physical environment impacts

Table 13.3 Models of Disability

Model	Explanation
Biomedical	The problem is with the individual and intervention is focused on addressing medical problems or symptoms with medication or other medical treatments.
Sociopolitical	The problem is with society and their expectations of individuals. Interventions are focused on providing civil and social rights for individuals with disabilities, as well as people with disabilities as a social group.
Functional	The problem is with the individual and interventions are designed to improve the individual's functioning.
Environmental	The problem lies within the environment of the person with a disability. Interventions are designed to change the person's environment, both the physical and the social.
Biopsychosocial	The problem is viewed as both biological and subjective, as well as the interaction between these factors. Interventions are designed to address both the disease and the experience of living with a disability or illness.

disability. The environment can cause, define, or exaggerate a person's disability. Interventions seek to change the individual's physical and social environments. In the sociopolitical model, disability is considered a societal concern. Advocates for this model suggest that many of the problems that people with disabilities face are caused by society and disability is both a social and political construction. Interventions seek to address providing civil and social rights to the individual with a disability, as well as people with disabilities as a whole group.

The newest, and most comprehensive, model of disability is the biopsychosocial model. This model was created by George Engel in 1977. The model tries to understand disability and chronic illness and the complex interaction between biological factors, psychological factors, and social factors. The biopsychosocial model examines both the objective biological event that is disease and the subjective experience of illness.

RELEVANT LEGISLATION

This section will cover a brief history of disability rights and relevant legislation. Entire books have been written on this topic, so this section will briefly discuss important movements and laws. For more detailed information, the books Disabled Rights: American Disability Policy and the Fight for Equity by Jacqueline Vaughn Switzer and No Pity: People with Disabilities Forging a New Civil

Rights Movement by Joseph Shapiro. This link also contains a detailed timeline of important events and legislation in the history of disability rights: https://www.paec.org/disabilityhistoryawareness/pdfs/Timeline.pdf.

REHABILITATION ACT OF 1973 (SECTION 504)

The U.S. Department of Justice summarizes the Rehabilitation Act of 1973 as the following: "The Rehabilitation Act prohibits discrimination on the basis of disability in programs conducted by Federal agencies, in programs receiving Federal financial assistance, in Federal employment, and in the employment practices of Federal contractors" (2009, p.1). Section 504 is the Equal Opportunities section. This section of the law states that:

No otherwise qualified individual with a disability . . . shall, solely by reason of his or her disability, be excluded from participation in, be denied the benefits of, or be subjected to discrimination under any program or activity receiving Federal financial assistance or under any program or activity conducted by any Executive agency. (U.S. Department of Labor, 2018b, para 1).

Examples of programs or activities receiving federal financial assistance include school districts, colleges or universities, nursing homes, hospitals, and day care centers.

Strongly emphasizing accessibility of buildings and programs for persons with disabilities, Section 504 has tremendous implications because of the many social institutions receiving some type of federal assistance. It is also important to note that under Section 504 a person with a disability cannot 'be found unqualified without considering whether a reasonable accommodation would render the individual qualified (Rubin, Roessler, & Rumrill, 2016, p. 51).

Section 504, in combination with the Americans with Disabilities Act, are supposed to prevent discrimination in hiring practices and admittance to colleges and universities for people with disabilities. Otherwise qualified individuals cannot be turned away from a job or denied admission to an institution of higher education. This is also allows individuals with disabilities to request reasonable academic accommodations in order to complete necessary coursework.

AMERICANS WITH DISABILITIES ACT

The Americans with Disabilities Act (ADA) was signed into law by President George H. W. Bush on July 26, 1990. At the ceremony, President Bush said, "With today's signing of the landmark Americans with Disabilities Act, every man, woman, and child with a disability can now pass through once-closed doors into a bright new era of equality, independence, and freedom" (U.S. Equal Employment Opportunity Commission (EEOC), 2018a, para 4). Switzer provides the following commentary on the ADA: "Whatever the act says legally, the clearly communicated promise of the ADA is that all people with disabilities will be fully equal, fully productive, fully prosperous, and fully welcome participants in the mainstream" (2003, p. 112). The U.S. Department of Justice provides the following summary of the ADA:

> The ADA prohibits discrimination on the basis of disability in employment, State and local government, public accommodations, commercial facilities, transportation, and telecommunications. It also applies to the United States Congress. To be protected by the ADA, one must have a disability or have a relationship or association with an individual with a disability. An individual with a disability is defined by the ADA as a person who has a physical or mental impairment that substantially limits one or more major life activities, a person who has a history or record of such an impairment, or a person who is perceived by others as having such an impairment. The ADA does not specifically name all of the impairments that are covered (2009, p.1).

There are five titles of the ADA. Title I covers employment and legally mandates that covered employers (employers with 15 or more employees) provide reasonable accommodations for employees and applicants with disabilities and prohibits discrimination based on disability. Title II covers public services and states that people with disabilities cannot be denied services or participation in programs or activities. Additionally, public transportation must be accessible for people with disabilities. Title III covers public accommodations, such as restaurants, hotels, and stores. This title requires that any new buildings that are constructed must be accessible for individuals with disabilities and barriers to services must be removed for existing facilities. Title IV covers telecommunications. This title requires that telephone services must have a telephone relay system in place to serve people who use telecommunication devise such as TTYs. Title V is the miscellaneous title, which "includes a provision prohibiting either (a) coercing or threatening or (b) retaliating against individuals with disabilities or those attempting to aid people with disabilities in asserting their rights under the ADA (Job Accommodation Network (JAN), 2012, para 6).

It is a common thought, especially among people without disabilities, that the passage and implementation of the ADA has fixed all problems for people with disabilities. A survey conducted by The Kessler Foundation and Harris Interactive in 2010 asked a nationally representative sample of 1,001 people with disabilities the question "Do you think the Americans with Disabilities Act has made your life better, worse, or made no difference?". 23% of the respondents indicated that the ADA had made their life better. But a shocking 61% of respondents indicated that the ADA had made no difference in their lives. Regarding the passage of the ADA, Switzer states:

> Advocates for persons with disabilities seldom argue that the ADA is a cure-all for unemployment, lack of affordable housing, social isolation, or other problems faced by the population at large. They do believe, however, that the statute is the only way of starting to end patterns of discrimination that have persisted for decades . . . even persons with disabilities are likely to admit that they do not expect decades of stereotypes to vanish overnight; if anything, they often talk of "another century of struggle." (Switzer, 2003, pp. 142–143).

The passage of the ADA was significant in many ways, but it is not the end of the fight for disability rights, it is the beginning, and we still have a long way to go. "More than ten years after the signing of the ADA, efforts to ensure equal access continues on the local, state, and national levels—evidence that much remains to be done" (Switzer, 2003, p. 173).

> Given the limitations of existing research, one can easily dismiss the impact of the ADA and other disability policies by arguing that the glass is half-full or half-empty. For activists who demand and expect immediate inclusion and economic and social parity, the glass is half-empty, and the tap is not even running . . . those who are veterans of disability rights activism, the glass is half-full—an improvement over the glass that was once virtually empty (Switzer, 2003, p. 205).

THE AMERICANS WITH DISABILITIES ACT AMENDMENT ACT

The ADA Amendment Act (ADAAA) was enacted on September 25, 2008 and became effective January 1, 2009. This law was significant because it made a number of substantial changes to how disability is defined under the ADA. One of the most major components of this law was that Congress made it easier than it was previously for an individual seeking protection from discrimination to establish having a disability within the meaning of the law. The definition of disability was to be construed more broadly rather than narrowly. Another addition to the law with the ADAAA is that an "impairment that is episodic or in remission is a disability if it would substantially limit a major life activity when active (EEOC, 2018b). "Clearly the ADAAA represents significant progress toward actualizing the original spirit of the ADA, with its reversal of mitigating measures exclusions and its list of presumptively disabling impairments. Many more people with impairments are now considered individuals with disabilities . . . " (Rubin et al., 2016, p. 93).

WORKFORCE INNOVATION AND OPPORTUNITY ACT

The Workforce Innovation and Opportunity Act (WIOA) was signed into law on July 22, 2014. "WIOA is designed to help job seeker access employment, education, training, and support services to succeed in the labor market and to match employers with the skilled workers they need to compete in the global economy" (U.S. Department of Labor, 2018a, para 1). This legislation supersedes the Workforce Investment Act of 1998 (WIA) and amends several previous acts, including the Rehabilitation Act of 1973. This is the first legislative reform of the public workforce system in 15 years. Roessler et al. (2016) captured this legislation best with the following summary:

> Specifically, the WIOA redoubles the federal commitment to provide effective and responsive transition services to students with disabilities exiting public school programs, emphasizes integrated community employment by closing access to most long-term sheltered workshops . . . promotes access for people with disabilities to the American job center system that provides employment services to 20 million people annually, and requires state VR agencies to emphasize employment opportunities for people with disabilities that include health insurance benefits and provide entry to the middle class. The WIOA also emphasizes employer engagement in all aspects of the VR process and calls for improvements in the quality and intensity of job-seeking services for Americans with disabilities (pp. 70–71).

One of the most significant components of WIOA is that vocational rehabilitation agencies are now required to allocate at least 15% of their federal funds to provide pre-employment transition services to students with disabilities. This will be covered further in the next section of this chapter.

INDIVIDUALS WITH DISABILITIES EDUCATION ACT

In 1975, a law was passed called the Education of Handicapped Children Act. In 1990, amendments to the law were passed and the name was changed to the Individuals with Disabilities Education Act (IDEA). Additional amendments were passed in 1997, 2004, and 2015 to continue to ensure that students with disabilities had equal access to education. IDEA is a law "that makes available a free appropriate public education to eligible children with disabilities throughout the nation and ensures special education and related services to those children" (U.S. Department of Education, 2018, para 1). Under IDEA Part C, infants and toddlers ages birth to two, receive early intervention services. Under

IDEA Part B, children and youth ages three to 21 are eligible to receive special education and related services. This law also governs how state and federal agencies provide education for all children with disabilities.

Relevant Disability Services

When working with individuals with disabilities, it is important to be aware of resources and agencies that are available to help and provide services for individuals with disabilities. This section will cover a brief overview of some of these services and agencies that speech language pathologists may need to refer to when working with adolescents or adults with disabilities.

VOCATIONAL REHABILITATION

Vocational rehabilitation (VR) is a federal-state program that helps people who have disabilities find or maintain gainful, competitive employment. Each state has their own vocational rehabilitation program and provides services in different ways. Rehabilitation counselors work on state VR agencies,

and they have many roles. They are responsible for meeting with potential clients and completing intake interviews, determining eligibility for services, developing and completing individualized plans for employment, providing services, assisting with job placement, building relationships with employers, and making appropriate referrals for additional services such as mental health counseling. Some rehabilitation counselors may also complete vocational and psychological assessments. Many times, the rehabilitation counselor is an important link between employers and clients, as well as other service providers and clients.

TRANSITION SERVICES

As previously stated, because of WIOA, vocational rehabilitation agencies are now required to allocate at least 15% of their federal funds to provide pre-employment transition services to students with disabilities. Pre-employment transition services is a wide umbrella and many services are required and recommended under this umbrella. Many VR agencies now have

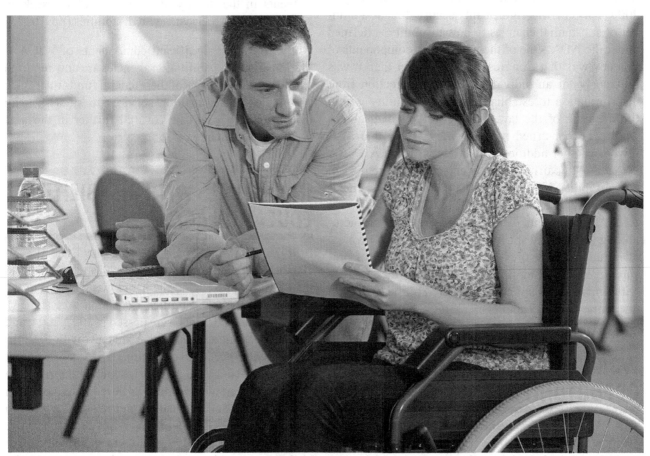

Phovoir/Shutterstock.com

or are in the process of creating a position for a VR counselor that specifically focuses on transition. The transition counselor may attend individualized education program (IEP) meetings, develop work opportunities for students with disabilities such as internships and summer employment, and work with schools to coordinate the provision of pre-employment transition services. Transition planning should begin before students turn 16, and any student that has an IEP should also have an individualized transition plan (ITP) in place by the time he/she turns 16. This plan should be developed by the IEP team, the student, parents, and a transition counselor may also be involved. Under the law, VR agencies are required to provide the following pre-employment transition services under WIOA: counseling for job exploration, work-based learning experiences, counseling about postsecondary educational programs, social skills and independent living training, and self-advocacy instruction.

COLLEGE DISABILITY SERVICES

As previously discussed, Section 504 of the Rehabilitation Act of 1973 and the Americans with Disabilities Act prevent colleges and universities from discriminating against individuals with disabilities in regards to admission. These laws also allow students with disabilities access to reasonable academic accommodations in order to be able to complete required coursework. Many students with disabilities and their families experience a bit of shock when transitioning from K-12 education and special education services to a college or university setting. The big difference in these two academic settings is that in K-12 settings, the goal is SUCCESS, and in higher education, the goal is ACCESS. In K-12 settings, assignments could be changed, exams could be modified, and nearly any accommodations or modifications could be put in place to ensure that the student succeeded in school. This is not the case in higher education. In this setting, students with disabilities must complete the same assignments, take the same exams, and participate in the same classrooms as students without disabilities. Academic accommodations promote access, essentially leveling the playing field so that all students have the same access to education. Examples of common academic accommodations include attendance flexibility, extended time on exams, distraction reduced testing environment, use of a note taker, and digital textbooks. In order to request academic accommodations, students must use the disability services office on campus. See **Table 13.4**, Questions to Ask the Disability Services Officer. Documentation of a disability must be provided to this office to facilitate the use of academic accommodations. However, details about the student's disability will not be disclosed to faculty and staff; typically a letter will be sent to faculty and staff in charge of classes stating that the student has a documented disability and is entitled to reasonable academic accommodations and the accommodations will be listed in the letter.

Table 13.4 Questions to Ask the Disability Services Office

10 Questions to Ask the Disability Services Office
What sort of documentation do I need?
How current does my testing (psychological, academic) need to be when applying for accommodations?
What accommodations am I eligible for? What are the procedure and timelines to put accommodations in place?
If a professor does not comply with necessary accommodations, how is the situation resolved?
Where do students take exams and who proctors the exams?
Will I have an assigned advisor in the disability services office? How often do I need to meet with someone from disability services? Once a year? Once a semester?
What assistive technology options are available?
How are my accommodations communicated to professors?
What is the role of the accommodations counselor/staff?
Can I change my accommodations as needed throughout my time in college?

Workplace Accommodations

According to the 2010 census report, approximately 18,525,862 people with disabilities are employed. This means that about 55.8% of people with disabilities ages 16–64 are working; 60% of men with disabilities are employed and 51% of women with disabilities are employed. Many disabilities will necessitate requesting job accommodations to be able to successfully complete the necessary tasks of the job. Reasonable accommodations can range from an ergonomic keyboard to modified work duties to flexible hours to telecommuting to accessible parking. At most workplaces, there is a designated person in human resources that handles job accommodations. The JAN provides helpful guidelines for going about requesting reasonable accommodations:

> According to the EEOC, you only have to let your employer know that you need an adjustment or change at work for a reason related to a medical condition. You can use "plain English" to make your request and you do not have to mention the ADA or use the phrase "reasonable accommodation" (JAN, 2018, para 2).

In order to request job accommodations, a person does need to disclose having a disability, but extensive details about the disability are not usually required, but this will depend on the accommodations being requested. JAN offers this advice, "you may want to tell your employer what you are having trouble doing, that the problem is related to a disability, and what your accommodation ideas are" (2018, para 9). There are no specific guidelines on a time frame for employers complying with an accommodation request, but unnecessary delays can result in a violation of the ADA.

CONCLUSION

The purpose of this chapter was to provide a basic overview of disability, important disability legislation, and relevant disability services. The different definitions, categories and models of disability were laid out. Important disability legislation, including the ADA, IDEA, and WIOA were explained. Lastly, important disability services such as vocational rehabilitation, transition services, and college disability services were discussed. Professionals in communication disorders may need to refer individuals with who they are working to receive disability services. It is important that school-based professionals be aware of the categories of

disability under IDEA as this information is pertinent in determining the types of services a child receives in the school setting. This chapter reviewed relevant legislation and definitions of disability to assist the professional in communication disorders to be able to make appropriate recommendations and referrals when proving quality, holistic services to individuals with disabilities.

REFERENCES

Americans with Disabilities Act National Network. (2018). *What is the definition of disability under the ADA?* Retrieved from https://adata.org/faq/what-definition-disability-under-ada

American Association of Intellectual and Developmental Disabilities (AAIDD). (2018). *Frequently asked questions on intellectual disability*. Retrieved from https://aaidd.org/intellectual-disability/definition/faqs-on-intellectual-disability

Bialik, K. (2017). *7 facts about Americans with disabilities*. Retrieved from http://www.pewresearch.org/fact-tank/2017/07/27/7-facts-about-americans-with-disabilities/

Job Accommodation Network (JAN). (2012). *The Americans with disabilities act: A brief overview*. Retrieved from https://askjan.org/links/adasummary.htm

National Dissemination Center for Children with Disabilities. (2012). *Categories of disability under IDEA*. Retrieved from https://www.parentcenterhub.org/wp-content/uploads/repo_items/gr3.pdf

Rubin, S., Roessler, R., & Rumrill, P. (2016). *Foundations of the vocational rehabilitation process* (7th ed.). Austin, TX: Pro-Ed.

Shapiro. J. S. (1994). *No pity: People with disabilities forging a new civil rights movement*. New York, NY: Three Rivers Press.

Smart, J. (2009a). *Disability, society, and the individual* (2nd ed.). Austin, TX: Pro-Ed.

Smart, J. (2009b). The power of models of disability. *Journal of Rehabilitation, 75*(2), 3–11.

Switzer, J. V. (2003). *Disabled rights: American disability policy and the fight for equality*. Washington, DC: Georgetown University Press.

U.S. Department of Education. (2018). *About IDEA*. Retrieved from https://sites.ed.gov/idea/about-idea/#IDEA-Purpose

U.S. Department of Labor. (2018a). *WIOA overview*. Retrieved from https://www.doleta.gov/WIOA/Overview.cfm

U.S. Department of Labor. (2018b). *Section 504, Rehabilitation Act of 1973*. Retrieved from https://www.dol.gov/oasam/regs/statutes/sec504.htm

U.S. Department of Justice. (2009). *A guide to disability rights laws*. Retrieved from https://www.ada.gov/cguide.htm#anchor62335

U.S. Equal Employment Opportunity Commission (2018a). Remarks of President George Bush at the signing of the Americans with Disabilities Act. Retrieved from https://www.eeoc.gov/eeoc/history/35th/videos/ada_signing_text.html

U.S. Equal Employment Opportunity Commission. (2018b). *Fact sheet on the EEOC's final regulations implementing the ADAAA*. Retrieved from https://www.eeoc.gov/laws/regulations/adaaa_fact_sheet.cfm

World Health Organization (WHO). (2018). *Disabilities*. Retrieved from http://www.who.int/topics/disabilities/en/

Study Questions

1. What is the EEOC and what role does it play in employment for individuals with disabilities?

2. Compare and contrast disability services in high school and college. What are 3 similarities and 3 differences?

3. What are the categories of disability under IDEA? Why is it important for SLPs and audiologists to understand the categories of disability under IDEA?

4. Describe the biopsychosocial model. How might this model benefit a young adult with a communication disorder who is looking to transition to the workforce in the coming year?

5. Describe the ADA. Why was the ADAAA so important for individuals with disabilities?

CHAPTER 14

Introduction to Language and Cognition in Adulthood

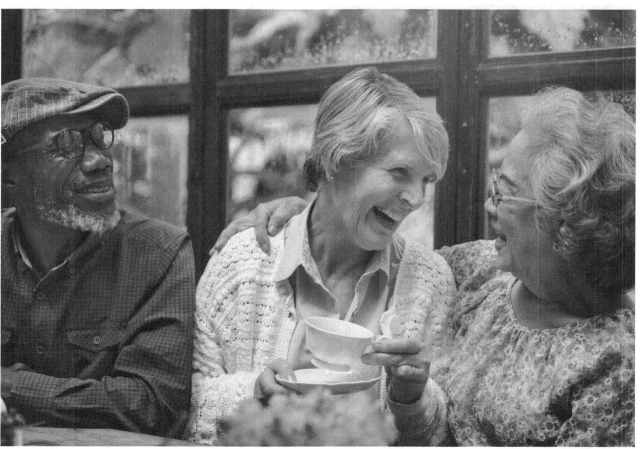

Rawpixel.com / Shutterstock.com

"Do what you can, with what you have, where you are."

—Theodore Roosevelt

OVERVIEW

The purpose of this chapter is to review common factors impacting communication in the aging population and to discuss recommendations for intervention with this group of individuals. The language skills that are targeted in speech therapy sessions with older adults can be quite similar to language skills targeted in speech therapy sessions with children at times. Clinicians need a working knowledge of language development and an ability to adapt therapy materials so they are functional and motivating when working with adults. This chapter serves as a resource to build a foundation for working on language and cognitive skills with adults.

DEMOGRAPHICS

There is no question that the population in the United States is aging, creating an even greater need for professionals in health related fields to provide intervention for this group of individuals. By 2030, the older population (over 65 years of age) in the United States is projected to be double that of the older population in 2000, growing from just over 35 million to over 73 million (Forum, 2016). According to the National Aphasia Association, approximately 180,000 Americans acquire a language disorder, also called *aphasia* (a loss in the ability to comprehend or express communication), every year (2016). The National Institute on Deafness and Other Communication Disorders (NIDCD, 2018) reports that one third of all older adults (age 65–74) have hearing loss and almost half of adults over the age of 75 have some degree of hearing loss. Additionally, nearly 2 million individuals (across all age groups) experience a traumatic brain injury (TBI) each year in the United States with adolescents and older adults being most likely to sustain a TBI (Faul, Xu, Walk, &

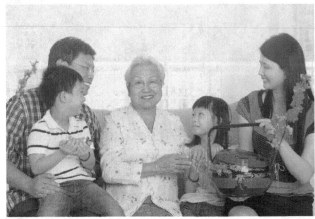

Coronado, 2010). Be it a language disorder, cognitive communication disorder resulting from brain injury, or hearing loss, chances are that if a clinician is working with individuals over the age of 65, he or she will need to be familiar with resources and appropriate interventions for these diagnoses.

AGING BRAIN

As the human body ages, so too does the brain. Theories about brain development across the lifespan continue to be debated. Generally, it is accepted that the brain completes its most rapid growth in the first few years of life. The ability of the brain to grow and form new connections (or *synapses*) is termed *neuroplasticity*. Contrary to previous hypotheses, the brain never stops developing. The idea that the brain reorganizes as it ages is not a new concept and is supported in the literature (Cabeza, Anderson, Locantore, & McIntosh, 2002; Park, & Reuter-Lorenz, 2009; Sala-Llonch, Bartrés-Faz, & Junqué, 2015). *Neurogenesis*, the development of neurons in the brain, continues throughout life (Galvan & Jin, 2007). Neuropsychologist Elkhonon Goldberg first discussed the Wisdom Paradox in 2006. This is the hypothesis that even though skills like short-term memory diminish with age; attributes associated with wisdom such as the ability to recognize patterns and make decisions actually improve with age. In 2006, Hubert reported that reorganization of the brain actually occurs twice, once during the aging process and again during the treatment of age related changes. Reorganization of the aging brain is something for intervention providers to be aware of as they consider the development of appropriate plans of care for individuals who are aging.

Jaul & Barron (2017) described relevant age-related changes for individuals over the age of 85 as including one or more the following components:

- Sensory changes (hearing, vision)
- Physical changes (muscle composition)
- Somatic Disease and Chronic Conditions
  - Cardiovascular disease
  - Hypertension
  - Cancer
  - Osteoarthritis
  - Diabetes
  - Osteoporosis
- Physical Function

- Psychological and Cognitive Factors
    - ○ Cognitive aging
    - ○ Dementia
    - ○ Depression
- Social Function
- Medical Decisions
    - ○ Polypharmacy (using 5+ medications)
    - ○ Hospitalization
    - ○ Institutional placement
    - ○ End of Life Care

As health-related professionals, it is important to consider the above listed components, to ask the individual with whom we are working (as well as his/her caregiver(s)) about these areas, and to refer for additional evaluations and care management as needed.

An area often neglected when working with adults is that of mental health. Depression is not uncommon in adulthood, but it is especially prominent in adults over the age of 80 (Forum, 2016). Adults often experience loss which can be followed by grief and strong emotions that are difficult to process. It is not within the scope of practice of a speech–language pathologist, speech–language pathology assistant, or an audiologist to provide treatment for depression. Depression is typically managed with medications, psychotherapy, or through services provided by a mental health professional. In 2011, Cohen and Eisdorfer's *Integrated Textbook of Geriatric Mental Health* outlined the challenges and recommended training and treatment for clinicians and health-related professionals who work with the geriatric population. It is expected that professionals in the field of communication disorders make appropriate referrals when providing intervention for an individual exhibiting depressive symptoms or mental health concerns.

Research has established addressing caregiver needs as well as educating caregivers of older adults can lead to a reduction in nursing home placement (Mittelman, Haley, Clay, & Roth, 2006) and an improvement in overall quality of life for the individual and the caregiver (Callahan et al., 2006). It is important that healthcare professionals take time to address caregiver needs, and educate them on the diagnosis, plan of care, and prognosis of their loved one. This may also include informational counseling regarding accommodations for activities of daily living.

LANGUAGE vs. COGNITION

In his book, *Communication Disorders in Aging*, Dr. Raymond Hull listed the following as being prominent disorders of communication among adults: laryngectomy (removal of the vocal mechanism) and other disorders affect the vocal mechanism, aphasia, Parkinson's disease, acquired cognitive disorders (confusion, disorientation, dementia), and hearing loss (2017). For the purposes of this chapter, the focus will

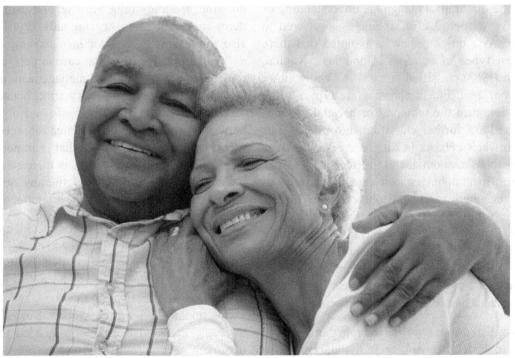

Monkey Business Images/Shutterstock.com

be on the intervention for language and cognitive-communication disorders. In 2011, the American Speech Language Hearing Associate (ASHA) reported that speech–language pathologists who worked with adults spent approximately 17% of intervention time treating in the area of aphasia and approximately 31% of intervention time treating in cognitive-communication disorder areas (e.g., dementia, traumatic brain injury (TBI), etc.). Professionals must first understand the difference between a language disorder and a cognitive-communication disorder before proceeding with an evaluation or treatment.

Language is defined as skills related to comprehending communication and expressing one's thoughts, feelings and desires. Skills such as generating grammatically correct sentences, understanding and expressing vocabulary, reading, spelling, using numbers or doing math, and writing are all considered language skills. *Cognition* is the process through which individuals know and interact with their environment. Skills such as problem solving, working memory tasks, reasoning, and the ability to be flexible in social situations (e.g., adapt behavior for a given situation or switch perspectives) are cognitive communication processes. Clinicians are directed to www.asha.org/slp/cognitive-referral/ for ASHA's referral guidelines for adults with cognitive-communication concerns. According to ASHA, the most common etiologies of cognitive communication disorders at Alzheimer's disease, brain tumors, stroke, and TBI (2018).

As has already been mentioned, a language disorder in adults, one that impacts language understanding or expressive or written use of language, is referred to as *aphasia*. As a quick review, it is noted that there are different types of aphasias. Goodglass, Kaplan, and Barresi (1983) classified aphasias as being either *fluent* or *nonfluent*. Fluent aphasias are typically the result of a lesion in the temporal or parietal lobes of the brain and are further classified into one of four types: Wernicke's aphasia (a.k.a., *receptive aphasia*), conduction aphasia, anomia, and transcortical sensory aphasia. Nonfluent aphasias are typically the result of a lesion in the anterior left hemisphere and are further classified into one of four types: Broca's aphasia (a.k.a., *expressive aphasia*), global aphasia, mixed nonfluent aphasia, or transcortical motor aphasia. For additional information on the classification system of aphasias, readers are encouraged to visit the following website: https://www.aphasia.org/aphasia-definitions/.

The aphasias listed above are due to brain damage most commonly in the left hemisphere. Individuals may also experience brain damage in the right hemisphere of the brain. A right-sided cerebrovascular accident (CVA) is most commonly associated with difficulties in memory, left-neglect (e.g., unable to see left side of page or clock, may neglect left side of body), attention, perseveration (repetition of word, response or question), and spatial awareness (e.g., unable to identify how parts relate to the whole). Understanding how the site of lesion of brain damage may impact subsequent deficits can be critical to identifying appropriate objectives for an individual's plan of care.

TREATMENT

Communication is key for optimal outcomes when working with adults. This includes communication not only with the individual who is receiving direct treatment, but also the caregivers and frequent communication partners of that individual. Including caregivers in the therapeutic process has been shown to be advantageous for individuals with aphasia as well as individuals with cognitive communication disorders (Bayles & Tomoeda, 2013; Egan, Bérubé, Racine, Leonard, & Rochon, 2010; Fox, Poulsen, Clark Bawden, & Packard, 2004; Lyon et al., 1997; Purdy & Hindenlang, 2005). Table 14.1 provides suggestions for interventionists when communicating with older adults.

When developing a plan of care, it is important to consider what *activities of daily living* (ADLs), sometimes referred to as basic activities of daily living (BADLs). These include skills like self-care tasks (bathing, dressing, feeding, toilet hygiene, and care of personal items such as glasses, hearing aids, or orthotics). It is also important to consider *instrumental activities of daily living* (IADLs) such as care of pets, communication management, financial management, and problem solving life events (e.g., leaky sink, house fire, need for exterminator). Therapy goals and objectives can be written to address communication needs for these specific activities based on what is important for the individual's quality of life. As is the case when working with children, functional therapy objectives are optimal when working with the adult population.

After the evaluation has been completed, it is then up to the speech–language pathologist to establish long-term goals and short-term objectives that are appropriate for the individual. Things like psychosocial impact, physical fatigue, and motivation may be taken into account as treatment plans are developed. Review Chapter 1 for basic knowledge and skills needed to develop a treatment plan across the lifespan. Sample language

Table 14.1 Accommodations When Communicating with Older Adults

• Minimize background noise (e.g., turn television off, avoid treatment when multiple people are talking in the room)	• Use basic language rather than medical terminology
• Face the individual when providing instruction or descriptions	• Speak slowly, but do not speak so slowly that speech is distorted or exaggerated. Reduce your rate of speech, not clarity. Avoid speaking loudly as this can distort speech clarity.
• *Make sure sensory aids (e.g., glasses, hearing aids, cochlear implants, communication devices) are functional and in place prior to initiating treatment*	• Discuss the purpose of your meeting at the forefront of the session
• Confirm understanding of expectations of tasks or information given by asking individual (and/or caregiver) to demonstrate comprehension (e.g., through recall or response to yes/no prompts if applicable)	• Inform the patient of any topic changes before they happen (e.g., "We have been working on problem solving, but now we are going to work on memory tasks.)
• Encourage family or caregiver participation in therapy sessions to aid in carry over of objectives and also education of family members and caregivers	• Provide important information or resources in writing or in a preferred reading format (e.g., large font, use informative headings, use bulleted lists when possible)
• Make sure the room has good lighting to allow for lip-reading and view of materials needed in the session	• Use positive statements (e.g., "We are working to improve your language to help you communicate.")

Adapted from a variety of sources.

and cognitive-communication short-term objectives are provided in Table 14.2, Sample Language and Cognition Short-Term Objectives.

GOALS AND OBJECTIVES

When writing treatment goals and objectives, it is important to remember the definition of each component of professional documentation. The *evaluation* is the document that summarizes the individual's strengths and weaknesses in communication skills. It is from the evaluation, that a *treatment plan or plan of care* (POC) is developed. It is important to note that the *goals* and *objectives* listed on the POC must correlate with the weaknesses listed in the evaluation report. POC documents typically consist of long-term goals and short-term objectives. *Long-term goals* (LTGs) are broad goals that aim to change a facet of communication within a pre-determined allotment of time. *Short-term objectives* (Also sometimes termed "behavioral objectives" or "objectives") are the specific steps by which the interventionist plans to achieve the long-term goals. Short-term objectives must be specific, measurable, and time-driven. For additional information on how to generate long- and short-term goals, please refer to Chapter 1. Sample goal and objectives for working with adults with

Table 14.2 Accommodations When Communicating with Older Adults

www.aphasia.org	**www.asha.org**
www.stroke.org	**www.nia.nih.gov**
www.alz.org	**www.strokeassociation.org**
www.ninds.nih.gov	**www.biausa.org**
www.brainline.org	**www.ancds.org**

language and cognitive-communication disorders follow. It is important to note there are a variety of ways to write goals and objectives. The list provided below is not a comprehensive list and should not be treated as such.

Sample Long-Term Goals:

1. The individual will improve receptive language skills to aid in communication.
2. The individual will improve expressive language skills to aid in activities of daily living.

3. The individual will improve cognitive communication to aid in activities of daily living.

Sample *Do* and *Condition* Statements for Short-Term Objectives:

It should be noted that for the short-term objective to be complete a *criterion* statement for mastery would need to be added to the sample short-term objectives listed in Table 14.3, Sample Language

Table 14.3   Sample Language and Cognition Short-Term Objectives

Expressive Language	Receptive Language	Cognition
• Given a familiar phrase, the individual will produce phrase completions • The individual will complete concrete divergent naming tasks • The individual will identify synonyms • The individual will identify antonym • Given a 1 sentence description, the individual will name familiar objects • The individual will label familiar objects in a closed set of 2 to 4 pictures • The individual will demonstrate written expression for single syllable words (CVC) words • The individual will demonstrate written expression for labeling familiar items/objects • Given a picture, the individual will generate a basic sentence (subject-verb-object) • The individual will identify absurdities in basic statements • The individual will label familiar categories • The individual will complete automatic verbal sequences (e.g., counting, days of the week (DOW), months of the year (MOY)) • The individual will answer "what" and "where" questions	• The individual will demonstrate reading comprehension of 1 sentence stories through picture matching • The individual will follow basic 2-step commands • The individual will demonstrate comprehension of familiar items/objects in a closed set of 2–4 pictures • Given a description of item/–4 pictures • The individual will demonstrate comprehension of multiple meaning words through picture matching • The individual will demonstrate comprehension of rhyming words through word matching tasks • Given a list of category items, the individual will identify the targeted category in pictures • The individual will identify emotions in closed set of 3–5 pictures • The individual will identify body parts in a closed set of 2–4 pictures • Given a closed set of 4 pictures, the individual will identify the targeted action/verb • The individual will identify written words when named by the clinician • The individual will demonstrate comprehension by answering moderately difficult yes/no questions	• The individual will state personally relevant information (e.g., first and last name, birthdate) • The individual will improve short-term memory by completing a word retrieval task with a 10 second delay • The individual will demonstrate function of familiar items/objects through role play • The individual will complete situational problem solving for instrumental activities of daily living. • The individual will sequence 3-step picture stimuli to increase safety common with basic activities of daily living tasks • The individual will demonstration orientation to time, place and person • The individual will complete divergent naming tasks (e.g., given the category "fruit" list 5 additional fruits) • The individual will complete convergent naming tasks (e.g., given a description, name the item/object being described) • The patient will define idioms • The patient will complete basic analogies

and Cognition Short-Term Objectives below. See the example provided below.

Given a description,	= Condition Statement
the individual will label the associated item/object	= Do Statement
with 80% accuracy across three consecutive sessions.	= Criterion Statement

The final draft of the short-term objective would be:

Given a description, the individual will label the associated item/object with 80% accuracy across three consecutive sessions.

For additional information on the development of criterion statements, please see Chapter 1.

SUMMARY

This chapter was intended to provide a brief review of communication as it relates to working with older adults. A review of the difference between language and cognition was provided as well as a discussion of the characteristics of communication disorders in aging. This foundational chapter is beneficial for emerging clinicians who would like guidance for where to start when providing treatment for adults with language and/or cognitive communication disorders.

REFERENCES

American Speech Language Hearing Association (ASHA). (2011). *SLP health care survey report: Patient caseload characteristics trends 2005-2011*. Retrieved from https://www.asha.org/uploadedFiles/HC11-Caseload-Characteristics-Trends.pdf

American Speech Language Hearing Association (ASHA). (2018). *Cognitive communication referral guidelines for adults*. Retrieved from https://www.asha.org/slp/cognitive-referral/

Bayles, K. A., & Tomoeda, C. K. (2013). *Cognitive-communication disorders of dementia: Definition, diagnosis, and treatment*. San Diego, CA: Plural Publishing.

Cabeza, R., Anderson, N. D., Locantore, J. K., & McIntosh, A. R. (2002). Aging gracefully: compensatory brain activity in high-performing older adults. *Neuroimage, 17*(3), 1394–1402.

Callahan, C. M., Boustani, M. A., Unverzagt, F. W., Austrom, M. G., Damush, T. M., Perkins, A. J., . . . & Hendrie, H. C. (2006). Effectiveness of collaborative care for older adults with Alzheimer disease in primary care: a randomized controlled trial. *Journal of the American Medical Assoication, 295*(18), 2148–2157.

Cohen, D., & Eisdorfer, C. (2011). *Integrated textbook of geriatric mental health*. Baltimore, MD: JHU Press.

Egan, M., Bérubé, D., Racine, G., Leonard, C., & Rochon, E. (2010). Methods to enhance verbal communication between individuals with Alzheimer's d isease and their formal and informal caregivers: a systematic review. *International Journal of Alzheimer's Disease, 2010*. doi:0.4061/2010/906818.

Faul, M., Xu, L., Wald, M. M., & Coronado, V. G. (2010). *Traumatic brain injury in the United States: Emergency department visits, hospitalizations and deaths 2002–2006*. Atlanta, GA: Centers for Disease Control and Prevention, National Center for Injury Prevention and Control.

Federal Interagency Forum on Aging-Related Statistics (Forum), (2016). *Older Americans: Key indicators of well-being*. Retrieved from https://agingstats.gov/docs/latestreport/older-americans-2016-key-indicators-of-wellbeing.pdf

Fox, L., Poulsen, S., Clark Bawden, K., & Packard, D. (2004). Critical elements and outcomes of a residential family-based intervention for aphasia caregivers. *Aphasiology, 18*(12), 1177–1199.

Galvan, V., & Jin, K. (2007). Neurogenesis in the aging brain. *Clinical Interventions in Aging, 2*(4), 605.

Goldberg, E. (2006). *The wisdom paradox: How your mind can grow stronger as your brain grows older*. USA: Penguin.

Goodglass, H., Kaplan, E., & Barresi, B. (1983). *The assessment of aphasia and related disorders* (Vol. 2). Philadelphia, PA: Lippincott Williams & Wilkins.

Hull, R. (2017). *Communication disorders in aging*. San Diego, CA: Plural Publications.

Jaul, E., & Barron, J. (2017). Age-Related Diseases and Clinical and Public Health Implications for the 85 Years Old and Over Population. *Frontiers in Public Health, 5*, 335.

Lyon, J. G., Cariski, D., Keisler, L., Rosenbek, J., Levine, R., Kumpula, J., Ryff, C., & Blanc, M. (1997). Communication partners: Enhancing participation in life and communication for adults with aphasia in natural settings. *Aphasiology, 11*(7), 693–708.

Mittelman, M. S., Haley, W. E., Clay, O. J., & Roth, D. L. (2006). Improving caregiver well-being delays nursing home placement of patients with Alzheimer disease. *Neurology, 67*(9), 1592–1599.

National Aphasia Association. (2016). *Aphasia FAQs*. Retrieved from https://www.aphasia.org/aphasia-faqs/

National Institute on Deafness and Other Communication Disorders (NIDCD). (2018). *Hearing loss in older adults*. Retrieved from https://www.nidcd.nih.gov/health/hearing-loss-older-adults

Park, D. C., & Reuter-Lorenz, P. (2009). The adaptive brain: Aging and neurocognitive scaffolding. *Annual Review of Psychology, 60*, 173–196.

Purdy, M., & Hindenlang, J. (2005). Educating and training caregivers of persons with aphasia. *Aphasiology, 19* (3-5), 377–388.

Sala-Llonch, R., Bartrés-Faz, D., & Junqué, C. (2015). Reorganization of brain networks in aging: A review of functional connectivity studies. *Frontiers in Psychology, 6*, 663.

PRACTICE

This purpose of this section is to provide emerging clinicians an opportunity to practice utilizing the information provided in the aforementioned chapter. Case scenarios provided are meant to facilitate discussion between emerging clinicians and educators to provide a foundation for competent clinical practice. There is often more than one way to answer the case scenario questions provided in this section. Long-term goals are meant to be over-arching goals for therapy during the current reporting period. Short-term objectives are to correlate with long-term goals and are to be utilized as steps to achieve the long-term goal. Emerging clinicians need always be mindful that short-term objectives are to be clearly stated, measurable, and time driven. Tasks are to be developmentally appropriate for the individual with which the clinician is working (which may not necessarily correlate with the individual's chronological age).

Case Scenario 14-1 Worksheet

NAME: _____ DATE: _____

Henry is an 83-year-old male who recently experienced a left cerebrovascular accident (LCVA). His recent evaluation indicated he is currently receiving occupational therapy and physical therapy to address mobility and independence secondary to right hemiparesis (right sided weakness). Moderate nonfluent (expressive) aphasia was noted in his report (*Strengths: auditory comprehension, reading comprehension, and automatic verbal sequences (e.g., counting, days of the week). Weaknesses: repetition of words, repetition of sentences, producing grammatically correct sentences (syntax), and impaired written expression*). There are currently no concerns with swallowing. Henry wears glasses and has a moderate hearing loss for which he wears bilateral, behind-the-ear (BTE hearing aids).

1. What is an appropriate LONG-TERM GOAL?

   _____

2. What are <u>three</u> appropriate SHORT-TERM OBJECTIVES? (Hint: Short-term objectives should correlate with the long-term goal listed above.)

   A.

   _____

   _____

   B.

   _____

   _____

   C.

   _____

   _____

3. List the TASK you would use to target the short-term objectives listed above. The task for 3A should pair with the short-term objective listed for 2A. Please list MATERIALS you plan to utilize.

A.

_____

_____

B.

_____

_____

C.

_____

_____

4. How would you introduce and explain the purpose of each short-term objective and task in the therapy session to the individual and/or caregiver?

A.

_____

_____

B.

_____

_____

C.

_____

_____

Case Scenario 14-2 Worksheet

NAME: _____ DATE: _____

James is a 65-year-old male who recently experienced a traumatic brain injury due to a car wreck. Prior to his injury, James was actively involved in his community and worked part-time as a greeter at the local grocery store. The speech–language evaluation report revealed a moderate delay in cognitive communication skills (*Strengths: automatic verbal sequences, repetition of words, labeling of body parts, and orientation (person, place, and time). Weaknesses: problem solving, social communication and short-term memory tasks*). There are currently no concerns with swallowing, vision, or hearing. James has a history of hypertension that is managed through medication.

1. What additional referrals might be needed?

   _____

2. What is an appropriate LONG-TERM GOAL?

   _____

3. What are <u>three</u> appropriate SHORT-TERM OBJECTIVES? (Hint: Short-term objectives should correlate with the long-term goal listed above.)

   A.

   _____

   _____

   B.

   _____

   _____

   C.

   _____

   _____

4. List the TASK you would use to target the short-term objectives listed above. The task for 3A should pair with the short-term objective listed for 2A. Please list MATERIALS you plan to utilize.

A.

_____

_____

B.

_____

_____

C.

_____

_____

5. How would you introduce and explain the purpose of each short-term objective and task in the therapy session to the individual or caregiver?

A.

_____

_____

B.

_____

_____

C.

_____

Case Scenario 14-3 Worksheet

NAME: _____   DATE: _____

Lauren is a 24-year-old female who recently experienced a right cerebrovascular accident (RCVA). Prior to this experience, Lauren was a senior in college with plans of attending graduate school in the fall. A moderate delay in language skills (*Strengths: auditory and reading comprehension, and sequencing familiar tasks in pictures. Weaknesses: left-neglect (unable to write check or read analog clock), attention for 1 minute task, labeling familiar items/objects, and understanding part-to-whole relationships (e.g., wheels on car, leaves on tree))* was noted in her report. Her vision and hearing are within normal limits (WNL) and there are no concerns with swallowing at this time.

1. What is an appropriate LONG-TERM GOAL?
   _____

2. What are <u>three</u> appropriate SHORT-TERM OBJECTIVES? (Hint: Short-term objectives should correlate with the long-term goal listed above.)

   A.

   _____

   _____

   B.

   _____

   _____

   C.

   _____

   _____

3. List the TASK you would use to target the short-term objectives listed above. The task for 3A should pair with the short-term objective listed for 2A. Please list MATERIALS you plan to utilize.

A.

_____

_____

B.

_____

_____

C.

_____

_____

4. How would you introduce and explain the purpose of each short-term objective and task in the therapy session to the individual or caregiver?

A.

_____

_____

B.

_____

_____

C.

_____

_____

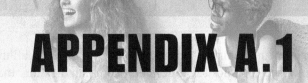

APPENDIX A.1

Code of Ethics in Speech-Language Pathology

Established by: American Speech-Language Hearing Association

Code of Ethics Effective March 1, 2016

Table of Contents

PREAMBLE

The American Speech-Language-Hearing Association (ASHA; hereafter, also known as "The Association") has been committed to a framework of common principles and standards of practice since ASHA's inception in 1925. This commitment was formalized in 1952 as the Association's first Code of Ethics. This Code has been modified and adapted as society and the professions have changed. The Code of Ethics reflects what we value as professionals and establishes expectations for our scientific and clinical practice based on principles of duty, accountability, fairness, and responsibility. The ASHA Code of Ethics is intended to ensure the welfare of the consumer and to protect the reputation and integrity of the professions.

The ASHA Code of Ethics is a framework and focused guide for professionals in support of day-to-day decision making related to professional conduct. The Code is partly obligatory and disciplinary and partly aspirational and descriptive in that it defines the professional's role. The Code educates professionals in the discipline, as well as students, other professionals, and the public, regarding ethical principles and standards that direct professional conduct.

The preservation of the highest standards of integrity and ethical principles is vital to the responsible discharge of obligations by audiologists, speech-language pathologists, and speech, language, and hearing scientists who serve as clinicians, educators, mentors, researchers, supervisors, and administrators. This Code of Ethics sets forth the fundamental principles and rules considered essential to this purpose and is applicable to the following individuals:

- A member of the American Speech-Language-Hearing Association holding the Certificate of Clinical Competence (CCC)
- A member of the Association not holding the CCC
- A nonmember of the Association holding the CCC
- An applicant for certification, or for membership and certification

By holding ASHA certification or membership, or through application for such, all individuals are automatically subject to the jurisdiction of the Board of Ethics for ethics complaint adjudication. Individuals who provide clinical services and who also desire membership in the Association must hold the CCC.

The fundamentals of ethical conduct are described by Principles of Ethics and by Rules of Ethics. The four Principles of Ethics form the underlying philosophical basis for the Code of Ethics and are reflected in the following areas: (I) responsibility to persons served professionally and to research participants, both human and animal; (II) responsibility for one's professional competence; (III) responsibility to the public; and (IV) responsibility for professional relationships. Individuals shall honor and abide by these Principles as affirmative obligations under all conditions of applicable professional activity. Rules of Ethics are specific statements of minimally acceptable as well as unacceptable professional conduct.

The Code is designed to provide guidance to members, applicants, and certified individuals as they make professional decisions. Because the Code is not intended to address specific situations and is not inclusive of all possible ethical dilemmas, professionals are expected to follow the written provisions and to uphold the spirit and purpose of the Code. Adherence to the Code of Ethics and its enforcement results in respect for the professions and positive outcomes for individuals who benefit from the work of audiologists, speech-language pathologists, and speech, language, and hearing scientists.

TERMINOLOGY

advertising   Any form of communication with the public about services, therapies, products, or publications.

ASHA Standards and Ethics   The mailing address for self-reporting in writing is American Speech-Language-Hearing Association, Standards and Ethics, 2200 Research Blvd., #313, Rockville, MD 20850.

conflict of interest   An opposition between the private interests and the official or professional responsibilities of a person in a position of trust, power, and/or authority.

crime   Any felony; or any misdemeanor involving dishonesty, physical harm to the person or property of another, or a threat of physical harm to the person or property of another. For more details, see the "Disclosure Information" section of applications for ASHA certification found on www.asha.org/certification/AudCertification/ and www.asha.org/certification/SLPCertification/.

diminished decision-making ability   Any condition that renders a person unable to form the specific intent necessary to determine a reasonable course of action.

fraud   Any act, expression, omission, or concealment—the intent of which is either actual or constructive—calculated to deceive others to their disadvantage.

impaired practitioner   An individual whose professional practice is adversely affected by addiction, substance abuse, or health-related and/or mental health–related conditions.

individuals   Members and/or certificate holders, including applicants for certification.

informed consent   May be verbal, unless written consent is required; constitutes consent by persons served, research participants engaged, or parents and/or guardians of persons served to a proposed course of action after the communication of adequate information regarding expected outcomes and potential risks.

jurisdiction   The "personal jurisdiction" and authority of the ASHA Board of Ethics over an individual holding ASHA certification and/or membership, regardless of the individual's geographic location.

know, known, or knowingly   Having or reflecting knowledge.

may versus shall   *May* denotes an allowance for discretion; *shall* denotes no discretion.

misrepresentation   Any statement by words or other conduct that, under the circumstances, amounts to an assertion that is false or erroneous (i.e., not in accordance with the facts); any statement made with conscious ignorance or a reckless disregard for the truth.

negligence   Breaching of a duty owed to another, which occurs because of a failure to conform to a requirement, and this failure has caused harm to another individual, which led to damages to this person(s); failure to exercise the care toward others that a reasonable or prudent person would take in the circumstances, or taking actions that such a reasonable person would not.

nolo contendere   No contest.

plagiarism   False representation of another person's idea, research, presentation, result, or product as one's own through irresponsible citation, attribution, or paraphrasing; ethical misconduct does not include honest error or differences of opinion.

publicly sanctioned   A formal disciplinary action of public record, excluding actions due to insufficient continuing education, checks returned for insufficient funds, or late payment of fees not resulting in unlicensed practice.

reasonable or reasonably   Supported or justified by fact or circumstance and being in accordance with reason, fairness, duty, or prudence.

self-report   A professional obligation of self-disclosure that requires (a) notifying ASHA Standards and Ethics and (b) mailing a hard copy of a certified document to ASHA Standards and Ethics (see term above). All self-reports are subject to a separate ASHA Certification review process, which, depending on the seriousness of the self-reported information, takes additional processing time.

shall versus may   *Shall* denotes no discretion; *may* denotes an allowance for discretion.

support personnel   Those providing support to audiologists, speech-language pathologists, or speech, language, and hearing scientists (e.g., technician, paraprofessional, aide, or assistant in audiology, speech-language pathology, or communication sciences and disorders). For more information, read the Issues in Ethics Statements on Audiology Assistants and/or Speech-Language Pathology Assistants.

telepractice, teletherapy   Application of telecommunications technology to the delivery of audiology and speech-language pathology professional services at a distance by linking clinician to client/patient or clinician to clinician for assessment, intervention, and/or consultation. The quality of the service should be equivalent to in-person service. For more information, see the telepractice section on the ASHA Practice Portal.

written   Encompasses both electronic and hard copy writings or communications.

Principle of Ethics I

Individuals shall honor their responsibility to hold paramount the welfare of persons they serve professionally or who are participants in research and scholarly activities, and they shall treat animals involved in research in a humane manner.

Rules of Ethics

A. Individuals shall provide all clinical services and scientific activities competently.

B. Individuals shall use every resource, including referral and/or interprofessional collaboration when appropriate, to ensure that quality service is provided.

C. Individuals shall not discriminate in the delivery of professional services or in the conduct of research and scholarly activities on the basis of race, ethnicity, sex, gender identity/gender expression, sexual orientation, age, religion, national origin, disability, culture, language, or dialect.

D. Individuals shall not misrepresent the credentials of aides, assistants, technicians, support personnel, students, research interns, Clinical Fellows, or any others under their supervision, and they shall inform those they serve professionally of the name, role, and professional credentials of persons providing services.

E. Individuals who hold the CCC may delegate tasks related to the provision of clinical services to aides, assistants, technicians, support personnel, or any other persons only if those persons are adequately prepared and are appropriately supervised. The responsibility for the welfare of those being served remains with the certified individual.

F. Individuals who hold the CCC shall not delegate tasks that require the unique skills, knowledge, judgment, or credentials that are within the scope of their profession to aides, assistants, technicians, support personnel, or any nonprofessionals over whom they have supervisory responsibility.

G. Individuals who hold the CCC may delegate to students tasks related to the provision of clinical services that require the unique skills, knowledge, and judgment that are within the scope of practice of their profession only if those students are adequately prepared and are appropriately supervised. The responsibility for the welfare of those being served remains with the certified individual.

H. Individuals shall obtain informed consent from the persons they serve about the nature and possible risks and effects of services provided, technology employed, and products dispensed. This obligation also includes informing persons served about possible effects of not engaging in treatment or not following clinical recommendations. If diminished decision-making ability of persons served is suspected, individuals should seek appropriate authorization for services, such as authorization from a spouse, other family member, or legally authorized/appointed representative.

I. Individuals shall enroll and include persons as participants in research or teaching demonstrations only if participation is voluntary, without coercion, and with informed consent.

J. Individuals shall accurately represent the intended purpose of a service, product, or research endeavor and shall abide by established guidelines for clinical practice and the responsible conduct of research.

K. Individuals who hold the CCC shall evaluate the effectiveness of services provided, technology employed, and products dispensed, and they shall provide services or dispense products only when benefit can reasonably be expected.

L. Individuals may make a reasonable statement of prognosis, but they shall not guarantee—directly or by implication—the results of any treatment or procedure.

M. Individuals who hold the CCC shall use independent and evidence-based clinical judgment, keeping paramount the best interests of those being served.

N. Individuals who hold the CCC shall not provide clinical services solely by correspondence, but may provide services via telepractice consistent with professional standards and state and federal regulations.

O. Individuals shall protect the confidentiality and security of records of professional services provided, research and scholarly activities conducted, and products dispensed. Access to these records shall be allowed only when doing so is necessary to protect the welfare of the person or of the community, is legally authorized, or is otherwise required by law.

P. Individuals shall protect the confidentiality of any professional or personal information about persons served professionally or participants involved in research and scholarly activities and may disclose confidential information only when doing so is necessary to protect the welfare of the person or of the community, is legally authorized, or is otherwise required by law.

Q. Individuals shall maintain timely records and accurately record and bill for services provided and products dispensed and shall not misrepresent services provided, products dispensed, or research and scholarly activities conducted.

R. Individuals whose professional practice is adversely affected by substance abuse, addiction, or other health-related conditions are impaired practitioners and shall seek professional assistance and, where appropriate, withdraw from the affected areas of practice.

S. Individuals who have knowledge that a colleague is unable to provide professional services with reasonable skill and safety shall report this information to the appropriate authority, internally if a mechanism exists and, otherwise, externally.

T. Individuals shall provide reasonable notice and information about alternatives for obtaining care in the event that they can no longer provide professional services.

PRINCIPLE OF ETHICS II

Individuals shall honor their responsibility to achieve and maintain the highest level of professional competence and performance.

Rules of Ethics

A. Individuals who hold the CCC shall engage in only those aspects of the professions that are within the scope of their professional practice and competence, considering their certification status, education, training, and experience.

B. Members who do not hold the CCC may not engage in the provision of clinical services; however, individuals who are in the certification application process may engage in the provision of clinical services consistent with current local and state laws and regulations and with ASHA certification requirements.

C. Individuals who engage in research shall comply with all institutional, state, and federal regulations that address any aspects of research, including those that involve human participants and animals.

D. Individuals shall enhance and refine their professional competence and expertise through engagement in lifelong learning applicable to their professional activities and skills.

E. Individuals in administrative or supervisory roles shall not require or permit their professional staff to provide services or conduct research activities that exceed the staff member's certification status, competence, education, training, and experience.

F. Individuals in administrative or supervisory roles shall not require or permit their professional staff to provide services or conduct clinical activities that compromise the staff member's independent and objective professional judgment.

G. Individuals shall make use of technology and instrumentation consistent with accepted professional guidelines in their areas of practice. When such technology is not available, an appropriate referral may be made.

H. Individuals shall ensure that all technology and instrumentation used to provide services or to conduct research and scholarly activities are in proper working order and are properly calibrated.

PRINCIPLE OF ETHICS III

Individuals shall honor their responsibility to the public when advocating for the unmet communication and swallowing needs of the public and shall provide accurate information involving any aspect of the professions.

Rules of Ethics

A. Individuals shall not misrepresent their credentials, competence, education, training, experience, and scholarly contributions.

B. Individuals shall avoid engaging in conflicts of interest whereby personal, financial, or other considerations have the potential to influence or compromise professional judgment and objectivity.

C. Individuals shall not misrepresent research and scholarly activities, diagnostic information, services provided, results of services provided, products dispensed, or the effects of products dispensed.

D. Individuals shall not defraud through intent, ignorance, or negligence or engage in any scheme to defraud in connection with obtaining payment, reimbursement, or grants and contracts for services provided, research conducted, or products dispensed.

E. Individuals' statements to the public shall provide accurate and complete information about the nature and management of communication disorders, about the professions, about professional services, about products for sale, and about research and scholarly activities.

F. Individuals' statements to the public shall adhere to prevailing professional norms and shall not contain misrepresentations when advertising, announcing, and promoting their professional services and products and when reporting research results.

G. Individuals shall not knowingly make false financial or nonfinancial statements and shall complete all materials honestly and without omission.

PRINCIPLE OF ETHICS IV

Individuals shall uphold the dignity and autonomy of the professions, maintain collaborative and harmonious interprofessional and intraprofessional relationships, and accept the professions' self-imposed standards.

Rules of Ethics

A. Individuals shall work collaboratively, when appropriate, with members of one's own profession and/or members of other professions to deliver the highest quality of care.

B. Individuals shall exercise independent professional judgment in recommending and providing professional services when an administrative mandate, referral source, or prescription prevents keeping the welfare of persons served paramount.

C. Individuals' statements to colleagues about professional services, research results, and products shall adhere to prevailing professional standards and shall contain no misrepresentations.

D. Individuals shall not engage in any form of conduct that adversely reflects on the professions or on the individual's fitness to serve persons professionally.

E. Individuals shall not engage in dishonesty, negligence, fraud, deceit, or misrepresentation.

F. Applicants for certification or membership, and individuals making disclosures, shall not knowingly make false statements and shall complete all application and disclosure materials honestly and without omission.

G. Individuals shall not engage in any form of harassment, power abuse, or sexual harassment.

H. Individuals shall not engage in sexual activities with individuals (other than a spouse or other individual with whom a prior consensual relationship exists) over whom they exercise professional authority or power, including persons receiving services, assistants, students, or research participants.

I. Individuals shall not knowingly allow anyone under their supervision to engage in any practice that violates the Code of Ethics.

J. Individuals shall assign credit only to those who have contributed to a publication, presentation, process, or product. Credit shall be assigned in proportion to the contribution and only with the contributor's consent.

K. Individuals shall reference the source when using other persons' ideas, research, presentations, results, or products in written, oral, or any other media presentation or summary. To do otherwise constitutes plagiarism.

L. Individuals shall not discriminate in their relationships with colleagues, assistants, students, support personnel, and members of other professions and disciplines on the basis of race, ethnicity, sex, gender identity/gender expression, sexual orientation, age, religion, national origin, disability, culture, language, dialect, or socioeconomic status.

M. Individuals with evidence that the Code of Ethics may have been violated have the responsibility to work collaboratively to resolve the situation where possible or to inform the Board of Ethics through its established procedures.

N. Individuals shall report members of other professions who they know have violated standards of care to the appropriate professional licensing authority or board, other professional regulatory body, or professional association when such violation compromises the welfare of persons served and/or research participants.

O. Individuals shall not file or encourage others to file complaints that disregard or ignore facts that would disprove the allegation; the Code of Ethics shall not be used for personal reprisal, as a means of addressing personal animosity, or as a vehicle for retaliation.

P. Individuals making and responding to complaints shall comply fully with the policies of the Board of Ethics in its consideration, adjudication, and resolution of complaints of alleged violations of the Code of Ethics.

Q. Individuals involved in ethics complaints shall not knowingly make false statements of fact or withhold relevant facts necessary to fairly adjudicate the complaints.

R. Individuals shall comply with local, state, and federal laws and regulations applicable to professional practice, research ethics, and the responsible conduct of research.

S. Individuals who have been convicted; been found guilty; or entered a plea of guilty or nolo contendere to (1) any misdemeanor involving dishonesty, physical harm—or the threat of physical harm—to the person or property of another, or (2) any felony, shall self-report by notifying ASHA Standards and Ethics (see Terminology for mailing address) in writing within 30 days of the conviction, plea, or finding of guilt. Individuals shall also provide a certified copy of the conviction, plea, nolo contendere record, or docket entry to ASHA Standards and Ethics within 30 days of self-reporting.

T. Individuals who have been publicly sanctioned or denied a license or a professional credential by any professional association, professional licensing authority or board, or other professional regulatory body shall self-report by notifying ASHA Standards and Ethics (see Terminology for mailing address) in writing within 30 days of the final action or disposition. Individuals shall also provide a certified copy of the final action, sanction, or disposition to ASHA Standards and Ethics within 30 days of self-reporting.

APPENDIX A.2

Code of Ethics in Audiology

Established by: American Academy of Audiology

PREAMBLE:

The Code of Ethics of the American Academy of Audiology specifies professional standards that allow for the proper discharge of audiologists' responsibilities to those served, and that protect the integrity of the profession. The Code of Ethics consists of two parts. The first part, the Statement of Principles and Rules, presents precepts that members (all categories of members including Student Members) effective January 1, 2009 of the Academy agree to uphold. The second part, the Procedures, provides the process that enables enforcement of the Principles and Rules.

PART I. STATEMENT OF PRINCIPLES AND RULES

PRINCIPLE 1: Members shall provide professional services and conduct research with honesty and compassion, and shall respect the dignity, worth, and rights of those served.

Rule 1a: Individuals shall not limit the delivery of professional services on any basis that is unjustifiable or irrelevant to the need for the potential benefit from such services.

Rule 1b: Individuals shall not provide services except in a professional relationship and shall not discriminate in the provision of services to individuals on the basis of sex, race, religion, national origin, sexual orientation, or general health.

PRINCIPLE 2: Members shall maintain the highest standards of professional competence in rendering services.

Rule 2a: Members shall provide only those professional services for which they are qualified by education and experience.

Rule 2b: Individuals shall use available resources, including referrals to other specialists, and shall not give or accept benefits or items of value for receiving or making referrals.

Rule 2c: Individuals shall exercise all reasonable precautions to avoid injury to persons in the delivery of professional services or execution of research.

Rule 2d: Individuals shall provide appropriate supervision and assume full responsibility for services delegated to supportive personnel. Individuals shall not delegate any service requiring professional competence to unqualified persons.

Rule 2e: Individuals shall not knowingly permit personnel under their direct or indirect supervision to engage in any practice that is not in compliance with the Code of Ethics.

Rule 2f: Individuals shall maintain professional competence, including participation in continuing education.

PRINCIPLE 3: Members shall maintain the confidentiality of the information and records of those receiving services or involved in research.

Rule 3a: Individuals shall not reveal to unauthorized persons any professional or personal information obtained from the person served professionally, unless required by law.

PRINCIPLE 4: Members shall provide only services and products that are in the best interest of those served.

Rule 4a: Individuals shall not exploit persons in the delivery of professional services.

Rule 4b: Individuals shall not charge for services not rendered.

Rule 4c: Individuals shall not participate in activities that constitute a conflict of professional interest.

Rule 4d: Individuals using investigational procedures with human participants or prospectively collecting research data from human participants shall obtain full informed consent from the participants or legal representatives. Members conducting research with human participants or animals shall follow accepted standards, such as those promulgated in the current Responsible Conduct of Research by the U.S. Office of Research Integrity.

PRINCIPLE 5: Members shall provide accurate information about the nature and management of communicative disorders and about the services and products offered.

Rule 5a: Individuals shall provide persons served with the information a reasonable person would want to know about the nature and possible effects of services rendered or products provided or research being conducted.

Rule 5b: Individuals may make a statement of prognosis, but shall not guarantee results, mislead, or misinform persons served or studied.

Rule 5c: Individuals shall conduct and report product-related research only according to accepted standards of research practice.

Rule 5d: Individuals shall not carry out teaching or research activities in a manner that constitutes an invasion of privacy or that fails to inform persons fully about the nature and possible effects of these activities, affording all persons informed free choice of participation.

Rule 5e: Individuals shall maintain accurate documentation of services rendered according to accepted medical, legal, and professional standards and requirements.

PRINCIPLE 6: Members shall comply with the ethical standards of the Academy with regard to public statements or publication.

Rule 6a: Individuals shall not misrepresent their educational degrees, training, credentials, or competence. Only degrees earned from regionally accredited institutions in which training was obtained in audiology, or a directly related discipline, may be used in public statements concerning professional services.

Rule 6b: Individuals' public statements about professional services, products or research results shall not contain representations or claims that are false, misleading, or deceptive.

PRINCIPLE 7: Members shall honor their responsibilities to the public and to professional colleagues.

Rule 7a: Individuals shall not use professional or commercial affiliations in any way that would limit services to or mislead patients or colleagues.

Rule 7b: Individuals shall inform colleagues and the public in an objective manner consistent with professional standards about products and services they have developed or research they have conducted.

PRINCIPLE 8: Members shall uphold the dignity of the profession and freely accept the Academy's self-imposed standards.

Rule 8a: Individuals shall not violate these Principles and Rules nor attempt to circumvent them.

Rule 8b: Individuals shall not engage in dishonesty or illegal conduct that adversely reflects on the profession.

Rule 8c: Individuals shall inform the Ethical Practices Committee when there are reasons to believe that a member of the Academy may have been in noncompliance with the Code of Ethics.

Rule 8d: Individuals shall fully cooperate with reviews being conducted by the Ethical Practices Committee in any matter related to the Code of Ethics.

PART II. PROCEDURES FOR THE MANAGEMENT OF ALLEGED NONCOMPLIANCE

INTRODUCTION

Members of the American Academy of Audiology are obligated to uphold the Code of Ethics of the Academy in their personal conduct and in the performance of their professional duties. To this end, it is the responsibility of each Academy member to inform the Ethical Practice Committee (EPC) of possible noncompliance with the Ethics Code. The processing of alleged noncompliance with the Code of Ethics will follow the procedures specified below in an expeditious manner to ensure that behaviors of noncompliant ethical conduct by members of the Academy are halted in the shortest time possible.

PROCEDURES

1. Suspected noncompliance with the Code of Ethics shall be reported in letter format, giving documentation sufficient to support the alleged noncompliance. Letters must be addressed to: American Academy of Audiology Chair, Ethical Practices Committee 11480 Commerce Park Dr. Suite 220 Reston, VA 20191.

2. Following receipt of a report of suspected noncompliance, at the discretion of the Chair, the Ethical Practices Committee will request a signed Waiver of Confidentiality from the complainant indicating that the complainant will allow the Ethical Practice Board to disclose his/her name and complaint details should become necessary during investigation of the allegation.
   a. The Committee may, under special circumstances, act in the absence of a signed Waiver of Confidentiality. For example, in cases where the EPC has received information from a state licensure board of a member having his or her license suspended or revoked, then the EPC will proceed without a complainant.
   b. The Chair may communicate with other individuals, agencies, and/or programs for additional information as may be required for Committee review at any time during the deliberation.

3. The EPC will convene to review the merit of the alleged noncompliance as it relates to the Code of Ethics
   a. The EPC shall meet to discuss the case, either in person, by electronic means, or by teleconference. The meeting will occur within 60 days of receipt of the Waiver of Confidentiality, or of notification by the complainant of refusal to sign the waiver. In cases where another form of notification brings the complaint to the attention of the EPC, the Committee will convene within 60 days of notification.
   b. If the alleged noncompliance has a high probability of being legally actionable, the case may be referred to the appropriate agency. The EPC will postpone member notification and further deliberation until the legal process has been completed.

4. If there is sufficient evidence that indicates noncompliance with the Code of Ethics has occurred, upon majority vote, the member will be forwarded a Notification of Potential Ethics Concern.
   a. The circumstances of the alleged noncompliance will be described.
   b. The member will be informed of the specific Code of Ethics principle(s) and/or rule(s) that may conflict with member behavior.
   c. Supporting AAA documents that may serve to further educate the member about the ethical implications will be included, as appropriate.
   d. The member will be asked to respond fully to the allegation and submit all supporting evidence within 30 calendar days.

5. The Ethical Practices Committee will meet either in person or by teleconference:
   a. Within 60 calendar days of receiving a response from the member to the Notification of Potential Ethics Concern to review the response and all information pertaining to the alleged noncompliance, or
   b. Within 60 calendar days of notification to member if no response is received from the member to review the information received from the complainant.

6. If the EPC determines that the evidence supports the allegation of noncompliance, the member will be provided written notice containing the following information:
   a. The right to a hearing in person or by teleconference before the EPC;
   b. The date, time, and place of the hearing;
   c. The ethical noncompliance being charged and the potential sanction;

    d. The right to present a defense to the charges. At this time the member should provide any additional relevant information. As this is the final opportunity for a member to provide new information, the member should carefully prepare all documentation.

7. Potential Rulings.

    a. When the Ethical Practices Committee determines there is insufficient evidence of ethical noncompliance, the parties to the complaint will be notified that the case will be closed.

    b. If the evidence supports the allegation of Code noncompliance, the Code(s)/Rule(s) will be cited and the sanction(s) will be specified.

8. The Committee shall sanction members based on the severity of the noncompliance and history of prior ethical noncompliance. A simple majority of voting members is required to institute a sanction unless otherwise noted. Sanctions may include one or more of the following:

    a. Educative Letter. This sanction alone is appropriate when:

        1. The ethics noncompliance appears to have been inadvertent.

        2. The member's response to Notification of Potential Ethics Concern indicates a new awareness of the problem and the member resolves to refrain from future ethical noncompliance.

    b. Cease and Desist Order. The member signs a consent agreement to immediately halt the practice(s) that were found to be in noncompliance with the Code of Ethics

    c. Reprimand. The member will be formally reprimanded for the noncompliance with of the Code of Ethics.

    d. Mandatory continuing education.

        1. The EPC will determine the type of education needed to reduce chances of recurrence of noncompliance.

        2. The member will be responsible for submitting documentation of continuing education within the period of time designated by the Ethical Practices Committee.

        3. All costs associated with compliance will be borne by the member.

    e. Probation of Suspension. The member signs a consent agreement in acknowledgment of the EPC decision and is allowed to retain membership benefits during a defined probationary period.

        1. The duration of probation and the terms for avoiding suspension will be determined by the EPC.

        2. Failure of the member to meet the terms for probation will result in the suspension of membership.

    f. Suspension of Membership.

        1. The duration of suspension will be determined by the EPC.

        2. The member may not receive membership benefits during the period of suspension.

        3. Members suspended are not entitled to a refund of dues or fees.

    g. Revocation of Membership. Revocation of membership is considered the maximum consequence for noncompliance with the Code of Ethics.

        1. Revocation requires a two-thirds majority of the voting members of the EPC.

        2. Individuals whose memberships are revoked are not entitled to a refund of dues or fees.

        3. One year following the date of membership revocation the individual may reapply for, but is not guaranteed, membership through normal channels, and must meet the membership qualifications in effect at the time of reapplication.

9. The member may appeal the Final Finding and Decision of the EPC to the Academy Board of Directors. The route of Appeal is by letter format through the EPC to the Board of Directors of the Academy. Requests for Appeal must:

    a. be received by the Chair of the EPC within 30 days of the EPC notification of the Final Finding and Decision,

    b. state the basis for the appeal and the reason(s) that the Final Finding and Decision of the EPC should be changed,

    c. not offer new documentation. The EPC chair will communicate with the Executive Director of the Academy to schedule the appeal at the earliest feasible Board of Director's meeting. The Board of Directors will review the documents and written summaries and deliberate the case. The decision of the Board of Directors regarding the member's appeal shall be final.

10. In order to educate the membership, upon majority vote of the EPC, the circumstances and nature of cases shall be presented in Audiology Today and in the Professional Resource area of the AAA website. The member's identity will not be made public.

11. No EPC member shall give access to records, act or speak independently, or on behalf of the EPC, without the expressed permission of the members then active. No member may impose the sanction of the EPC or interpret the findings of the EPC in any manner that may place members of the EPC or Board of Directors, collectively or singly, at financial, professional, or personal risk

12. The EPC Chair and Staff Liaison shall maintain electronic records that shall form the basis for future findings of the Committee.

CONFIDENTIALITY AND RECORDS

Confidentiality shall be maintained in all EPC discussion, correspondence, communication, deliberation, and records pertaining to members reviewed by the EPC.

1. Complaints and suspected noncompliance with the Code of Ethics are assigned a case number.
2. Identity of members involved in complaints and suspected noncompliance cases and access to EPC files is restricted to the following:
   a. EPC members
   b. Executive Director
   c. Agent(s) of the Executive Director
   d. Other(s), following majority vote of EPC
3. Original records shall be maintained at the Central Records Repository at the Academy office in a locked cabinet.
   a. One copy will be sent to the EPC Chair or member designated by the Chair.
   b. Redacted copies will be sent to members.
4. Communications shall be sent to the members involved in complaints by the Academy office via certified or registered mail, after review by Legal Counsel, as needed.
5. When a case is closed,
   a. The Chair will forward all documentation to the Staff Liaison to be maintained at the Academy Central Records Repository.
   b. Members shall destroy all material pertaining to the case.
6. Complete records generally shall be maintained at the Academy Central Records Repository for a period of 5 years.
   a. Records will be destroyed 5 years after a member receives a sanction less than suspension, or 5 years after the end of a suspension, or after membership is reinstated.
   b. Records of membership revocations for persons who have not returned to membership status will be maintained indefinitely.

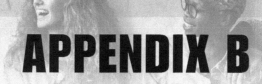

APPENDIX B

Tips for the Emerging Clinician

Before the session:
- Prepare for therapy sessions in advance. Write down therapy objectives to be directly targeted.
- Consider setting a timing goal for each objective. (e.g., objective #1: 8:00–8:10 am, objective #2: 8:11–8:20 am).
- Make sure games/toys/activities have all the pieces/content and batteries (if applicable).
- For crafts and creations, consider providing a picture or model of the final creation so the child or individual is aware of the expectations for the craft/creation.
- Carefully clean toys, items, and materials prior to the session. This may include disinfecting spray or sanitizing wipes.
- In an effort to protect the child/individual and the clinician, sanitize surfaces in the therapy room (e.g., table, door knob, counter tops, etc.).
- Provide parents/caregivers a list of known stimulus items for targeted objectives to encourage participation in therapy as well as carryover of therapy objectives.
- Consider writing down the stimulus items for each objective (or pulling specific desired prompt cards/items) in advance.

During the session:
- Check to make sure all technologies and sensory devices are in working order prior to starting the session (e.g., clean glasses, check for hearing aid or cochlear implant function, check to make sure AAC device is in working order, etc.)
- Obtain the child/individual's attention prior to providing instructions or descriptions.
- Use "specific language." Rather than using words like, "Here, there, this, that," use more descriptive language to encourage the child/individual to use more descriptive language too.
- Provide specific feedback. Positive reinforcement phrases like "good job" do not provide detail regarding what was done well. Positive phrases are encouraged; however, consider adding description (e.g., "You are learning new words today!" "Your speech is sounding clearer because of your hard work.").
- Consider providing homework of objectives to be targeted at home or outside therapy time in written form for parents/caregivers.
- Consider starting the session with a brief review of the outline of the session (e.g., "First we will read a book, then we will practice your sounds, and last we will practice using plural /s/.).
- Help the client/individual to set goals within each objective (e.g., "Should we practice 3 more to 5 more before we move on to a new task?").
- Consider using a timer to help set a goal for how long an objective will be targeted. Explain the use of the timer to the child/individual so they are aware of the goal too.
- Provide an introduction of each objective to the child/individual and parent/caregiver (if applicable) so they are aware of what is to be targeted and the purpose of each objective.

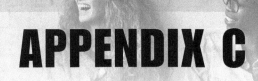

APPENDIX C

Sample SOAP Note

Speech Pathology Clinic Note

Name: Jane Doe

Date of Birth (DOB): 3/14/15

Chronological Age (CA): 3 years, 2 months

Date of Service (DOS): 5/18/2018

Time: 10:00 am–11:00 am

Subjective:

Jane was seen for an individual, speech-language therapy session at Changing the World Clinic. She was accompanied to this session by her mother, who actively participated in all structured therapy activities. Jane's mother provided verbal and written report of Jane's progress this past week. She reported Jane consistently used 2 words to request and that the clarity of her speech continues to improve. Jane participated well with moderate prompts and redirections from her mother and this clinician. She had a good session.

Objective:

1. **Expressive language, produce plural /s/:** (5/10) 50% accuracy in structured play. Additional work is needed. Continue to target this objective.

2. **Expressive language, produce subject pronouns:** (13/20) 66% accuracy in semi-structured play. "I, He, She" targeted today. Jane most consistently substituted her name for "I" (e.g., "Jane do it."). Additional work is needed.

3. **Receptive language, identify quantity "one":** (3/10) 30% accuracy in structured play. This objective was introduced on this date. Additional work is needed. Continue to target this objective.

4. **Receptive language, identify "on top, under":** (10/20) 50% accuracy. This is improved from previous sessions. Additional work is needed. Continue to target this objective.

5. **Receptive language, comprehension of basic question forms:**

   "What happened?" – (10/200 50% accuracy
   "How many?" – (3/10) 30% accuracy
   Questions were targeted indirectly throughout the session in structured and semi-structured play activities. Additional work is needed. Continue to target this objective.

** Materials/activities for this session included: Fisher Price Little People, toy food items, Weebles Tree house toy, toy dishes, toy farm animals

**Jane's mother was provided homework in written form and reported she had no questions. She reported she would target all objectives at home with Jane this week.

Assessment: Jane's receptive identification of "on top, under" improved from 30% accuracy to 50% accuracy on this date. Receptive identification of "one" was introduced. Jane was in a good mood and participated well for all activities today. Additional work is needed for all targeted therapy objectives. Jane continues to present with a receptive and expressive language delay.

Plan: Continue with current plan of care. Return to this clinic in 1 week.

Jack Smith, M.S., CCC-SLP
Speech Language Pathologist
Changing the World Clinic

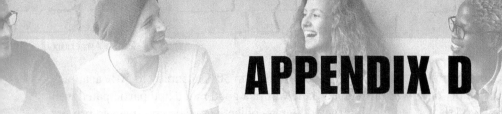

APPENDIX D

Sample Plan of Care

Speech Language Plan of Care

January 1, 2017–December 30, 2017

Name: Jackson Thunder

Date of Birth (DOB): 4/22/2013

Chronological Age (CA): 3 years, 8 months

Diagnosis: Severe Articulation & Expressive Language Delay

Examiner (s): Wanda Getresults

LONG TERM GOAL(S):

1. Jackson will improve speech sound production to aid in communication.
2. Jackson will improve expressive language skills to a level commensurate with his same aged peers.

SHORT TERM OBJECTIVES:

**Achievement of objective completion is measured by performance of 80% accuracy across 3 consecutive sessions.

** All baselines are 0% indicating no experience with the objective unless otherwise noted.

Articulation/Speech Sound Objectives:

Jackson will:

1. Produce [h, n, w, b] in isolation.
2. Produce [h, n, w, b] in the initial position of single syllables.
3. Produce [h, n, w, b] in the initial position of 2–3 repetitive syllables.
4. Produce [h, n, w, b] in the initial position of 2–3 alternating syllables.
5. Produce [h, n, w, b] in the initial position of words.
6. Produce [h, n, w, b] in the initial position of words in phrases.
7. Produce [h, n, w, b] in the initial position of words in sentences.
8. Produce [h, n, w, b] in the initial position of words in spontaneous speech.

Expressive Language Objectives:

Jackson will:

1. Produce 2 words to: comment, greet, request and protest.
2. Use the possessive pronoun "mine".
3. Label familiar action words/verbs in play.
4. Label familiar action words/verbs in pictures.

5. Use plural /s/
6. Label familiar toys/items in play.
7. Label familiar toys/items in pictures.
8. Use regular past tense verbs (e.g., jump<u>ed</u>).

Wanda Getresults, M.S., CCC-SLP
Speech Language Pathologist
Changing the World Clinic

APPENDIX E

Sample Lesson Plan Template

Client:

Session Date:

Clinician:

Start Time: 10:00 am, **End Time:** 11:00 am

Theme: Take care of baby at home

Order of tasks in session	Objective	Data	Procedure/ Activity	Materials	Introduction of task & objective to parent and/or child
1	**Expressive language – labeling body parts.** **Target:** Eyes Hands Nose Ears Mouth Hair		Give baby doll a bath	Small container of water, tear-free soap, doll brush, towel, lotion	Child: We are going to talk about body parts while we give your baby a bath. Parent: Labeling body parts is an important expressive language skill. Bath time is a great time to talk about body parts.
2					Child: Parent:
3					Child: Parent:
4					Child: Parent:
5					Child: Parent:
6					Child: Parent:
7					Child: Parent:
8					Client: Parent:

Notes:

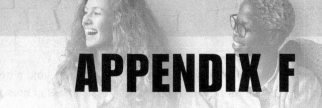

APPENDIX F

Sample Pediatric Evaluation Report

April 4–6th, 2017

NAME: Jessica Jones

DOB:

CA: 6 years, 6 months

PARENTS:

ADDRESS:

PHONE:

PRIMARY CARE PHYSICIAN:

EXAMINER: N'tasha James, M.S., CCC-SLP

DIAGNOSIS:

BACKGROUND INFORMATION:

Jessica Jones, a six year, 6 month old female, was seen at Changing the World Clinic on this date for an evaluation of her communication skills. She was accompanied to this clinic visit by her mother, who provided background information and a verbal report on Jessica's current communication skills. Jessica was referred for this evaluation by her primary care physician. The following appears to be significant in her case:

Prenatal: Nothing significant was reported.
Birth: Full term birth (38 weeks gestation), weighing 7 pounds, 3 ounces, 19 inches in length.
Neonatal: Nothing significant was reported.
Medical: Significant for pressure equalization (PE) tube placement at 3 years of age. PE tubes have not been in place for the past 2 years and mom reports no addition concerns with middle ear function. Jessica currently takes no medications.
Developmental: Jessica has met all developmental milestones, with the exception of communication, at expected rates, per guardian report. Ms. Jones did not report concern about other areas of development.
Communication: Jessica uses single words, short phrases, and simple sentences to communicate with others. In both familiar and unfamiliar contexts, Jessica's speech is difficult to understand, especially to the unfamiliar listener. Ms. Jones reported that she is very concerned about Jessica's communication development and feels that she is behind other children of the same age. Mrs. Jones reported it is her goal for Jessica to use spoken language as a primary means of communication.
Social: Jessica lives at home with both parents. She will be entering the first grade at Washington Elementary in city, state this fall. Ms. Jones reported Jessica interacts well at school and has many friends.

Audiology: No concerns with hearing were reported. Otoscopy, tympanometry, and a hearing screening were performed prior to the speech-language evaluation by this clinician. Jessica passed otoscopy and tympanometry as well as her hearing screening.

Vision: No concerns with vision were reported. Mrs. Jones reported Jessica passed her vision screening at school last month.

BEHAVIORAL OBSERVATIONS:

Jessica, her mother, and this SLP participated in this evaluation session. Jessica was in a great mood and participated well for all evaluation tasks. She displayed appropriate attention and was very interactive during this evaluation session. She demonstrated pretend play skills that were commensurate with her chronological age. This evaluation was conducted in Jessica's primary language, English.

ASSESSMENT BATTERY:

The Clinical Evaluation of Language Fundamentals, Preschool, Second Edition (CELF-P2)
The Goldman Fristoe Test of Articulation, Second Edition (GFTA-2)
The Arizona Articulation Proficiency Scale, Third Revision (AAPS-3)
The Receptive One-Word Vocabulary Test, Fourth Edition (ROWPVT-4)
The Expressive One-Word Vocabulary Test, Fourth Edition (EOWPVT-4)
Voice/Resonance
Fluency
Oral-Peripheral Examination
Hearing (see background information)

EVALUATION:

LANGUAGE:

The Clinical Evaluation of Language Fundamentals was attempted but discontinued due to Jessica's limited language skills at this time. The Clinical Evaluation of Language Fundamentals—Preschool, Second Edition (CELF-P2) is an updated diagnostic language assessment used to assess the foundations of language form and content, word meanings (semantics), word and sentence structure (morphology and syntax), and recall of spoken language (auditory memory). The Core Language Score is a measure of general language ability and is derived by summing the scaled scores from the subtests that best discriminate typical language performance from disordered language performance. The index scores are based on a mean of 100 with a standard deviation of +/−15. Therefore, scores between 85 and 115 are considered to be within the average range of performance for the child's chronological age. This assessment was normed on children of the same chronological age. The following CELF-P2 index scores were obtained:

Administered: April 4, 2017

Index	Index Score	Percentile Rank
Core Language	53	0.1
Receptive Language	51	0.1
Expressive Language	50	<0.1

The CELF-P2 subtests are given on a mean of 10 with a standard deviation of +/−3. Therefore, scaled scores between 7 and 13 indicate performance in the average range. The following scores were obtained on the individual subtests:

Subtest	Scaled Score	Percentile Rank
Sentence Structure	4	2
Word Structure	1	0.1
Expressive Vocabulary	1	0.1
Concepts & Following Directions	1	0.1
Recalling Sentences	3	1
Word Classes - Receptive	1	0.1
Word Classes - Expressive	3	1
Word Classes - Total	2	0.4

On the _Sentence Structure_ subtest, Jessica was asked to interpret sentences that make comparisons, identify location or direction, specify time relationships, include serial order, or are expressed in passive voice. She was able to correctly answer 11 of 22 questions on this subtest. In the classroom, interpretation of relationships presented verbally and in text materials is required in curriculum areas such as English, language arts, math, science and vocational training. Jessica's performance on this subtest is within the severely delayed range of performance for her chronological age.

On the _Word Structure_ subtest, Jessica had difficulty identifying the following syntactical structures: present progressive verb+ing (walking, sleeping, running), regular plurals (dogs), irregular plural (1 child, 2 children), possessive nouns, possessive pronouns (i.e. hers, his, yours), regular past tense verbs, objective pronouns (i.e. them, us, him), future tense verbs (i.e. will do, will say), comparatives/superlatives (i.e. fast, faster, fastest), uncontractible auxiliary verbs (i.e. is, are), derivation of adjectives (i.e. all the luck - lucky), reflexive pronouns (i.e. himself, herself), subjective pronouns (i.e. she, he, they, we), and irregular past tense verbs (i.e. drew, ran). The ability to determine appropriate word structure is required for reading comprehension, writing narratives, learning vocabulary, and developing grammar. Jessica's performance on this subtest is within the severely delayed range of performance for her chronological age.

On the _Expressive Vocabulary_ subtest, Jessica was asked to label illustrations of people, objects, and actions. In the classroom, the precise use of words to create meaning is emphasized in telling stories, giving descriptions of events and labeling pictured references. Jessica's score on this subtest is the severely delayed range of performance for her chronological age.

The _Concepts and Following Directions_ subtest evaluates a child's ability to interpret spoken directions of increasing length and complexity. In the classroom, comprehension, recall, and ability to act upon spoken directions is essential for following directions for classroom assignments and projects, remembering assigned tasks, and following teacher instructions for managing classroom activities and interactions. Jessica struggled to consistently follow commands with more than one unit or step. Her performance on this subtest is in the severely delayed range for her chronological age.

The _Recalling Sentences_ subtest evaluates a child's ability to listen to spoken sentences of increasing length and complexity and repeat sentences without changing word meanings, inflections, derivations or comparisons, or sentence structure. At home and in the classroom, the ability to remember spoken sentences of increasing complexity in meaning and structure is required in following directions and academic instructions, learning vocabulary, understanding subjects content, playing imitation games and role playing. Jessica was able to consistently repeat sentences up to 3 words in length. Her performance on this subtest is in the severely delayed range of performance for her chronological age.

The _Word Classes_ subtest evaluates a child's ability to perceive relationships between words that are related by semantic class features and to express those relationships. The use of semantic relationships is important in daily activities such as rephrasing utterances, storytelling, role playing, and developing categorization skills. Jessica's receptive and expressive vocabulary were noted to be severely delayed on these subtests.

The Expressive One-Word Picture Vocabulary Test (EOWPVT) is a norm-referenced test designed to offer a quick and reliable measure of an individual's speaking vocabulary, which is assessed by asking the individual to identify a picture or group of pictures. This assessment was standardized on a group of children having the same chronological age. The assessment yields standard scores with a mean of 100 and a standard deviation of +/−15. Standard scores between 85 and 115 are considered to be within the average range of performance for this child's chronological age. Obtained results are listed below:

Raw Score: 46
Standard Score: 74
Percentile: 4
Test Age Equivalent: 3 years, 11 months

Results on the EOWPVT support findings on the CELF-P2 that indicate a severe delay in expressive language skills for Jessica's chronological age at this time.

The Receptive One-Word Picture Vocabulary Test (ROWPVT) is a norm-referenced test designed to offer a quick and reliable measure of an individual's English vocabulary, which is assessed by asking the individual to identify an illustration that depicts the meaning of a word presented orally by the examiner. This assessment was standardized on a group of children having the same chronological age, but no peripheral hearing impairment. This should be considered when interpreting test results. Standard scores between 85 and 115 are considered to be within the average range of performance for this child's chronological age. Obtained results are listed below:

Raw Score: 58
Standard Score: 83
Percentile: 13
Test Age Equivalent: 4 years, 6 months

Results of the ROWPVT indicate receptive language skills are below average for Jessica's chronological age at this time.

ARTICULATION:

The Goldman Fristoe Test of Articulation, Second Edition (GFTA-2) was administered on April 6th, 2017, to sample Jessica's ability to co-articulate sounds when presented in single words. A comparison of results is provided below. This assessment is normed on children having the same chronological age. Results are represented in standard scores having a mean of 100 and a standard deviation of +/−15 points. Therefore, standard scores between 85 and 115 are considered to be within the average range of performance for the child's chronological age. Obtained results are reported below:

April 6th, 2017

Type of Score	
Raw Score	47
Standard Score	< 40
Percentile Rank	< 1

The following errors were obtained:

* = Omission

Initial: p/f, l/"y", s/ "sh", t/"ch", "y"/l, w/r, d/ "j", "y"/ "voiceless th", b/v, "y"/z, d/"voiced th"

Medial: distortion/g, t/k, p/f, distortion/"sh", t/"ch", */r, d/ "j", */"voiceless th", b/v, d/ "voiced th"

Final: */k, p/f, */d, */t, distortion/ "sh", */"ch", */l. */"j", */"voiceless th", */v

Initial Blends: b/bl, b/br, d/dr, f/fl, w/fr, g/gl, w/gr, k/kl, k/kr, w/kw, p/pl, s/sl, p/sp, s/st, s/sw, t/tr

Results indicate Jessia's articulation skills fall within the severely delayed range of performance for her chronological age.

The Arizona Articulation Proficiency Scale, Third Revision (AAPS-3) is designed to provide a useful assessment measure of articulatory proficiency in children. This assessment is normed on children having the same chronological age. Results provide the child's level of correct articulation. The AAPS-3 standard scores have a mean of 100 and a standard deviation of +/−15. Therefore, scores between 85 and 115 are within the normal range of performance. Obtained results are reported below.

April 6th, 2017

Total Score	Standard Score	Percentile Rank
74.5	73	4

Results of the AAPS-3 indicate articulation skills at this time that fall within the severely delayed range of performance for Jessica's chronological age. This supports findings on the GFTA-2. An inventory of errors is reported below.

Initial: distortion/g, d/ "j", b/v, "y"/l, l/"y", w/r, d/ "voiced th", s/"ch", s/ "voiceless th", "y"/z

Final: omission/k, omission/g, omission/d, s/"sh", b/v, omission/l, s/f, omission/ "ch", s/ "voiceless th", omission/z

Blends: p/pl, p/tr, g/gr, s/st-, s/-st, omission/ks, omission/ld

ORAL MECHANISM EVALUATION: Observation of oral-facial structures was done to assess the structure and function of Jessica's oral mechanism. Facial features were judged to be symmetrical. No drooling, anterior tongue carriage or open mouth posture were observed. Tongue size and shape as well as mobility appeared to be normal. No concerns with shape and contour of hard and soft palates were noted. No deviation or bifid in the uvula was noted and no concerns with velopharyngeal closure were noted. Overall, oral motor structures/ functioning appeared to be adequate to support continued speech and language development.

VOICE AND FLUENCY: No formal assessment was conducted due to Jessica's age and language abilities. All parameters are considered to be appropriate for her chronological age and gender.

IMPRESSIONS:

- Expressive language skills are judged to be severely delayed.
- Receptive language skills are judged to be severely delayed on the CELF-P2.
- Receptive language skills are judged to be in the low average on the ROWPVT-4.
- Articulation skills are judged to be severely delayed on the GFTA-2 and the AAPS-3.
- Structure and function of the oral mechanism are judged to be within normal limits.
- Attending skills are judged to be age appropriate for structured tasks directed by others.

RECOMMENDATIONS:

1. It is the informed clinical opinion that Jessica be referred for direct speech therapy services to address the above listed deficits. Due to the nature and severity of this child's delay, 60 minutes of therapy per week (1 session, 60 minutes each session) is recommended.

2. It is recommended that Jessica's family participate actively in her speech therapy program. It is recommended that the family be assisted in learning techniques, which can be used in the home to further develop her articulation, receptive, expressive language skills. In order for Jessica to progress optimally, a conscious emphasis on therapy goals should be incorporated into the child's daily activities.

Prognosis for improvement in Jessica's communication skills is considered to be good with appropriate intervention. Her strong family support for therapy, ability to participate in structured tasks, desire to communicate and interact with persons in her environment, positive responses to stimulability testing in today's session, and good imitation skills are all indications that she will continue to do well in therapy.

Potential barriers to progress may include decreased attending skills for structured activities, unknown factors related to cognitive functioning or other unknown diagnoses at this time.

Following today's evaluation, a brief verbal summary of results and proposed recommendations were discussed with Mrs. Jones. An opportunity was given to provide feedback and to ask questions. Ms. Jones indicated she was in agreement with today's recommendations and expressed appreciation for this evaluation. If there are any questions concerning this report, please feel free to contact this clinician at (555) 123-4567 or by email at njames@changingtheworldclinic.com

N'Tasha James, M.S., CCC-SLP
Speech Language Pathologist
Changing the World Clinic

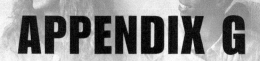

APPENDIX G

Sample Speech Sound Disorder Evaluation

Lovelytown Public Schools

305 Mockingbird Road

Anywhere, USA 45962

(479) 333-3399

Name:	Sally Sample
Birthdate:	03/20/2014
CA:	5 years, 0 months
Parent(s):	John Sample & Fredia Sample
Evaluation date(s):	04/05/2019
Evaluated by:	Ms. Sarah Verysmart, M.S., CCC-SLP

SPEECH-LANGUAGE ASSESSMENT

STATEMENT OF CONCERN

Sally was referred for a speech-language evaluation as part of her transition from preschool services to school-age services. Testing was necessary to determine Sally's current speech and language needs and eligibility for services as a kindergarten student. The results of the evaluation follow. For additional information, refer to her folder.

BACKGROUND INFORMATION

An updated social history was not available at the time of this report. According to previous reports and social history forms, Sally is a preschool student in the ABC preK program at Lovelytown Elementary School. Before attending ABC preschool, Sally attended Children's World preschool. Sally's parents are divorced and she spends time with both parents. Previous reports indicate Ms. Sample had an unremarkable pregnancy with spontaneous preterm labor at 35 weeks. Sally was born weighing 5 pounds. Ms. Braswell indicated on previous social history forms that Sally had difficulty eating due to poor oral muscle strength as an infant. All developmental milestones were reportedly attained within normal limits with the exception of using first words at 12-18 months.

Sally has been receiving speech therapy services through the local Head Start program since July 2017. Therapy has focused on articulation. Currently, Sally receives speech therapy 45 minutes weekly.

ASSESSMENT BATTERY

Sally was assessed using the following tools:

Pure Tone Hearing Screening

Vision Screening

Arizona Articulation Proficiency Scale-3rd Edition (AAPS-3)

Goldman-Fristoe Test of Articulation-3rd Edition (GFTA-3)

Oral and Written Language Scales-2nd Edition (OWLS-2)

Oral-Peripheral Examination

Informal Systematic Observation of Voice and Fluency

GENERAL OBSERVATIONS

Sally was tested in the speech room at Lovelytown Elementary. Testing was conducted over one session with frequent breaks to accommodate Sally's attention and to minimize testing fatigue. She was pleasant and cooperative during the evaluation sessions. She was observed to use single words, phrases, and sentences throughout the evaluation. Test results are considered valid and reliable indicators of her current speech and language abilities.

EVALUATION RESULTS AND CLINICAL IMPRESSIONS

SENSORY

A pure tone hearing screening was administered bilaterally at 25dB at 1000, 2000, and 4000 HZ on September 13, 2019. Sally's hearing acuity appears to be within normal limits.

Sally's visual acuity on February 13, 2019. Sally passed the screening.

ARIZONA ARTICULATION PROFICIENCY SCALE-3RD REVISION (AAPS-3)

The AAPS-3 assesses an individual's articulation of both consonant and vowels sound in the initial and final positions in words. The frequency of occurrence of each speech sound is used in the AAPS-3 to determine the severity of a communication disorder. Error scores are totaled and compared to other speakers of the same age. Standard scores between 85 and 115 are considered to be within normal limits. Sally received an AAPS-3 standard score of 70 for a percentile rank of 2. Sally's score on the AAPS-3 fell two standard deviations below the mean, suggesting severely delayed articulation skills when compared to other children of her chronological age. The corresponding description of speech intelligibility for this score is "Speech intelligibility is difficult."

Test Results

Arizona-3 Total Score	64.5
Standard Score	**70**
Percentile	2
Impairment Rating	Severe

Errors:

X/Y – X = sound made by child, Y = target sound
(UV = unvoiced, V = voiced) ("j" is as in 'judge', "y" is as in 'yellow')

Initial Position	Final Position	Vowel
b/p	t/k	Distorted vocalic-r
d/t	d/g	
d/g	n/ng	
d/t	h/sh	
d/j	d/v	
h/sh	omitted l	
w/l	wd/ld	
pw/pl	t/f	
w/r	t/ch	
dw/tr	t/th (UV)	
d/th (V)	d/z	
d/ch	t/s	
dw/gr	t/st	
h/th (UV)	t/ts	
v/z	t/ks	
h/s		
t/st		

GOLDMAN-FRISTOE TEST OF ARTICULATION-3RD EDITION (GFTA-3)

The GFTA-3 was administered to assess Sally's articulatory skills. This test samples all English consonants and some blends in one-word utterances. Percentile ranks of 17th percentile or higher are considered to be within the normal range. Sally's raw score of 103 yielded a percentile of <.1 and a standard score of 40. Sally's percentile rank on the GFTA-3 suggests articulatory skills are significantly delayed.

Test Results

GFTA-3 Raw Score	102
Standard Score	**40**
Percentile	**<.1**
Impairment Rating	Severe

Errors:

X/Y – X = sound made by child, Y = target sound
(UV = unvoiced, V = voiced) ("j" is as in 'judge', "y" is as in 'yellow')

Initial Position	Medial Position	Final Position
d/k	n/ng	Omitted s
d/g	t/k	Distorted r
tw/kw	h/s	d/g
d/t	d/g	omitted l
h/f	d/z	t/k
p/sp	w/l	distorted l
dw/dr	h/f	t/sh

Initial Position	Medial Position	Final Position
pw/pl	omitted y	t/ch
hw/hl	h/ch	n/ng
hw/sw	bw/br	ts/z
d/g	w/r	nd/ng
w/l	t/j	h/f
t/ch	h/sh	n/ng
f/s	d/th (V)	d/g
gw/gl	d/j	t/f
h/f	t/s	d/z
w/r	b/v	f/th (UV)
h/th (UV)		t/s
b/v		d/v
v/z		
d/j		
bw/br		
bl/bw		
fw/fr		
dw/gr		
d/th (V)		
t/k		
t/ch		
pw/pr		
tw/tr		
h/z		
t/st		
h/f		

ORAL AND WRITTEN LANGUAGE SCALES-2ND EDITION (OWLS-2)

The OWLS-2 is an assessment of receptive and expressive language. Oral language skills are assessed using the Listening Comprehension and Oral Expression subtests of the OWLS-2. The Listening Comprehension subtest measures the understanding of spoken language and the Oral Expression subtest measures the understanding and use of spoken language. Both subtests yield a raw score, which is converted into a standard score with a mean of 100 and a standard deviation of 15. Scores between 85 and 115 are considered to be within normal range.

Sally obtained a Listening Comprehension standard score of 122, an Oral Expression standard score of 116, and an Oral Composite standard score of 119 yielding a percentile rank of 90. Sally's scores on both subtests as well as the Oral Language composite suggest above average language skills.

Test Results

Subtest	Raw Score	Standard Score	Percentile Rank
Listening Comp.	63	122	93
Oral Exp.	42	116	86
Oral Composite	238	119	90

ORAL-PERIPHERAL

An oral peripheral examination revealed adequate structure and function for effective speech production.

OBSERVATION OF VOICE AND FLUENCY

Systematic observation of fluency revealed no significant dysfluencies. Voice and resonance are within normal limits

DIAGNOSTIC IMPRESSIONS AND CONCLUSIONS

Sally is a five-year old female whose articulation and language were assessed to determine her current speech-language needs and eligibility for special services. Test results indicate severely delayed articulation skills. Language skills, voice, and speech fluency are within normal limits.

RECOMMENDATIONS

The results of this assessment should be considered when determining the best educational programming and placement for Sally. Improved articulation skills may be beneficial to Sally's academic success and continued speech-language therapy is an appropriate educational consideration.

_____

Sarah Verysmart, M.S., CCC-SLP

Speech-Language Pathologist

APPENDIX H.1

Scope of Practice in Speech-Language Pathology

About this Document: This scope of practice document is an official policy of the American Speech-Language-Hearing Association (ASHA) defining the breadth of practice within the profession of speech-language pathology. This document was developed by the ASHA Ad Hoc Committee on the Scope of Practice in Speech- Language Pathology. Committee members were Mark DeRuiter (chair), Michael Campbell, Craig Coleman, Charlette Green, Diane Kendall, Judith Montgomery, Bernard Rousseau, Nancy Swigert, Sandra Gillam (board liaison), and Lemmietta McNeilly (ex officio). This document was approved by the ASHA Board of Directors on February 4, 2016 (BOD 01-2016). The BOD approved a revision in the prevention of hearing section of the document on May 9, 2016 (Motion 07-2016).

Table of Contents

INTRODUCTION

The *Scope of Practice in Speech-Language Pathology* of the American Speech-Language-Hearing Association (ASHA) includes the following: a statement of purpose, definitions of *speech-language pathologist* and *speech-language pathology*, a framework for speech-language pathology practice, a description of the domains of speech-language pathology service delivery, delineation of speech-language pathology service delivery areas, domains of professional practice, references, and resources.

The *speech-language pathologist (SLP)* is defined as the professional who engages in professional practice in the areas of communication and swallowing across the life span. *Communication* and *swallowing* are broad terms encompassing many facets of function. *Communication* includes speech production and fluency, language, cognition, voice, resonance, and hearing. *Swallowing* includes all aspects of *swallowing*, including related feeding behaviors. Throughout this document, the terms *communication* and *swallowing* are used to reflect all areas. This document is a guide for SLPs across all clinical and educational settings to promote best practice. The term *individuals* is used throughout the document to refer to students, clients, and patients who are served by the SLP.

As part of the review process for updating the *Scope of Practice in Speech-Language Pathology*, the committee revised the previous scope of practice document to reflect recent advances in knowledge and research in the discipline. One of the biggest changes to the document includes the delineation of practice areas in the context of eight domains of speech-language pathology service delivery: collaboration; counseling; prevention and wellness; screening; assessment; treatment; modalities, technology, and instrumentation; and population and systems. In addition, five domains of professional practice are delineated: advocacy and outreach, supervision, education, research, and administration/leadership.

Service delivery areas include all aspects of communication and swallowing and related areas that impact communication and swallowing: speech production, fluency, language, cognition, voice, resonance, feeding, swallowing, and hearing. The practice of speech-language pathology continually evolves. SLPs play critical roles in health literacy; screening, diagnosis, and treatment of autism spectrum disorder; and use of the *International Classification of Functioning, Disability and Health* (ICF; World Health Organization [WHO], 2014) to develop functional goals and collaborative practice. As technology and science advance, the areas of assessment and intervention related to communication and swallowing disorders grow accordingly. Clinicians should stay current with advances in speech-language pathology practice by regularly reviewing the research literature, consulting the Practice Management section of the ASHA website, including the Practice Portal, and regularly participating in continuing education to supplement advances in the profession and information in the scope of practice.

STATEMENT OF PURPOSE

The purpose of the *Scope of Practice in Speech-Language Pathology* is to:

1. Delineate areas of professional practice;
2. Inform others (e.g., health care providers, educators, consumers, payers, regulators, and the general public) about professional roles and responsibilities of qualified providers;
3. Support SLPs in the provision of high-quality, evidence-based services to individuals with communication, feeding, and/or swallowing concerns;
4. Support SLPs in the conduct and dissemination of research; and
5. Guide the educational preparation and professional development of SLPs to provide safe and effective services.

The scope of practice outlines the breadth of professional services offered within the profession of speech-language pathology. Levels of education, experience, skill, and proficiency in each practice area identified within this scope will vary among providers. An SLP typically does not practice in all areas of clinical service delivery across the life cycle. As the ASHA Code of Ethics specifies, professionals may practice only in areas in which they are competent, based on their education, training, and experience.

This scope of practice document describes evolving areas of practice. These include interdisciplinary work in both health care and educational settings, collaborative service delivery wherever appropriate, and telehealth/telepractice that are effective for the general public.

Speech-language pathology is a dynamic profession, and the overlapping of scopes of practice is a reality in rapidly changing health care, education, and other environments. Hence, SLPs in various settings work collaboratively with other school or health care professionals to make sound decisions for the benefit of individuals with communication and swallowing disorders. This *interprofessional collaborative practice* is defined as "members or students of two or more professions associated with health or social care, engaged in learning with, from and about each other" (Craddock, O'Halloran, Borthwick, & McPherson, 2006, p. 237). Similarly, "interprofessional education provides an ability to share skills and knowledge between professions and allows for a better understanding, shared values, and respect for the roles of other healthcare professionals" (Bridges, Davidson, Odegard, Maki, & Tomkowiak, 2011, para. 5).

This scope of practice does not supersede existing state licensure laws or affect the interpretation or implementation of such laws. However, it may serve as a model for the development or modification of licensure laws. Finally, in addition to this scope of practice document, other ASHA professional resources outline practice areas and address issues related to public protection (e.g., a guide to disability rights law and the Practice Portal). The highest standards of integrity and ethical conduct are held paramount in this profession.

DEFINITIONS OF SPEECH-LANGUAGE PATHOLOGIST AND SPEECH-LANGUAGE PATHOLOGY

Speech-language pathologists (SLPs), as defined by ASHA, are professionals who hold the ASHA Certificate of Clinical Competence in Speech-Language Pathology (CCC-SLP), which requires a master's, doctoral, or other recognized postbaccalaureate degree. ASHA-certified SLPs complete a supervised postgraduate professional experience and pass a national examination as described in the ASHA certification standards (2014). Demonstration of continued professional development is mandated for the maintenance of the CCC-SLP. SLPs hold other required credentials where applicable (e.g., state licensure, teaching certification, specialty certification).

Each practitioner evaluates his or her own experiences with preservice education, practice, mentorship and supervision, and continuing professional development. As a whole, these experiences define the scope of competence for each individual. The SLP should engage in only those aspects of the profession that are within her or his professional competence.

SLPs are autonomous professionals who are the primary care providers of speech-language pathology services. Speech-language pathology services are not prescribed or supervised by another professional. Additional requirements may dictate that speech-language pathology services are prescribed and required to meet specific eligibility criteria in certain work settings, or as required by certain payers. SLPs use professional judgment to determine if additional requirements are indicated. Individuals with communication and/or swallowing disorders benefit from services that include collaboration by SLPs with other professionals.

The profession of speech-language pathology contains a broad area of speech-language pathology practice that includes both speech-language pathology service delivery and professional practice domains. These domains are defined in subsequent sections of this document and are represented schematically in **Figure 1**.

FRAMEWORK FOR SPEECH-LANGUAGE PATHOLOGY PRACTICE

The overall objective of speech-language pathology services is to optimize individuals' abilities to communicate and to swallow, thereby improving quality of life. As the population of the United States continues to become increasingly diverse, SLPs are committed to the provision of culturally and linguistically appropriate services and to the consideration of diversity in scientific investigations of human communication and swallowing.

An important characteristic of the practice of speech-language pathology is that, to the extent possible, decisions are based on best available evidence. ASHA defines *evidence-based practice* in speech-language pathology as an approach in which current, high-quality research evidence is integrated with practitioner expertise, along with the client's values and preferences (ASHA, 2005). A high-quality basic and applied research base in communication sciences and disorders and related disciplines is essential to providing evidence-based practice and high-quality services. Increased national and international interchange of professional knowledge,

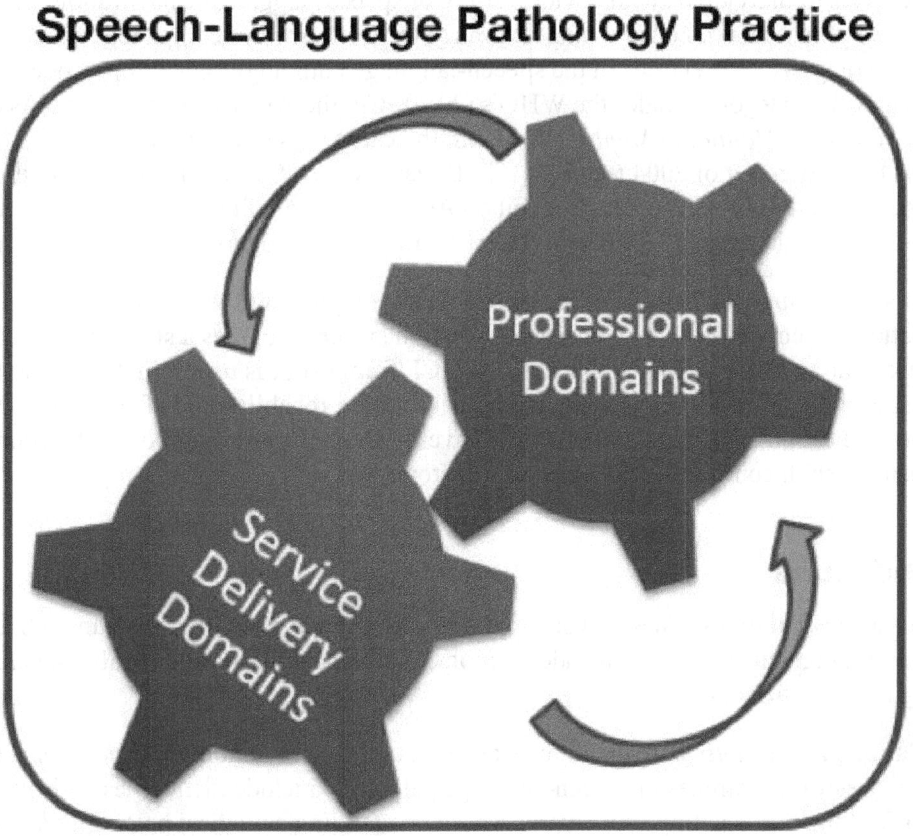

Speech-Language Pathology Practice

Figure 1   Schematic Representation of Speech-Language Pathology Practice, Including Both Service Delivery and Professional Domains.

information, and education in communication sciences and disorders is a means to strengthen research collaboration and improve services. ASHA has provided a resource for evidence-based research via the Practice Portal.

The scope of practice in speech-language pathology comprises five domains of professional practice and eight domains of service delivery.

Professional practice domains:

- Supervision
- Education
- Administration/Leadership
- Research

Service delivery domains:

- Counseling
- Prevention and Wellness
- Screening
- Assessment
- Treatment
- Modalities, Technology, and Instrumentation
- Population and Systems

SLPs provide services to individuals with a wide variety of speech, language, and swallowing differences and disorders within the above-mentioned domains that range in function from completely intact to completely compromised. The diagnostic categories in the speech-language pathology scope of practice are consistent with relevant diagnostic categories under the WHO's (2014) *ICF*, the American Psychiatric Association's (2013) *Diagnostic and Statistical Manual of Mental Disorders*, the categories of disability under the Individuals with Disabilities Education Act of 2004 (see also U.S. Department of Education, 2004), and those defined by two semiautonomous bodies of ASHA: the Council on Academic Accreditation in Audiology and Speech-Language Pathology and the Council for Clinical Certification in Audiology and Speech-Language Pathology.

The domains of speech-language pathology service delivery complement the *ICF*, the WHO's multipurpose health classification system (WHO, 2014). The classification system provides a standard language and framework for the description of functioning and health. The ICF framework is useful in describing the breadth of the role of the SLP in the prevention, assessment, and habilitation/rehabilitation of communication and swallowing disorders and the enhancement and scientific investigation of those functions. The framework consists of two components: health conditions and contextual factors.

Health Conditions

Body Functions and Structures: These involve the anatomy and physiology of the human body. Relevant examples in speech-language pathology include craniofacial anomaly, vocal fold paralysis, cerebral palsy, stuttering, and language impairment.

Activity and Participation: *Activity* refers to the execution of a task or action. *Participation* is the involvement in a life situation. Relevant examples in speech-language pathology include difficulties with swallowing safely for independent feeding, participating actively in class, understanding a medical prescription, and accessing the general education curriculum.

Contextual Factors

Environmental Factors: These make up the physical, social, and attitudinal environments in which people live and conduct their lives. Relevant examples in speech-language pathology include the role of the communication partner in augmentative and alternative communication (AAC), the influence of classroom acoustics on communication, and the impact of institutional dining environments on individuals' ability to safely maintain nutrition and hydration.

Personal Factors: These are the internal influences on an individual's functioning and disability and are not part of the health condition. Personal factors may include, but are not limited to, age, gender, ethnicity, educational level, social background, and profession. Relevant examples in speech-language pathology might include an individual's background or culture, if one or both influence his or her reaction to communication or swallowing.

The framework in speech-language pathology encompasses these health conditions and contextual factors across individuals and populations. **Figure 2** illustrates the interaction of the various components of the ICF. The health condition component is expressed on a continuum of functioning. On one end of the continuum is intact functioning; at the opposite end of the continuum is completely compromised function. The contextual factors interact with each other and with the health conditions and may serve as facilitators or barriers to functioning. SLPs influence contextual factors through education and advocacy efforts at local, state, and national levels.

DOMAINS OF SPEECH-LANGUAGE PATHOLOGY SERVICE DELIVERY

The eight domains of speech-language pathology service delivery are collaboration; counseling; prevention and wellness; screening; assessment; treatment; modalities, technology, and instrumentation; and population and systems.

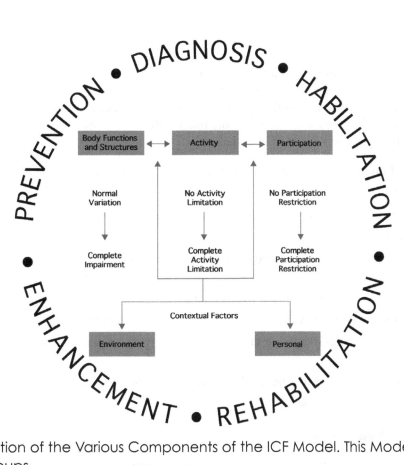

Figure 2   Interaction of the Various Components of the ICF Model. This Model Applies to Individuals or Groups.

Collaboration

SLPs share responsibility with other professionals for creating a collaborative culture. Collaboration requires joint communication and shared decision making among all members of the team, including the individual and family, to accomplish improved service delivery and functional outcomes for the individuals served. When discussing specific roles of team members, professionals are ethically and legally obligated to determine whether they have the knowledge and skills necessary to perform such services. Collaboration occurs across all speech-language pathology practice domains.

As our global society is becoming more connected, integrated, and interdependent, SLPs have access to a variety of resources, information technology, diverse perspectives and influences (see, e.g., Lipinski, Lombardo, Dominy, & Feeney, 1997). Increased national and international interchange of professional knowledge, information, and education in communication sciences and disorders is a means to strengthen research collaboration and improve services. SLPs:

- Educate stakeholders regarding interprofessional education (IPE) and interprofessional practice (IPP; ASHA, 2014) principles and competencies;
- Partner with other professions/organizations to enhance the value of speech-language pathology services;
- Share responsibilities to achieve functional outcomes;
- Consult with other professionals to meet the needs of individuals with communication and swallowing disorders;
- Serve as case managers, service delivery coordinators, members of collaborative and patient care conference teams; and
- Serve on early intervention and school prereferral and intervention teams to assist with the development and implementation of individualized family service plans (IFSPs) and individualized education programs (IEPs).

Counseling

SLPs counsel by providing education, guidance, and support. Individuals, their families, and their caregivers are counseled regarding acceptance, adaptation, and decision making about communication, feeding and swallowing, and related disorders. The role of the SLP in the counseling process includes interactions related to emotional reactions, thoughts, feelings, and behaviors that result from living with the communication disorder, feeding and swallowing disorder, or related disorders.

SLPs engage in the following activities in counseling persons with communication and feeding and swallowing disorders and their families:

- Empower the individual and family to make informed decisions related to communication or feeding and swallowing issues.

- Educate the individual, family, and related community members about communication or feeding and swallowing disorders.

- Provide support and/or peer-to-peer groups for individuals with disorders and their families.

- Provide individuals and families with skills that enable them to become self-advocates.

- Discuss, evaluate, and address negative emotions and thoughts related to communication or feeding and swallowing disorders.

- Refer individuals with disorders to other professionals when counseling needs fall outside of those related to (a) communication and (b) feeding and swallowing.

Prevention and Wellness

SLPs are involved in prevention and wellness activities that are geared toward reducing the incidence of a new disorder or disease, identifying disorders at an early stage, and decreasing the severity or impact of a disability associated with an existing disorder or disease. Involvement is directed toward individuals who are vulnerable or at risk for limited participation in communication, hearing, feeding and swallowing, and related abilities. Activities are directed toward enhancing or improving general well-being and quality of life. Education efforts focus on identifying and increasing awareness of risk behaviors that lead to communication disorders and feeding and swallowing problems. SLPs promote programs to increase public awareness, which are aimed at positively changing behaviors or attitudes.

Effective prevention programs are often community based and enable the SLP to help reduce the incidence of spoken and written communication and swallowing disorders as a public health and public education concern.

Examples of prevention and wellness programs include, but are not limited to, the following:

- *Language impairment:* Educate parents, teachers and other school-based professionals about the clinical markers of language impairment and the ways in which these impairments can impact a student's reading and writing skills to facilitate early referral for evaluation and assessment services.

- *Language-based literacy disorders:* Educate parents, school personnel, and health care providers about the SLP's role in addressing the semantic, syntactic, morphological, and phonological aspects of literacy disorders across the lifespan.

- *Feeding:* Educate parents of infants at risk for feeding problems about techniques to minimize long-term feeding challenges.

- *Stroke prevention:* Educate individuals about risk factors associated with stroke.

- *Serve on teams:* Participate on multitiered systems of support (MTSS)/response to intervention (RTI) teams to help students successfully communicate within academic, classroom, and social settings.

- *Fluency:* Educate parents about risk factors associated with early stuttering.

- *Early childhood:* Encourage parents to participate in early screening and to collaborate with physicians, educators, child care providers, and others to recognize warning signs of developmental disorders during routine wellness checks and to promote healthy communication development practices.

- *Prenatal care:* Educate parents to decrease the incidence of speech, hearing, feeding and swallowing, and related disorders due to problems during pregnancy.

- *Genetic counseling:* Refer individuals to appropriate professionals and professional services if there is a concern or need for genetic counseling.

- *Environmental change:* Modify environments to decrease the risk of occurrence (e.g., decrease noise exposure).

- *Vocal hygiene:* Target prevention of voice disorders (e.g., encourage activities that minimize phonotrauma and the development of benign vocal fold pathology and that curb the use of smoking and smokeless tobacco products).

- *Hearing:* Educate individuals about risk factors associated with noise-induced hearing loss and preventive measures that may help to decrease the risk.

- *Concussion /traumatic brain injury awareness:* Educate parents of children involved in contact sports about the risk of concussion.

- *Accent/dialect modification:* Address sound pronunciation, stress, rhythm, and intonation of speech to enhance effective communication.

- *Transgender (TG) and transsexual (TS) voice and communication:* Educate and treat individuals about appropriate verbal, nonverbal, and voice characteristics (feminization or masculinization) that are congruent with their targeted gender identity.

- *Business communication:* Educate individuals about the importance of effective business communication, including oral, written, and interpersonal communication.

- *Swallowing:* Educate individuals who are at risk for aspiration about oral hygiene techniques.

Screening

SLPs are experts at screening individuals for possible communication, hearing, and/or feeding and swallowing disorders. SLPs have the knowledge of—and skills to treat—these disorders; they can design and implement effective screening programs and make appropriate referrals. These screenings facilitate referral for appropriate follow-up in a timely and cost-effective manner. SLPs:

- Select and use appropriate screening instrumentation;

- Develop screening procedures and tools based on existing evidence;

- Coordinate and conduct screening programs in a wide variety of educational, community, and health care settings;

- Participate in public school MTSS/RTI team meetings to review data and recommend interventions to satisfy federal and state requirements (e.g., Individuals with Disabilities Education Improvement Act of 2004 [IDEIA] and Section 504 of the Rehabilitation Act of 1973);

- Review and analyze records (e.g., educational, medical);

- Review, analyze, and make appropriate referrals based on results of screenings;

- Consult with others about the results of screenings conducted by other professionals; and

- Utilize data to inform decisions about the health of populations.

Assessment

SLPs have expertise in the differential diagnosis of disorders of communication and swallowing. Communication, speech, language, and swallowing disorders can occur developmentally, as part of a medical condition, or in isolation, without an apparent underlying medical condition. Competent SLPs can diagnose communication and swallowing disorders but do not differentially diagnose medical conditions. The assessment process utilizes the

ICF framework, which includes evaluation of body function, structure, activity, and participation, within the context of environmental and personal factors. The assessment process can include, but is not limited to, culturally and linguistically appropriate behavioral observation and standardized and/or criterion-referenced tools; use of instrumentation; review of records, case history, and prior test results; and interview of the individual and/or family to guide decision making. The assessment process can be carried out in collaboration with other professionals. SLPs:

- Administer standardized and/or criterion-referenced tools to compare individuals with their peers;
- Review medical records to determine relevant health, medical, and pharmacological information;
- Interview individuals and/or family to obtain case history to determine specific concerns;
- Utilize culturally and linguistically appropriate assessment protocols;
- Engage in behavioral observation to determine the individual's skills in a naturalistic setting/context;
- Diagnose communication and swallowing disorders;
- Use endoscopy, videofluoroscopy, and other instrumentation to assess aspects of voice, resonance, velopharyngeal function, and swallowing;
- Document assessment and trial results for selecting AAC interventions and technology, including speech-generating devices (SGDs);
- Participate in meetings adhering to required federal and state laws and regulations (e.g., IDEIA [2004] and Section 504 of the Rehabilitation Act of 1973).
- Document assessment results, including discharge planning;
- Formulate impressions to develop a plan of treatment and recommendations; and
- Discuss eligibility and criteria for dismissal from early intervention and school-based services.

Treatment

Speech-language services are designed to optimize individuals' ability to communicate and swallow, thereby improving quality of life. SLPs develop and implement treatment to address the presenting symptoms or concerns of a communication or swallowing problem or related functional issue. Treatment establishes a new skill or ability or remediates or restores an impaired skill or ability. The ultimate goal of therapy is to improve an individual's functional outcomes. To this end, SLPs:

- Design, implement, and document delivery of service in accordance with best available practice appropriate to the practice setting;
- Provide culturally and linguistically appropriate services;
- Integrate the highest quality available research evidence with practitioner expertise and individual preferences and values in establishing treatment goals;
- Utilize treatment data to guide decisions and determine effectiveness of services;
- Integrate academic materials and goals into treatment;
- Deliver the appropriate frequency and intensity of treatment utilizing best available practice;
- Engage in treatment activities that are within the scope of the professional's competence;
- Utilize AAC performance data to guide clinical decisions and determine the effectiveness of treatment; and
- Collaborate with other professionals in the delivery of services.

Modalities, Technology, and Instrumentation

SLPs use advanced instrumentation and technologies in the evaluation, management, and care of individuals with communication, feeding and swallowing, and related disorders. SLPs are also involved in the research and development of emerging technologies and apply their knowledge in the use of advanced instrumentation and technologies to enhance the quality of the services provided. Some examples of services that SLPs offer in this domain include, but are not limited to, the use of:

- The full range of AAC technologies to help individuals who have impaired ability to communicate verbally on a consistent basis—AAC devices make it possible for many individuals to successfully communicate within their environment and community;

- Endoscopy, videofluoroscopy, fiber-optic evaluation of swallowing (voice, velopharyngeal function, swallowing) and other instrumentation to assess aspects of voice, resonance, and swallowing;

- Telehealth/telepractice to provide individuals with access to services or to provide access to a specialist;

- Ultrasound and other biofeedback systems for individuals with speech sound production, voice, or swallowing disorders; and

- Other modalities (e.g., American Sign Language), where appropriate.

Population and Systems

In addition to direct care responsibilities, SLPs have a role in (a) managing populations to improve overall health and education; (b) improving the experience of the individuals served; and, in some circumstances, (c) reducing the cost of care. SLPs also have a role in improving the efficiency and effectiveness of service delivery. SLPs serve in roles designed to meet the demands and expectations of a changing work environment. SLPs:

- Use plain language to facilitate clear communication for improved health and educationally relevant outcomes;

- Collaborate with other professionals about improving communication with individuals who have communication challenges;

- Improve the experience of care by analyzing and improving communication environments;

- Reduce the cost of care by designing and implementing case management strategies that focus on function and by helping individuals reach their goals through a combination of direct intervention, supervision of and collaboration with other service providers, and engagement of the individual and family in self-management strategies;

- Serve in roles designed to meet the demands and expectations of a changing work environment;

- Contribute to the management of specific populations by enhancing communication between professionals and individuals served;

- Coach families and early intervention providers about strategies and supports for facilitating prelinguistic and linguistic communication skills of infants and toddlers; and

- Support and collaborate with classroom teachers to implement strategies for supporting student access to the curriculum.

Speech-Language Pathology Service Delivery Areas

This list of practice areas and the bulleted examples are not comprehensive. Current areas of practice, such as literacy, have continued to evolve, whereas other new areas of practice are emerging. Please refer to the ASHA Practice Portal for a more extensive list of practice areas.

Fluency

- Stuttering
- Cluttering

Speech Production

- Motor planning and execution
- Articulation
- Phonological

Language: Spoken and written language (listening, processing, speaking, reading, writing, pragmatics)

- Phonology
- Morphology
- Syntax
- Semantics
- Pragmatics (language use and social aspects of communication)
- Prelinguistic communication (e.g., joint attention, intentionality, communicative signaling)
- Paralinguistic communication (e.g., gestures, signs, body language)
- Literacy (reading, writing, spelling)

Cognition

- Attention
- Memory
- Problem solving
- Executive functioning

Voice

- Phonation quality
- Pitch
- Loudness
- Alaryngeal voice

Resonance

- Hypernasality
- Hyponasality
- Cul-de-sac resonance
- Forward focus

Feeding and Swallowing

- Oral phase
- Pharyngeal phase
- Esophageal phase
- Atypical eating (e.g., food selectivity/refusal, negative physiologic response)

Auditory Habilitation/Rehabilitation

- Speech, language, communication, and listening skills impacted by hearing loss, deafness
- Auditory processing

Potential etiologies of communication and swallowing disorders include:

- Neonatal problems (e.g., prematurity, low birth weight, substance exposure);
- Developmental disabilities (e.g., specific language impairment, autism spectrum disorder, dyslexia, learning disabilities, attention-deficit disorder, intellectual disabilities, unspecified neurodevelopmental disorders);

- Disorders of aerodigestive tract function (e.g., irritable larynx, chronic cough, abnormal respiratory patterns or airway protection, paradoxical vocal fold motion, tracheostomy);
- Oral anomalies (e.g., cleft lip/palate, dental malocclusion, macroglossia, oral motor dysfunction);
- Respiratory patterns and compromise (e.g., bronchopulmonary dysplasia, chronic obstructive pulmonary disease);
- Pharyngeal anomalies (e.g., upper airway obstruction, velopharyngeal insufficiency/incompetence);
- Laryngeal anomalies (e.g., vocal fold pathology, tracheal stenosis);
- Neurological disease/dysfunction (e.g., traumatic brain injury, cerebral palsy, cerebrovascular accident, dementia, Parkinson's disease, and amyotrophic lateral sclerosis);
- Psychiatric disorder (e.g., psychosis, schizophrenia);
- Genetic disorders (e.g., Down syndrome, fragile X syndrome, Rett syndrome, velocardiofacial syndrome); and
- Orofacial myofunctional disorders (e.g., habitual open-mouth posture/nasal breathing, orofacial habits, tethered oral tissues, chewing and chewing muscles, lips and tongue resting position).

This list of etiologies is not comprehensive.

Elective services include:

- Transgender communication (e.g., voice, verbal and nonverbal communication);
- Preventive vocal hygiene;
- Business communication;
- Accent/dialect modification; and
- Professional voice use.

This list of elective services is not comprehensive.

DOMAINS OF PROFESSIONAL PRACTICE

This section delineates the domains of professional practice, that is, a set of skills and knowledge that goes beyond clinical practice. The domains of professional practice include advocacy and outreach, supervision, education, research, and administration and leadership.

Advocacy and Outreach

SLPs advocate for the discipline and for individuals through a variety of mechanisms, including community awareness, prevention activities, health literacy, academic literacy, education, political action, and training programs. Advocacy promotes and facilitates access to communication, including the reduction of societal, cultural, and linguistic barriers. SLPs perform a variety of activities, including the following:

- Advise regulatory and legislative agencies about the continuum of care. Examples of service delivery options across the continuum of care include telehealth/telepractice, the use of technology, the use of support personnel, and practicing at the top of the license.
- Engage decision makers at the local, state, and national levels for improved administrative and governmental policies affecting access to services and funding for communication and swallowing issues.
- Advocate at the local, state, and national levels for funding for services, education, and research.
- Participate in associations and organizations to advance the speech-language pathology profession.
- Promote and market professional services.
- Help to recruit and retain SLPs with diverse backgrounds and interests.
- Collaborate on advocacy objectives with other professionals/colleagues regarding mutual goals.

- Serve as expert witnesses, when appropriate.
- Educate consumers about communication disorders and speech-language pathology services.
- Advocate for fair and equitable services for all individuals, especially the most vulnerable.
- Inform state education agencies and local school districts about the various roles and responsibilities of school-based SLPs, including direct service, IEP development, Medicaid billing, planning and delivery of assessment and therapy, consultation with other team members, and attendance at required meetings.

Supervision

Supervision is a distinct area of practice; is the responsibility of SLPs; and crosses clinical, administrative, and technical spheres. SLPs are responsible for supervising Clinical Fellows, graduate externs, trainees, speech-language pathology assistants, and other personnel (e.g., clerical, technical, and other administrative support staff). SLPs may also supervise colleagues and peers. SLPs acknowledge that supervision is integral in the delivery of communication and swallowing services and advances the discipline. Supervision involves education, mentorship, encouragement, counseling, and support across all supervisory roles. SLPs:

- Possess service delivery and professional practice skills necessary to guide the supervisee;
- Apply the art and science of supervision to all stakeholders (i.e., those supervising and being supervised), recognizing that supervision contributes to efficiency in the workplace;
- Seek advanced knowledge in the practice of effective supervision;
- Establish supervisory relationships that are collegial in nature;
- Support supervisees as they learn to handle emotional reactions that may affect the therapeutic process; and
- Establish a supervisory relationship that promotes growth and independence while providing support and guidance.

Education

SLPs serve as educators, teaching students in academic institutions and teaching professionals through continuing education in professional development formats. This more formal teaching is in addition to the education that SLPs provide to individuals, families, caregivers, decision makers, and policy makers, which is described in other domains. SLPs:

- Serve as faculty at institutions of higher education, teaching courses at the undergraduate, graduate, and postgraduate levels;
- Mentor students who are completing academic programs at all levels;
- Provide academic training to students in related disciplines and students who are training to become speech-language pathology assistants; and
- Provide continuing professional education to SLPs and to professionals in related disciplines.

Research

SLPs conduct and participate in basic and applied/translational research related to cognition, verbal and nonverbal communication, pragmatics, literacy (reading, writing, and spelling), and feeding and swallowing. This research may be undertaken as a facility-specific effort or may be coordinated across multiple settings. SLPs engage in activities to ensure compliance with Institutional Review Boards and international laws pertaining to research. SLPs also collaborate with other researchers and may pursue research funding through grants.

Administration and Leadership

SLPs administer programs in education, higher education, schools, health care, private practice, and other settings. In this capacity, they are responsible for making administrative decisions related to fiscal and personnel management; leadership; program design; program growth and innovation; professional development; compliance with laws and regulations; and cooperation with outside agencies in education and health care. Their administrative roles are not limited to speech-language pathology, as they may administer programs across departments and at different levels within an institution. In addition, SLPs promote effective and manageable workloads in school settings, provide appropriate services under IDEIA (2004), and engage in program design and development.

Ad Hoc Committee on the Scope of Practice in Speech-Language Pathology

REFERENCES

American Psychiatric Association. (2013). *Diagnostic and statistical manual of mental disorders* (5th ed.). Washington, DC: Author.

American Speech-Language-Hearing Association (ASHA). (2005). *Evidence-based practice in communication disorders* [Position statement]. Retrieved from www.asha.org/policy/.

American Speech-Language-Hearing Association (ASHA). (2014). *Interprofessional education/interprofessional practice (IPE/IPP)*. Retrieved from www.asha.org/Practice/Interprofessional-Education-Practice/

Bridges, D. R., Davidson, R. A., Odegard, P. S., Maki, I. V., & Tomkowiak, J. (2011). Interprofessional collaboration: Three best practice models of interprofessional education. *Medical Education Online, 16.* doi:10.3402/meo.v16i0.6035. Retrieved from www.ncbi.nlm.nih.gov/pmc/articles/PMC3081249/

Craddock, D., O'Halloran, C., Borthwick, A., & McPherson, K. (2006). Interprofessional education in health and social care: Fashion or informed practice? *Learning in Health and Social Care, 5,* 220–242. Retrieved from http://onlinelibrary.wiley.com/doi/10.1111/j.1473-6861.2006.00135.x/abstract

Individuals with Disabilities Education Act of 2004, 20 U.S.C. § 1400 et seq. (2004).

Individuals with Disabilities Education Improvement Act of 2004, 20 U.S.C. § 1400 et seq. (2004).

Lipinski, C. A., Lombardo, F., Dominy, B. W., & Feeney, P. J. (1997). Experimental and computational approaches to estimate solubility and permeability in drug discovery and development settings. *Advanced Drug Delivery Reviews, 46*(1–3), 3–26. Retrieved from http://www.ncbi.nlm.nih.gov/pubmed/11259830

Rehabilitation Act of 1973, 29 U.S.C. § 701 et seq.

U.S. Department of Education. (2004). *Building the legacy: IDEA 2004*. Retrieved from http://idea.ed.gov/

World Health Organization (WHO). (2014). *International Classification of Functioning, Disability and Health.* Geneva, Switzerland: Author. Retrieved from www.who.int/classifications/icf/en/

Resources

American Speech-Language-Hearing Association. (n.d.). *Introduction to evidence-based practice.* Retrieved from www.asha.org/Research/EBP/Introduction-to-Evidence-Based-Practice/

American Speech-Language-Hearing Association. (n.d.). Practice Portal. Retrieved from http://www.asha.org/practice-portal/

American Speech-Language-Hearing Association. (1991). *A model for collaborative service delivery for students with language-learning disorders in the public schools* [Paper]. Retrieved from www.asha.org/policy/

American Speech-Language-Hearing Association. (2003). *Evaluating and treating communication and cognitive disorders: Approaches to referral and collaboration for speech-language pathology and clinical neuropsychology* [Technical report]. Retrieved from www.asha.org/policy/

Paul, D. (2013). A quick guide to DSM-V. *The ASHA Leader, 18,* 52–54. Retrieved from http://leader.pubs.asha.org/article.aspx?articleid=1785031

U.S. Department of Justice. (2009). *A guide to disability rights laws*. Retrieved from www.ada.gov/cguide.htm

Reference this material as: American Speech-Language-Hearing Association. (2016). *Scope of practice in speech-language pathology* [Scope of Practice]. Retrieved from www.asha.org/policy/.

APPENDIX H.2

Scope of Practice for a Speech-Language Pathology Assistant

Table of Contents

ABOUT THIS DOCUMENT

This scope of practice for the speech-language pathology assistant (SLPA) was developed by the American Speech-Language-Hearing Association (ASHA) Speech-Language Pathology Assistant Scope of Practice ad hoc committee. It was approved by ASHA's Board of Directors (January 2013). Members of the committee were DeAnne Wellman Owre (chair), Diane L. Eger, Ashley Northam, Mary Jo Schill, Rosemary Scott, Monica Marruffo, and Lemmietta McNeilly (ex officio). Gail J. Richard, vice president for speech-language pathology practice, served as the monitoring vice president. The composition of the ad hoc committee included ASHA-certified speech-language pathologists with specific knowledge and experience working with support personnel in clinical practice in schools, health care, and/or private practice, as well as two members who have served on the ASHA Board of Ethics (Diane L. Eger and Mary Jo Schill).

The document is intended to provide guidance for SLPAs and their supervisors regarding ethical considerations related to the SLPA practice parameters. The document addresses how SLPAs should be utilized and what specific responsibilities are within and outside their roles of clinical practice. Given that standards, licensure, and practice issues vary from state to state, this document delineates ASHA's policy for the use of SLPAs.

DEDICATION

In loving memory of Lisa Cabiale O'Connor (1937–2012), whose dedication, commitment, and perseverance contributed to ensuring integrity and quality in addressing the topic of SLPAs within the ASHA structure.

EXECUTIVE SUMMARY

This scope of practice presents a model for the training, use, and supervision of support personnel in speech-language pathology. Support personnel in speech-language pathology, or SLPAs (SLPAs), perform tasks as pre-scribed, directed, and supervised by ASHA-certified speech-language pathologists (SLPs). Support personnel can be used to increase the availability, frequency, and efficiency of services.

Some tasks, procedures, or activities used to treat individuals with communication and related disorders can be performed successfully by individuals other than SLPs if the persons conducting the activity are prop-erly trained and supervised by ASHA-certified and/or licensed SLPs. The decision to shift responsibility for implementation of the more repetitive, mechanical, or routine clinical activities to SLPAs should be made only by qualified professionals and only when the quality of care and level of professionalism will not be compro-mised. The utilization of evidence and ethical and professional judgment should be at the heart of the selection, management, training, supervision, and use of support personnel.

This scope of practice specifies the qualifications and responsibilities for an SLPA and indicates the tasks that are the exclusive responsibilities of the SLP. Additionally, the document provides guidance regarding ethical considerations when support personnel provide clinical services and outlines the supervisory responsibilities of the supervising SLP.

INTRODUCTION

The SLPA scope of practice provides information regarding the training, use, and supervision of assistants in speech-language pathology that was established by the American-Speech-Language-Hearing Association to be applicable in a variety of work settings. Training for SLPAs should be based on the type of tasks specified in their scope of responsibility. Specific education and on-the-job training may be necessary to prepare assistants for unique roles in professional settings (e.g., hospitals and schools).

ASHA has established an associate affiliation program for support personnel in speech-language pathology and audiology. Individuals who are working in this capacity under the direct supervision of ASHA-certified SLPs or audiologists are eligible for this category of affiliation with ASHA.

ASHA has addressed the topic of support personnel in speech-language pathology since the 1960s. In 1967, the Executive Board of ASHA established the Committee on Supportive Personnel and in 1969 the docu-ment *Guidelines on the Role, Training and Supervision of the Communicative Aide* was approved by the

Legislative Council (LC). In the 1990s, several entities—including committees, a task force, and a consensus panel—were established and the LC passed a position statement, technical report, guidelines, and curriculum content for support personnel. In 2002, ASHA developed an approval process for SLPA programs, and in 2003 a registration process for SLPAs was established. Both were discontinued by vote of the LC because of fiscal concerns. In 2004, a position statement on the training, use, and supervision of support personnel in speech-language pathology was passed by the LC. Since then, the number of SLPAs has increased primarily in schools and private practice settings. Specific guidance from ASHA continues to be requested by ASHA members in many states.

This document does not supersede federal legislation and regulation requirements or any existing state licensure laws, nor does it affect the interpretation or implementation of such laws. The document may serve, however, as a guide for the development of new laws or, at the appropriate time, for revising existing licensure laws.

STATEMENT OF PURPOSE

The purpose of this document is to define what is within and outside the scope of responsibilities for SLPAs who work under the supervision of properly credentialed SLPs. The following aspects are addressed:

a. Parameters for education and professional development for SLPAs;

b. SLPAs' responsibilities within and outside the scope of practice;

c. Examples of practice settings;

d. Information for others (e.g., special educators, parents, consumers, health professionals, payers, regulators, members of the general public) regarding services SLPAs perform;

e. Information regarding the ethical and liability considerations for the supervising SLP and the SLPA;

f. Supervisory requirements for the SLP and the SLPA.

QUALIFICATIONS FOR A SPEECH-LANGUAGE PATHOLOGY ASSISTANT

Minimum Recommended Qualifications for a Speech-Language Pathology Assistant

An SLPA must complete an approved course of academic study, field work under the supervision of an ASHA-certified and/or licensed SLP, and on-the-job training specific to SLPA responsibilities and workplace behaviors.

The academic course of study must include or be equivalent to:

a. An associate's degree in an SLPA program or a bachelor's degree in a speech-language pathology or communication disorders program, and

b. Successful completion of a minimum of one hundred (100) hours of supervised field work experience or its clinical experience equivalent and

c. Demonstration of competency in the skills required of an SLPA.

Expectations of a Speech-Language Pathology Assistant

a. Seek employment only in settings in which direct and indirect supervision are provided on a regular and systematic basis by an ASHA-certified and/or licensed SLP.

b. Adhere to the responsibilities for SLPAs specified in this document and refrain from performing tasks or activities that are the sole responsibility of the SLP.

c. Perform only those tasks prescribed by the supervising SLP.

d. Adhere to all applicable state licensure laws and rules regulating the practice of speech-language pathology, such as those requiring licensure or registration of support personnel.

e. Conduct oneself ethically within the scope of practice and responsibilities for an SLPA.

f. Actively participate with the SLP in the supervisory process.

g. Consider securing liability insurance.

h. Actively pursue continuing education and professional development activities.

RESPONSIBILITIES WITHIN THE SCOPE FOR SPEECH-LANGUAGE PATHOLOGY ASSISTANTS

The supervising SLP retains full legal and ethical responsibility for the students, patients, and clients he or she serves but may delegate specific tasks to the SLPA. The SLPA may execute specific components of a speech and language program as specified in treatment plans developed by the SLP. Goals and objectives listed on the treatment plan and implemented by the SLPA are only those within their scope of responsibilities and are tasks the SLP has determined the SLPA has the training and skill to perform. The SLP must provide at least the minimum specified level of supervision to ensure quality of care to all persons served. The amount of supervision may vary and must depend on the complexity of the case and the experience of the assistant. Under no circumstances should use of the ASHA Code of Ethics or the quality of services provided be diluted or circumvented by the use of an SLPA. Again, the use of an SLPA is optional, and an SLPA should be used only when appropriate.

Provided that the training, supervision, and planning are appropriate, tasks in the following areas of focus may be delegated to an SLPA.

Service Delivery

a. Self-identify as SLPAs to families, students, patients, clients, staff, and others. This may be done verbally, in writing, and/or with titles on name badges.

b. Exhibit compliance with The Health Insurance Portability and Accountability Act (HIPAA) and Family Educational Rights and Privacy Act (FERPA) regulations, reimbursement requirements, and SLPAs' responsibilities.

c. Assist the SLP with speech, language, and hearing screenings **without** clinical interpretation.

d. Assist the SLP during assessment of students, patients, and clients exclusive of administration and/or interpretation

e. Assist the SLP with bilingual translation during screening and assessment activities exclusive of interpretation; refer to *Knowledge and Skills Needed by Speech-Language Pathologists and Audiologists to Provide Culturally and Linguistically Appropriate Services* (ASHA 2004).

f. Follow documented treatment plans or protocols developed by the supervising SLP.

g. Provide guidance and treatment via telepractice to students, patients, and clients who are selected by the supervising SLP as appropriate for this service delivery model.

h. Document student, patient, and client performance (e.g., tallying data for the SLP to use; preparing charts, records, and graphs) and report this information to the supervising SLP.

i. Program and provide instruction in the use of augmentative and alternative communication devices.

j. Demonstrate or share information with patients, families, and staff regarding feeding strategies developed and directed by the SLP.

k. Serve as interpreter for patients/clients/students and families who do not speak English.

l. Provide services under SLP supervision in another language for individuals who do not speak English and English-language learners.

Administrative Support

a.   Assist with clerical duties, such as preparing materials and scheduling activities, as directed by the SLP.

b.   Perform checks and maintenance of equipment.

c.   Assist with departmental operations (scheduling, recordkeeping, safety/maintenance of supplies and equipment).

Prevention and Advocacy

a.   Present primary prevention information to individuals and groups known to be at risk for communication disorders and other appropriate groups; promote early identification and early intervention activities.

b.   Advocate for individuals and families through community awareness, health literacy, education, and training programs to promote and facilitate access to full participation in communication, including the elimination of societal, cultural, and linguistic barriers.

c.   Provide information to emergency response agencies for individuals who have communication and/or swallowing disorders.

d.   Advocate at the local, state, and national levels for improved public policies affecting access to services and research funding.

e.   Support the supervising SLP in research projects, in-service training, public relations programs, and marketing programs.

f.   Participate actively in professional organizations.

RESPONSIBILITIES OUTSIDE THE SCOPE FOR SPEECH-LANGUAGE PATHOLOGY ASSISTANTS

There is potential for misuse of an SLPA, particularly when responsibilities are delegated by administrative or nonclinical staff without the approval of the supervising SLP. It is highly recommended that the *ASHA Scope of Practice for Speech-Language Pathology Assistants* (ASHA, 2007) and the *ASHA Code of Ethics* (ASHA, 2010a) be reviewed with all personnel involved when employing an SLPA. It should be emphasized that an individual's communication or related disorder and/or other factors may preclude the use of services from anyone other than an ASHA-certified and/or licensed SLP. The SLPA should not perform any task without the approval of the supervising SLP. The student, patient, or client should be informed that he or she is receiving services from an SLPA under the supervision of an SLP.

The SLPA should *NOT* engage in the following:

a.   Represent himself or herself as an SLP;

b.   Perform standardized or nonstandardized diagnostic tests, formal or informal evaluations, or swallowing screenings/checklists;

c.   Perform procedures that require a high level of clinical acumen and technical skill (e.g., vocal tract prosthesis shaping or fitting, vocal tract imaging, and oral pharyngeal swallow therapy with bolus material);

d.   Tabulate or interpret results and observations of feeding and swallowing evaluations performed by SLPs;

e.   Participate in formal parent conferences, case conferences, or any interdisciplinary team without the presence of the supervising SLP or other designated SLP;

f.   Provide interpretative information to the student/patient/client, family, or others regarding the patient/client status or service;

g.   Write, develop, or modify a student's, patient's, or client's treatment plan in any way;

h.   Assist with students, patients, or clients without following the individualized treatment plan prepared by the certified SLP and/or without access to supervision;

i.   Sign any formal documents (e.g., treatment plans, reimbursement forms, or reports; the SLPA **should** sign initial informal treatment notes for review and cosign with the supervising SLP as requested);

j. Select students, patients, or clients for service;

k. Discharge a student, patient, or client from services;

l. Make referrals for additional service;

m. Disclose clinical or confidential information either orally or in writing to anyone other than the supervising SLP (the SLPA must comply with current HIPPA and FERPA guidelines) unless mandated by law;

n. Develop or determine the swallowing strategies or precautions for patients, family, or staff;

o. Treat medically fragile students/patients/clients independently;

p. Design or select augmentative and alternative communication systems or devices.

PRACTICE SETTINGS

Under the specified guidance and supervision of an ASHA-certified SLP, SLPAs may provide services in a wide variety of settings, which may include, but are not limited to, the following:

a. Public, private, and charter elementary and secondary schools;

b. Early intervention settings, preschools, and day care settings;

c. Hospitals (in- and outpatient);

d. Residential health care settings (e.g., long-term care and skilled nursing facilities);

e. Nonresidential health care settings (e.g., home health agencies, adult day care settings, clinics);

f. Private practice settings;

g. University/college clinics;

h. Research facilities;

i. Corporate and industrial settings;

j. Student/patient/client's residences.

ETHICAL CONSIDERATIONS

ASHA strives to ensure that its members and certificate holders preserve the highest standards of integrity and ethical practice. The *ASHA Code of Ethics* (2010a) sets forth the fundamental principles and rules considered essential to this purpose. The code applies to every individual who is (a) a member of ASHA, whether certified or not, (b) a nonmember holding the ASHA Certificate of Clinical Competence, (c) an applicant for membership or certification, or (d) a Clinical Fellow seeking to fulfill standards for certification.

Although some SLPAs may choose to affiliate with ASHA as associates, the Code of Ethics does not directly apply to associates. However, any individual who is working in a support role (technician, aide, assistant) under the supervision of an SLP or speech scientist must be knowledgeable about the provisions of the code. It is imperative that the supervising professional and the assistant behave in a manner that is consistent with the principles and rules outlined in the ASHA Code of Ethics. Since the ethical responsibility for patient care or for subjects in research studies cannot be delegated, the SLP or speech scientist takes overall responsibility for the actions of the assistants when they are performing assigned duties. If the assistant engages in activities that violate the Code of Ethics, the supervising professional may be found in violation of the code if adequate oversight has not been provided.

The following principles and rules of the ASHA Code of Ethics specifically address issues that are pertinent when an SLP supervises support personnel in the provision of services or when conducting research.

Principle of Ethics I: Individuals shall honor their responsibility to hold paramount the welfare of persons they serve professionally or who are participants in research and scholarly activities and they shall treat animals involved in research in a humane manner.

Guidance:

The supervising SLP remains responsible for the care and well-being of the client or research subject. If the supervisor fails to intervene when the assistant's behavior puts the client or subject at risk or when services or procedures are implemented inappropriately, the supervisor could be in violation of the Code of Ethics.

Principle of Ethics I, Rule A: Individuals shall provide all services competently.

Guidance:

The supervising SLP must ensure that all services, including those provided directly by the assistant, meet practice standards and are administered competently. If the supervisor fails to intervene or correct the actions of the assistant as needed, this could be a violation of the Code of Ethics.

Principle of Ethics I, Rule D: Individuals shall not misrepresent the credentials of assistants, technicians, support personnel, students, Clinical Fellows, or any others under their supervision, and they shall inform those they serve professionally of the name and professional credentials of persons providing services.

Guidance:

The supervising SLP must ensure that clients and subjects are informed of the title and qualifications of the assistant. This is not a passive responsibility; that is, the supervisor must make this information easily available and understandable to the clients or subjects and not rely on the individual to inquire about or ask directly for this information. Any misrepresentation of the assistant's qualifications or role could result in a violation of the Code of Ethics by the supervisor.

Principle of Ethics I, Rule E: Individuals who hold the Certificate of Clinical Competence shall not delegate tasks that require the unique skills, knowledge, and judgment that are within the scope of their profession to assistants, technicians, support personnel, or any nonprofessionals over whom they have supervisory responsibility.

Guidance:

The supervising SLP is responsible for monitoring and limiting the role of the assistant as described in these guidelines and in accordance with applicable licensure laws.

Principle of Ethics I, Rule F: Individuals who hold the Certificate of Clinical Competence may delegate tasks related to provision of clinical services to assistants, technicians, support personnel, or any other persons only if those services are appropriately supervised, realizing that the responsibility for client welfare remains with the certified individual.

Guidance:

The supervising SLP is responsible for providing appropriate and adequate direct and indirect supervision to ensure that the services provided are appropriate and meet practice standards. The SLP should document supervisory activities and adjust the amount and type of supervision to ensure that the Code of Ethics is not violated.

Principle of Ethics II, Rule B: Individuals shall engage in only those aspects of the professions that are within the scope of their professional practice and competence, considering their level of education, training, and experience.

Guidance:

The supervising SLP is responsible for ensuring that he or she has the skills and competencies needed in order to provide appropriate supervision. This may include seeking continuing education in the area of supervision practice.

Principle of Ethics II, Rule D: Individuals shall not require or permit their professional staff to provide services or conduct research activities that exceed the staff member's competence, level of education, training, and experience.

Guidance:

The supervising SLP must ensure that the assistant only performs those activities and duties that are defined as appropriate for the level of training and experience and in accordance with applicable licensure laws. If the assistant exceeds the practice role that has been defined for him or her, and the supervisor fails to correct this, the supervisor could be found in violation of the Code of Ethics.

Principle of Ethics IV, Rule B: Individuals shall prohibit anyone under their supervision from engaging in any practice that violates the Code of Ethics.

Guidance:

Because the assistant provides services as "an extension" of those provided by the professional, the SLP is responsible for informing the assistant about the Code of Ethics and monitoring the performance of the assistant. Failure to do so could result in the SLP's being found in violation of the Code.

LIABILITY ISSUES

Individuals who engage in the delivery of services to persons with communication disorders are potentially vulnerable to accusations of engaging in unprofessional practices. Therefore, liability insurance is recommended as a protection for malpractice. SLPAs should consider the need for liability coverage. Some employers provide it for all employees. Other employers defer to the employee to independently acquire liability insurance. Some universities provide coverage for students involved in practicum/fieldwork. Checking for liability insurance coverage is the responsibility of the SLPA and needs to be done prior to providing services.

SPEECH-LANGUAGE PATHOLOGIST'S SUPERVISORY ROLE

Qualifications for a Supervising Speech-Language Pathologist

Minimum qualifications for an SLP who will supervise an SLPA include:

a. Current ASHA certification and/or state licensure;
b. Completion of at least 2 years of practice following ASHA certification;
c. Completion of an academic course or at least 10 hours of continuing education credits in the area of supervision, completed prior to or concurrent with the first SLPA supervision experience.

Additional Expectations of the Supervising Speech-Language Pathologist

a. Conduct ongoing competency evaluations of the SLPAs.
b. Provide and encourage ongoing education and training opportunities for the SLPA consistent with competency and skills and needs of the students, patients, or clients served.
c. Develop, review, and modify treatment plans for students, patients, and clients that SLPAs implement under the supervision of the SLP.
d. Make all case management decisions.
e. Adhere to the supervisory responsibilities for SLPs.
f. Retain the legal and ethical responsibility for all students, patients, and clients served.
g. Adhere to the principles and rules of the ASHA Code of Ethics.
h. Adhere to applicable licensure laws and rules regulating the practice of speech-language pathology.

GUIDELINES FOR SLP SUPERVISION OF SPEECH-LANGUAGE PATHOLOGY ASSISTANTS

It is the SLP's responsibility to design and implement a supervision system that protects the students', patients', and clients' care and maintains the highest possible standards of quality. The amount and type of supervision should meet the minimum requirements and be increased as needed based on the needs, competencies, skills, expectations, philosophies, and experience of the SLPA and the supervisor; the needs of students, patients, and clients served; the service setting; the tasks assigned; and other factors. More intense supervision, for example, would be required in such instances as the orientation of a new SLPA; initiation of a new program, equipment, or task; or a change in student, patient, or client status (e.g., medical complications). Functional assessment of the SLPA's skills with assigned tasks should be an ongoing, regular, and integral element of supervision. SLPs and SLPAs should treat each other with respect and interact in a professional manner.

As the supervisory responsibility of the SLP increases, overall responsibilities will change because the SLP is responsible for the students, patients, and clients as well as for supervision of the SLPA. Therefore, adequate time for direct and indirect supervision of the SLPA(s) and caseload management must be allotted as a critical part of the SLP's workload. The purpose of the assistant level position is not to significantly increase the caseload size for SLPs. Assistants should be used to deliver services to individuals on the SLP's caseload. Under no circumstances should an assistant have his or her own caseload.

Diagnosis and treatment for the students, patients, and clients served remains the legal and ethical responsibility of the supervisor. Therefore, the level of supervision required is considered the minimum level necessary for the supervisor to retain direct contact with the students, patients, and clients. The supervising SLP is responsible for designing and implementing a supervisory plan that protects consumer care, maintains the highest quality of practice, and documents the supervisory activities.

The supervising SLP must:

a. Hold a Certificate of Clinical Competence in Speech-Language Pathology from ASHA and/or a state licensure (where applicable);
b. Have an active interest in use of and desire to use support personnel;
c. Have practiced speech-language pathology for at least 2 years following ASHA certification;
d. Have completed or be currently enrolled in at least one course or workshop in supervision for at least 1.0 CEUs (10 clock hours).

The relationship between the supervising SLP and the SLPA is paramount to the welfare of the client. Because the clinical supervision process is a close, interpersonal experience, the supervising SLP should participate in the selection of the SLPA when possible.

SLP to SLPA Ratio

Although more than one SLP may provide supervision of an SLPA, an SLP should not supervise or be listed as a supervisor for more than two full-time equivalent (FTE) SLPAs in any setting or combination thereof. The supervising SLP should assist in determining the appropriate number of assistants who can be managed within his or her workload. When multiple supervisors are used, it is critical that the supervisors coordinate and communicate with each other so that minimum supervisory requirements are met and that the quality of services is maintained.

Minimum Requirements for the Frequency and Amount of Supervision

First 90 workdays: A total of at least 30% supervision, including at least 20% direct and 10% indirect supervision, is required weekly. Direct supervision of student, patient, and client care should be no less than 20% of the actual student, patient, and client contact time weekly for each SLPA. This ensures that the supervisor will have direct contact time with the SLPA as well as with the student, patient, or client. During each week, data on every student, patient, and client seen by the SLPA should be reviewed by the supervisor. In addition, the direct supervision should be scheduled so that all students, patients, and clients seen by the assistant are directly supervised in a timely manner. Supervision days and time of day (morning/afternoon) may be alternated to ensure that all students, patients, and clients receive some direct contact with the SLP **at least once every 2 weeks**.

After first 90 workdays: The amount of supervision can be adjusted if the supervising SLP determines the SLPA has met appropriate competencies and skill levels with a variety of communication and related disorders.

Minimum ongoing supervision must always include documentation of direct supervision provided by the SLP to each student, patient, or client **at least every 60 calendar days.**

A minimum of 1 hour of direct supervision weekly and as much indirect supervision as needed to facilitate the delivery of quality services must be maintained.

Documentation of all supervisory activities, both direct and indirect, must be accurately recorded.

Further, 100% direct supervision of SLPAs for medically fragile students, patients, or clients is required.

The supervising SLP is responsible for designing and implementing a supervisory plan that ensures the highest standard of quality care can be maintained for students, patients, and clients. The amount and type of supervision required should be consistent with the skills and experience of the SLPA; the needs of the students, patients, and clients; the service setting; the tasks assigned; and the laws and regulations that govern SLPAs. Treatment of the student, patient, or client remains the responsibility of the supervisor.

Direct supervision means on-site, in-view observation and guidance while a clinical activity is performed by the assistant. This can include the supervising SLP viewing and communicating with the SLPA via telecommunication technology as the SLPA provides clinical services, because this allows the SLP to provide ongoing immediate feedback. Direct supervision does not include reviewing a taped session at a later time.

Supervision feedback should provide information about the quality of the SLPA's performance of assigned tasks and should verify that clinical activity is limited to tasks specified in the SLPA's ASHA-approved responsibilities. Information obtained during direct supervision may include, but is not limited to, data relative to (a) agreement (reliability) between the assistant and the supervisor on correct/incorrect recording of target behavior, (b) accuracy in implementation of assigned treatment procedures, (c) accuracy in recording data, and (d) ability to interact effectively with the patient, client, or student during presentation and application of assigned therapeutic procedures or activities.

Indirect supervision does not require the SLP to be physically present or available via telecommunication in real time while the SLPA is providing services. Indirect supervisory activities may include demonstration tapes, record review, review and evaluation of audio or videotaped sessions, and/or supervisory conferences that may be conducted by telephone and/or live, secure webcam via the Internet. The SLP will review each treatment plan as needed for timely implementation of modifications.

An SLPA may not perform tasks when a supervising SLP cannot be reached by personal contact, phone, pager, or other immediate or electronic means. If for any reason (i.e., maternity leave, illness, change of jobs) the supervisor is no longer available to provide the level of supervision stipulated, the SLPA may not perform assigned tasks until an ASHA-certified and/or state-licensed SLP with experience and training in supervision has been designated as the new supervising SLP.

Any supervising SLP who will not be able to supervise an SLPA for more than 1 week will need to (a) inform the SLPA of the planned absence and (b) make other arrangements for the SLPA's supervision of services while the SLP is unavailable or (c) inform the clients/student/patients that services will be rescheduled.

CONCLUSION

It is the intent of this document to provide guidance for the use of SLPAs in appropriate settings, thereby increasing access to timely and efficient speech-language services. It is the responsibility of the supervising speech-language pathologists to stay abreast of current guidelines and to ensure the quality of services rendered.

DEFINITIONS

Accountability

Accountability refers to being legally responsible and answerable for actions and inactions of self or others during the performance of a task by the SLPA.

Direct Supervision

Direct supervision means on-site, in-view observation and guidance by an SLP while an assigned activity is performed by support personnel. Direct supervision performed by the supervising SLP may include, but is not limited to, the following: observation of a portion of the screening or treatment procedures performed by the SLPA, coaching the SLPA, and modeling for the SLPA. The supervising SLP must be physically present during all services provided to a medically fragile client by the SLPA (e.g., general and telesupervision). The SLP can view and communicate with the patient and SLPA live via real-time telecommunication technology to supervise the SLPA, giving the SLP the opportunity to provide immediate feedback. This does not include reviewing a taped session later.

Indirect Supervision

Indirect supervision means the supervising SLP is not at the same facility or in close proximity to the SLPA, but is available to provide supervision by electronic means. Indirect supervision activities performed by the supervising SLP may include, but are not limited to, demonstration, record review, review and evaluation of audio or videotaped sessions, and interactive television and supervisory conferences that may be conducted by telephone, e-mail, or live webcam.

Interpretation

Summarizing, integrating, and using data for the purpose of clinical decision making, which may only be done by SLPs. SLPAs may summarize objective data from a session to the family or team members.

Medically Fragile

A term used to describe an individual who is acutely ill and in an unstable condition. If such an individual is treated by an SLPA, 100% direct supervision by an SLP is required.

Screening

A pass–fail procedure to identify, without interpretation, clients who may require further assessment following specified screening protocols developed by and/or approved by the supervising SLP.

Speech-Language Pathology Aides/Technician

Aides or technicians are individuals who have completed on-the-job training, workshops, and so forth and work under the direct supervision of ASHA-certified SLPs.

Speech-Language Pathology Assistant

Individuals who, following academic coursework, clinical practicum, and credentialing can perform tasks prescribed, directed, and supervised by ASHA-certified SLPs.

Supervising Speech-Language Pathologist

An SLP who is certified by ASHA and has been practicing for at least 2 years following ASHA certification, has completed not less than 10 hours of continuing professional development in supervision training prior to supervision of an SLPA, and who is licensed and/or credentialed by the state (where applicable).

Supervision

The provision of direction and evaluation of the tasks assigned to an SLPA. Methods for providing supervision include direct supervision, indirect supervision, and telesupervision.

Support Personnel

Support personnel in speech-language pathology perform tasks as prescribed, directed, and supervised by ASHA-certified SLPs. There are different levels of support personnel based on training and scope of responsibilities. Support personnel include SLPAs and speech-language pathology aides/technicians. ASHA is operationally defining these terms for ASHA resources. Some states use different terms and definitions for support personnel.

Telepractice

This refers to the application of telecommunications technology to delivery of professional services at a distance by linking clinician to client, or clinician to clinician, for assessment, intervention, and/or consultation.

Telesupervision

The SLP can view and communicate with the patient and SLPA in real time via Skype, webcam, and similar devices and services to supervise the SLPA, providing the opportunity for the SLP to give immediate feedback. This does not include reviewing a taped session later.

REFERENCES

American Speech-Language-Hearing Association (ASHA). (2004). *Knowledge and skills needed by speech-language pathologists and audiologists to provide culturally and linguistically appropriate services* [Knowledge and Skills]. Retrieved from www.asha.org/policy.

American Speech-Language-Hearing Association (ASHA). (2007). *Scope of practice in speech-language pathology* [Scope of Practice]. Available from www.asha.org/policy.

American Speech-Language-Hearing Association (ASHA). (2010). *Code of ethics* [Ethics]. Retrieved from www.asha.org/policy.

Reference this material as: American Speech-Language-Hearing Association. (2013). *Speech-language pathology assistant scope of practice* [Scope of Practice]. Retrieved from www.asha.org/policy.

APPENDIX H.3

Scope of Practice in Audiology

About This Document: This scope of practice document is an official policy of the American Speech Language Hearing Association (ASHA) defining the breadth of practice within the profession of audiology. The *Audiology Scope of Practice* document has not been updated since 2004. The aim of this document is to reflect the current and evolving clinical practice in audiology. Such changes include, but are not limited to, telehealth, discussion of hearing technologies beyond traditional hearing devices (e.g., over-the-counter [OTC]), and personal sound amplification products (PSAPs). Additional updates in advancements in hearing device implantation, vestibular assessment and rehabilitation, hearing preservation, educational audiology, and interoperative monitoring practice are included.

This document was developed by the ASHA Ad Hoc Committee on the Scope of Practice in Audiology. Committee members were Julie Honaker (chair), Robert Beiter, Kathleen Cienkowski, Gregory Mannarelli, Maryrose McInerney, Tena McNamara, Jessica Sullivan, Julie Verhoff, Robert Fifer (board liaison), and Pam Mason (ex officio). This document was approved by the ASHA Board of Directors on August 20, 2018.

Table of Contents

INTRODUCTION

Definition of Terms

Audiologist

By virtue of education, training, licensure, and certification, audiologists engage in professional practice in the areas of hearing and balance assessment, nonmedical treatment, and (re)habilitation. Audiologists provide patient-centered care in the prevention, identification, diagnosis, and evidence-based intervention and treatment of hearing, balance, and other related disorders for people of all ages. Hearing, balance, and other related disorders are complex, with medical, psychological, physical, social, educational, and employment implications. Treatment services require audiologists to know existing and emerging technologies, intervention strategies, and interpersonal skills to counsel and guide individuals and their family members through the (re)habilitative process. Audiologists provide professional and personalized services to minimize the negative impact of these disorders, leading to improved outcomes and quality of life. Audiologists are licensed and/or regulated in all 50 states and in the District of Columbia.

Balance

Includes all aspects of equilibrium, specific to the balance and vestibular systems, both peripheral and central. This includes management of symptoms and signs consistent with both peripheral and central etiologies.

Hearing

Includes all peripheral and central functional components of sound reception and analytic processing. This also includes management of symptoms and sequelae of disorders of the auditory system such as tinnitus, hyperacusis, misophonia, and other auditory perceptual disorders.

Hearing, balance, and other related disorders

Throughout this document, the broad term *hearing, balance, and other related disorders* is used to reflect all areas of assessment and intervention within the audiology scope of practice.

IEP/IFSP/504 Plan

The *Individualized Education Plan* (IEP) is a written statement that guides the educational plan for a child, ages 3 to 21, in accordance with the Individuals with Disabilities Education Act of 2004 (IDEA). The *Individual Family Service Plan* (IFSP) guides the early intervention services for a child with disabilities and their family. The IEP and IFSP are developed, reviewed, and revised in accordance with federal law. Also, under the IDEA, a student with disabilities is ensured a Free and Appropriate Public Education (FAPE) as well as monitoring the student's progress. The parents/guardians play a central role in the IEP/IFSP progress (IDEA, 2004). A *504 Plan* is a plan developed to ensure that a child with a disability receives accommodations for a general education classroom.

Individuals

The term *individuals* is used throughout the document to refer to students, clients, patients, children, adults, families, and caregivers who are served by the audiologist.

Interprofessional collaborative practice (IPP)

This term stems from the World Health Organization's (WHO) framework of looking at a health condition alongside a person's functional ability, social community, and personal goals, in concert with the perspective of other health care providers. Health care professionals must communicate and collaborate with each other and the individual receiving care, along with the individual's family or support system. This is called *interprofessional collaborative practice (IPP)*. The blending of skill sets results in better outcomes, improved quality of life, and greater satisfaction. It also minimizes the cost of care and improves the individual's safety and sense of well-being (Skevington, Lotfy, & O'Connell, 2004).

Management

This refers to the organization and coordination of activities in order to develop and provide relevant audiologic care for individuals. These activities include assessment techniques and treatment/intervention strategies. Appropriate management aids in the achievement of goals and objectives set forth for individuals with hearing and/or vestibular difficulties.

Other related disorders

This term is intended to reflect that audiologists with the appropriate training can use their skills and techniques to contribute to the knowledge, understanding, and overall care of individuals with other disorders outside the hearing and balance system. A few purely illustrative examples of this could include: (a) performing a battery of facial nerve function tests on a patient with a facial paresis or (b) performing a battery of auditory tests on a patient with a developmental or cognitive delay. This type of care is increasingly used as a part of an interprofessional collaborative practice team.

Person-centered care

This approach considers the whole person, taking into account more than the physical symptoms of a specific, discreet disorder. It includes psychological, social, cultural, and environmental factors. Optimal outcomes are achieved when working collaboratively—along with input and accountability—with the individual, supportive family members, and with fellow professionals.

Quality of life

WHO defines *quality of life* as an individual's perception of their position in life in the context of the culture and value systems in which they live and in relation to their goals, expectations, standards, and concerns. It is a broad-ranging concept affected in a complex way by the person's physical health, psychological state, personal beliefs, social relationships, and relationship to salient features of their environment (Skevington et al., 2004; WHOQOL Group, 1994).

Telehealth

The use of electronic information and telecommunications technologies to support long-distance clinical health care, patient and professional health-related education, public health, and health administration.

Treatment/Intervention

These terms refer to the application of care given to an individual to directly address hearing and/or vestibular difficulties. *Management* (defined above) is the overall coordination of activities that address the needs of individuals. *Treatment/intervention* is one of those direct activities.

Working at the top of license

This is the concept that audiologists should engage in patient care activities that require their (i.e., the audiologists') specialized level of expertise and skill. Other less skilled tasks may be delegated to other individuals (e.g., assistants, automated systems, and/or individuals and family members; Burkhard & Trembath, 2015). This would greatly decrease the cost of achieving outcomes (and also increase family satisfaction by decreasing the inconvenience, cost, and overall burden of care; ASHA, 2013). Working at the top of the license is not meant to imply nor does it prohibit audiologists from completing tasks that are not at the top of the license.

STATEMENT OF PURPOSE

The purpose of the *Scope of Practice in Audiology* is as follows:

1. Delineate areas of professional practice.
2. Inform others (e.g., health care providers, educators, consumers, payers, regulators, and the general public) about professional roles and responsibilities of qualified providers.
3. Support audiologists in the provision of high-quality, evidence-based services to individuals with hearing and balance concerns.
4. Support audiologists working at the top of their license.
5. Support audiologists in the conduct and dissemination of research.
6. Guide the educational preparation and professional development of audiologists to provide safe and effective services.

7. Inform members of ASHA, certificate holders, and students of the activities for which certification in audiology is required in accordance with the *ASHA Code of Ethics* (ASHA, 2016). Each practitioner evaluates his or her own experiences with preservice education, practice, mentorship and supervision, and continuing professional development. As a whole, these experiences define the scope of competence for each individual. Audiologists should engage in only those aspects of the profession that are within her or his professional competence. ASHA members and ASHA-certified professionals are bound by the *ASHA Code of Ethics* (ASHA, 2016) to provide services that are consistent with the scope of their competence, education, and experience.

By virtue of training and practice, audiology is a unique profession that specializes in and provides comprehensive diagnostic and nonmedical treatment services for hearing and balance disorders, and related impairments. These services are provided to individuals across the entire age span from birth through adulthood; these individuals include persons of different races, genders, religions, national origins, and sexual orientations. This position statement is not intended to be exhaustive; however, the activities described in this document reflect current practice within the profession. Practice activities related to emerging clinical, technological, and scientific developments are not precluded from consideration as part of the scope of practice of an audiologist. If the audiologist can document appropriate training for new and emerging clinical or technological procedures that fall under the heading of *auditory, balance, and other related disorders*, then such innovations and advances may be incorporated into the *Audiology Scope of Practice*. Audiologists are trained in all areas of clinical service delivery; however, they commonly have one or more specific areas of specialization. ASHA also recognizes that credentialed professionals in related disciplines have knowledge, skills, and experience that could be applied to some areas within the *Audiology Scope of Practice*. Defining the scope of practice of audiologists is not meant to exclude other appropriately credentialed postgraduate professionals from rendering services in overlapping practice areas. Often, these partially overlapping skill sets can result in excellent opportunities for IPP.

Audiologists must achieve required competencies in ancillary professional areas. These areas are distinct from but contribute to diagnostic and nonmedical treatment activities. They are very important areas in which to maintain high standards of clinical service. Examples include cultural and linguistic competencies, IPP, patient- and family-centered care, supervision, and mentoring and knowledge of federal and state statutes and regulations.

This scope of practice does not supersede existing state licensure laws or affect the interpretation or implementation of such laws. It should serve, however, as a model for the development or modification of licensure laws.

The goals of this updated *Scope of Practice in Audiology* of the American Speech-Language-Hearing Association (ASHA) are as follows:

1. Revise the current scope of practice for audiologists based on new and evolving training, skills, technology, and literature within the profession.
2. Align our professional activities with the evolving best practice models in audiology within the overall health care field.
3. Serve as a resource for other agencies, professional organizations, and the general public (e.g., federal, state, nongovernmental organizations, licensing and credentialing bodies, etc.).
4. Provide a language and framework that is applicable for all audiologists, regardless of professional setting.

AUDIOLOGY SERVICE DELIVERY AREAS

Clinical service delivery areas include all aspects of hearing, balance, and other related disorders that impact hearing and balance, including areas of tinnitus, cognition, and auditory processing for individuals across the lifespan. Audiologists play critical roles in health literacy; in the screening, diagnosis, and treatment of hearing, balance, and other related disorders; and in the use of the *International Classification of Functioning, Disability and Health* (ICF; WHO, 2014) to develop functional goals and collaborative practice. As technology and science advance, the areas of assessment and intervention related to hearing, balance, and other related disorders grow accordingly. Clinicians should stay current with advances in hearing and balance practice by regularly reviewing the research literature; regularly consulting the Practice Management section of the ASHA website, including the Practice Portal; and regularly participating in continuing education to supplement advances in the profession and to provide additional information that can inform the *Scope of Practice in Audiology.*

Diagnostics for Hearing, Balance, and Other Related Disorders

Audiologists are responsible for the assessment of hearing, balance, and other related disorders, including tinnitus and auditory processing, across the lifespan that includes the following:

- Administration and interpretation of clinical case history.
- Administration and interpretation of behavioral, electroacoustic, and electrophysiologic measures of the peripheral and central auditory, balance, and other related systems.
- Administration and interpretation of diagnostic screening that includes measures to detect the presence of hearing, balance, and other related disorders. Additional screening measures of mental health and cognitive impairment should be used to assess, treat, and refer (American Academy of Audiology, 2013; Beck & Clark, 2009; Li et al., 2014; Shen, Anderson, Arehart, & Souza, 2016; Sweetow, 2015; Weinstein, 2017, 2018).

This assessment includes measurement and professional interpretation of sensory and motor-evoked potentials, electromyography, and other electrodiagnostic tests for purposes of neurophysiologic intraoperative monitoring and cranial nerve assessment.

Diagnostic measures should be modified based on patient age and on cognitive and physical abilities of the individuals being assessed. Case findings of dementia, memory, vision, and balance (falling risk) should be used when difficulty in communication and/or change of behavior is evident (Beck & Clark, 2009; Li et al., 2014; Shen et al., 2016; Sweetow, 2015; Weinstein, 2017, 2018). Assessment extends beyond diagnostic evaluation and includes informational counseling, interpretation of results, and intervention.

Assessment is accomplished using quantitative and qualitative measurements—including standardized testing, observations, and procedures and appropriately calibrated instrumentation—and leads to the diagnosis of abnormal audiologic and/or balance function. Interpretation of test results includes diagnostic statements as to the probable locus of impairment and functional ability within the hearing, balance, and other related systems under assessment.

Audiologists collaborate with other professionals and serve on care teams to help reduce the perceived burden of hearing, balance, and other related disorders and maximize quality of life for individuals.

Treatment for Hearing, Balance, and Other Related Disorders

Audiologists provide comprehensive audiologic (re)habilitation services for individuals and their families across the lifespan who are experiencing hearing, balance, or other related disorders (e.g., tinnitus and auditory processing disorder). Intervention encompasses the following:

- Auditory training for sound identification and discrimination
- Cerumen management
- Communication strategies (e.g., environmental manipulation, mode of communication)
- Counseling

- Manual communication
- (Re)habilitation related to auditory disorders
- Self-advocacy for personal needs or systems change
- Speechreading
- Strategies to address other related disorders (tinnitus, misophonia)
- Technology interventions
- Vestibular rehabilitation to include management of benign paroxysmal positional vertigo as well as peripheral and/or central vestibular disorders

In this role, audiologists:

- Design, implement, and document delivery of service in accordance with best available practice;
- Screen for possible cognitive disorders;
- Case-finding for dementia;
- Provide culturally and linguistically appropriate services;
- Integrate the highest quality available research evidence with practitioner expertise as well as with individual preference and values in establishing treatment goals;
- Utilize treatment data to determine effectiveness of services and guide decisions;
- Deliver the appropriate frequency and intensity of treatment utilizing best available practice;
- Engage in treatment activities that are within the scope of the professional's competence; and
- Collaborate with other professionals in the delivery of services to ensure the highest quality of interventions.

As part of the comprehensive audiologic (re)habilitation program, audiologists evaluate, select, fit, verify, validate, and monitor the performance of a variety of technologies interventions for hearing, balance, and other related disorders. Audiologists provide individual counseling and public education about the benefits and/or limitations of various different classes of devices. Treatment utilizing technology interventions include but are not limited to other emerging technologies:

- Auditory brainstem implants (ABIs)
- Assistive listening devices
- Balance-related devices
- Classroom audio distribution systems
- Cochlear implants
- Custom ear impressions and molds for hearing devices, hearing protection, in-ear monitors, swim plugs, communication devices, stenosis stents, and so forth
- Hearing aids
- Hearing assistive technology
- Hearing protection
- Large-area amplification systems
- Middle ear implants
- Over-the-counter (OTC) hearing aids
- Osseointegrated devices (OIDs),bone-anchored devices, and bone conduction devices
- Personal sound amplification products (PSAPs)
- Remote microphone systems
- Tinnitus devices (both stand-alone and integrated with hearing aids)

Treatment for children also includes developmental and educational interventions such as the following:

- Participation in the development and implementation of an IEP/IFSP for school-aged children or implementation of an IFSP for children birth to 36 months of age
- Participation in the development and implementation of a 504 plan
- Measurement of noise levels in educational institutions and recommendations for noise reduction modification

Early Hearing Detection and Intervention (EHDI)

Audiologists provide screening, assessment, and treatment services for infants and young children with hearing-related disorders and their families. Services include the following:

- Apply Joint Committee on Infant Hearing (JCIH) protocols for early detection and intervention of infants and children with hearing loss (American Academy of Pediatrics, Joint Committee on Infant Hearing, 2007)
- Establish, manage, and/or review programs following the EHDI protocol
- Provide training and supervision to support personnel
- Monitor the program's outcome measures for quality assurance
- Perform audiological diagnostics to confirm or rule out the presence of a hearing loss
- Provide early intervention treatment for hearing loss to enhance communication and to improve cognitive and social skills
- Upon diagnosis of hearing loss, ensure that the child and family are enrolled in an appropriate early intervention program
- Provide comprehensive information about family support, training, and communication options
- Provide education to community/hospital personnel
- Collaborate with other professionals and with parent groups

Educational Audiology

Audiologists in educational settings provide a full spectrum of hearing services to support academic and social achievement for school-aged children, adolescents, young adults, and their families with hearing and related difficulties. Services include the following:

- Perform assessments and interpret the educational implications of the student's auditory needs. This also includes assessing and making appropriate recommendations as an advocate on behalf of students, ensuring least restrictive environments
- Collect data from classroom assessments and from observations of students in various environments, and assess the impact of audiologic interventions on academic and social performance
- Collect data on classroom acoustics, and assess the impact on auditory perception
- Ensure IPP with members of the school multidisciplinary team who facilitate listening, learning, and communication
- Collaborate with private sector/community-based audiologists and other professionals relative to the student's educational needs
- Provide instructional training for educators and staff for the development of skills needed in servicing students with hearing difficulties, which includes providing evidence and recommending support services and resources
- Provide (re)habilitative activities in collaboration with classroom teachers and other support personnel
- Monitor personal hearing instruments

- Recommend, fit, and manage hearing assistance technology
- Counsel children to promote personal responsibility, self-advocacy, and social awareness
- Counsel parents on management options, and provide resource information
- Assist with transitions between academic and vocational settings
- Manage school programs for the preservation of hearing and the prevention of hearing loss
- Manage and implement hearing screening programs

Hearing Conservation and Preservation

The terms *hearing conservation* and *hearing preservation* are often used interchangeably. Both terms focus on preventing noise-induced hearing loss, whether from occupational or recreational sources. *Hearing conservation programs* are most often, although not exclusively, associated with occupational noise exposure and with U.S. Occupational Safety and Health Administration (OSHA) regulations (OSHA, 2002). In addition, hearing conservation programs have additional elements not found in hearing preservation programs: engineering controls for reducing environmental noise levels, administrative controls for monitoring hearing sensitivity levels, mandated use of hearing protection devices when needed, employee training about noise, the potential synergistic effects of chemical exposure combined with hazardous noise, and requirements for communication about hazards (e.g., warning signs, posting of signs in required hearing protection environments).

Hearing preservation programs focus on nonoccupational settings and are most often intended to prevent hearing loss from occurring in individuals who enter the program with normal hearing sensitivity. Examples of hearing preservation programs may include (a) monitoring of auditory function for patients receiving chemotherapy or radiation therapy of the head or neck (University Health Network, 2018) or (b) providing education to students and young adults on the effects of recreational noise and methods to prevent hearing loss (see the Save Your Hearing Foundation at www.earpeacefoundation.org). Audiologists are uniquely qualified through education and training to design, establish, implement, and supervise hearing conservation programs for individuals of all ages in schools, in industry, and for the general public (Lipscomb, 1988).

Audiologists who engage in occupational hearing conservation must monitor current OSHA regulations (OSHA, 2002) regarding the impact of noise levels on hearing sensitivity. This extends to the distribution of, and instructions related to the use of, hearing protection devices.

Audiologists test hearing levels, determine functional hearing ability, measure noise levels, and assess the risk of incurring hearing loss from noise exposure from any source, including nonoccupational and recreational noise (Franks, Stephenson, & Merry, 1996a, 1996b, 1996c).

Audiologists implement and manage all aspects of hearing conservation activities—including education, testing, and the determination of program effectiveness—and serve as the supervisor for OSHA and other U.S. government–mandated hearing conservation programs (Suter, 2003).

Audiologists educate the public and other professionals on how to recognize hazardous noise, ways of preventing noise-induced hearing loss, and the risks associated with reduced audibility when exposed to high-level sound.

Telehealth

Telehealth, for audiology, is an alternative method of service delivery that encompasses both diagnostics and intervention services. Diagnostic services are provided using either synchronous or asynchronous protocols (i.e., *store and forward*, whereby data are collected, stored within a computer, and forwarded at a later time). Audiologists provide services using an evidence-based standard of care (American Telemedicine Association, 2017). When practicing via telehealth, audiologists provide care consistent with jurisdictional regulatory, licensing, credentialing and privileging, malpractice and insurance laws, and rules for their profession in both the jurisdiction in which they are practicing as well as the jurisdiction in which the patient is receiving care. The audiologists providing the service shall ensure compliance as required by appropriate regulatory and accrediting agencies (American Telemedicine Association, 2017).

Areas in which telehealth is a viable option include the following:

- Aural/auditory (re)habilitation
- Auditory evoked potentials
- Hearing aid and cochlear implant fitting/programming
- Hearing screening
- Otoacoustic emissions
- Otoscopy
- Pure-tone audiometry and speech recognition in noise
- Supervision of electrophysiology services (e.g., intraoperative monitoring and diagnostic examinations)
- Supervision of vestibular services (e.g., vestibular diagnostic examinations)
- Tympanometry
- Vestibular rehabilitation

Counseling

Audiologists counsel by providing information, education, guidance, and support to individuals and their families. Counseling includes discussion of assessment results and treatment options. Counseling facilitates decision making regarding intervention, management, educational environment, and mode of communication. The role of the audiologist in the counseling process includes interactions related to emotions, thoughts, feelings, and behaviors that result from living with hearing, balance, and other related disorders.

Audiologists engage in the following activities when counseling individuals and their families:

- Providing informational counseling regarding interpretation of assessment outcomes and treatment options
- Empowering individuals and their families to make informed decisions related to their plan of care
- Educating the individual, the family, and relevant community members
- Providing support and/or access to peer-to-peer groups for individuals and their families
- Providing individuals and their families with skills that enable them to become self-advocates
- Providing adjustment counseling related to the psychosocial impact on the individual
- Referring individuals to other professionals when counseling needs fall outside those related to auditory, balance, and other related disorders.

ADDITIONAL AREAS OF AUDIOLOGY PRACTICE

Audiology is a dynamic profession, and the fact that the audiology scope of practice overlaps with those of other professionals is a reality in rapidly changing health care, education, industrial, and other environments. Hence, audiologists in various settings work collaboratively with other academic and/or health care professionals to make appropriate decisions for the benefit of individuals with hearing, balance, and other related disorders. This is known as *IPP* and is defined as "members or students of two or more professions associated with health or social care, engaged in learning with, from and about each other" (Craddock, O'Halloran, Borthwick, & McPherson, 2006, p. 237). Similarly, "interprofessional education [often referred to as "IPE"] provides an ability to share skills and knowledge between professions and allows for a better understanding, shared values, and respect for the roles of other healthcare professionals" (Bridges, Davidson, Soule Odegard, Maki, & Tomkowiak, 2011, para. 5). The advantage of using IPP/IPE is that it broadens the care teams' depth of knowledge and understanding of the individual being evaluated and/or treated. This type of collaboration improves outcomes, efficiency, and safety through person-centered care.

Research

Audiologists conduct and participate in basic and applied/translational research related to auditory, balance, and other related disorders. This research is undertaken as a facility-specific effort or is coordinated across multiple settings. Audiologists engage in activities to ensure compliance with Institutional Review Boards, federal regulations, and international laws pertaining to research. Audiologists also collaborate with other researchers and pursue research funding through grants.

Administration and Leadership

Audiologists administer programs in education, higher education, schools, health care, private practice, and other settings. In this capacity, they are responsible for making administrative decisions related to fiscal and personnel management, leadership, program design, program growth and innovation, professional development, compliance with laws and regulations, and cooperation with outside agencies in education and health care. Their administrative roles are not limited to audiology, as they engage in program administration across departments and at different levels within an institution. In addition, audiologists promote effective and manageable workloads in school settings, provide appropriate services under the Individuals with Disabilities Education Improvement Act of 2004 (IDEA), and engage in program design and development.

Education

Audiologists serve as educators, teaching students in academic institutions and teaching professionals through continuing education in professional development formats. This more formal teaching is in addition to the education that audiologists provide to individuals, families, caregivers, decision makers, and policy makers, which is described in other domains. In this role, audiologists:

- Serve as faculty at institutions of higher education, teaching courses at the undergraduate, graduate, and postgraduate levels;

- Mentor students who are completing academic programs at all levels;

- Provide academic training to students in related disciplines and students who are training to become audiology assistants; and

- Provide continuing professional education to audiologists and to professionals in related disciplines.

Advocacy and Outreach

Audiologists focus on upholding person-centered care in our complex health care and educational systems. Audiologists advocate for hearing, balance, and other related disorders needs of the individuals and families whom they serve.

Audiologists advocate for the profession and for individuals through a variety of mechanisms, including community awareness, prevention activities, health literacy, academic literacy, education, political action, and training programs. Advocacy promotes and facilitates access to communication, including the reduction of societal, cultural, and linguistic barriers. Audiologists perform a variety of activities related to advocacy and outreach, including the following:

- Advising regulatory and legislative agencies about the continuum of care for hearing, balance, and other related disorders

- Engaging decision makers at the local, state, and national levels for improved administrative and governmental policies affecting access to services for the diagnosis and treatment of hearing, balance, and other related disorders

- Advocating at the local, state, and national levels for funding for services, education, and research
- Participating in associations and organizations to advance the audiology profession
- Promoting and marketing professional services
- Consulting with industry in the development of products and instrumentation related to hearing, balance, and other related disorders
- Helping to recruit and retain audiologists with diverse backgrounds and interests
- Collaborating on advocacy objectives with other professionals/colleagues regarding mutual goals
- Serving as expert witnesses, when appropriate
- Educating individuals about communication; development; disorders pertaining to auditory, balance, and other related systems; and audiology services
- Advocating for fair and equitable services, including accessibility for all individuals, especially the most vulnerable
- Providing case management and serving as a liaison for individuals and their families in order to meet educational and vocational programming needs
- Consulting with individuals, their families, professionals, public and private agencies, and governmental bodies on technology intervention, hearing assistive technology, interpreting services, and other relevant assistive technology needed to enhance communication
- Consulting with state education agencies, local school districts, and interdisciplinary teams on direct service and IFSP, IEP, and 504 plan development
- Advocating for appropriate reimbursement of services

Cultural Competency

Audiologists serve diverse populations, and this includes persons of different races, ages, genders, religions, national origins, and sexual orientations. Audiologists' caseloads include individuals from diverse ethnic, cultural, and linguistic backgrounds as well as persons with disabilities. Culturally based family and community dynamics should be included in the development of an appropriate treatment plan that includes consideration of diversity and evidence-based practice guidelines.

Clinical Supervision/Precepting

Supervision is broadly defined as overseeing and directing the work of others. The terms *clinical supervisor* and *clinical supervision* are often used in reference to the training and education of student clinicians, recognizing that supervision is part of the training and education process. However, clinical supervisors do more than oversee the work of the student clinician. They teach specific skills, clarify concepts, assist with critical thinking, conduct performance evaluations, mentor, advise, and model professional behavior (Council on Academic Programs in Communication Sciences and Disorders [CAPCSD], 2013). Supervision is a distinct area of practice; is the responsibility of audiologists; and crosses clinical, administrative, and technical spheres. Audiologists are responsible for supervising clinical externs/trainees, audiology assistants, credentialed technical staff, and other professional and administrative support personnel. Audiologists also supervise colleagues and peers. Audiologists acknowledge that supervision is integral in the delivery of hearing, balance, and other related services and that supervision advances the profession. Supervision involves education, mentorship, encouragement, counseling, and support across all supervisory roles. In this role, audiologists:

- Possess service delivery and professional practice skills necessary to guide the supervisee;
- Apply the art and science of supervision to all stakeholders (i.e., those supervising and being supervised), recognizing that supervision contributes to workplace efficiency;
- Seek advanced knowledge in the practice of effective supervision;
- Establish supervisory relationships that are collegial in nature; and
- Establish supervisory relationships that promote growth and independence while providing support and guidance.

Interprofessional Education and Interprofessional Practice (IPE/IPP)

According to ASHA's definition, *interprofessional education* (IPE) is an activity that occurs when two or more professions learn about, from, and with each other to enable effective collaboration and improve outcomes for individuals and families whom we serve (ASHA, n.d.-b). Similarly, IPP occurs when multiple service providers from different professional backgrounds jointly provide comprehensive health care or educational services by working with individuals and their families, caregivers, and communities to deliver the highest quality of care across settings. When both IPE and IPP are used, we refer to this combined term as *IPE/IPP*.

Business Management

Audiology is a service profession to which principles of business must be applied for success in educational, health care, and industrial settings. For a business entity (profit or nonprofit) to be successful, good business practices are essential. Providing high-quality services that are consistent in type and amount with a person's needs and with professional and ethical standards is good business practice. It is important that revenues collected for services cover and exceed all expenses (e.g., salary, benefits, overhead). Audiologists must understand their individual responsibility for adhering to practice standards that financially support their organization. Each audiologist's daily decisions (clinical and nonclinical) affect the financial viability of his or her organization. Audiologists must remain compliant and current on policy changes related to billing and coding.

Legal/Professional Consulting

Audiologists may be called upon to provide expertise to other professionals, business, industry, courts, attorneys, public and private agencies, and/or individuals in all areas related to the profession of audiology. Consulting services include but are not limited to:

- Recommendations for occupational and recreational hearing preservation and conservation, education, and advocacy for policy development;
- Quality assessment and improvement; and
- Expert witness testimony or second opinion and/or independent evaluation for educational, health, worker's compensation, or other legal purposes.

Ad Hoc Committee on the Scope of Practice in Audiology

RESOURCES

American Speech-Language-Hearing Association. (n.d.-a). Evidence-based practice. Retrieved from https://www.asha.org/Research/EBP

American Speech-Language-Hearing Association. (n.d.-b). Practice portal. Retrieved from https://www.asha.org/practice-portal

American Speech-Language-Hearing Association. (1991). *A model for collaborative service delivery for students with language-learning disorders in the public schools* [Relevant Paper]. Retrieved from https://www.asha.org/policy/RP1991-00123/

American Speech-Language-Hearing Association. (2003). *Evaluating and treating communication and cognitive disorders: Approaches to referral and collaboration for speech-language pathology and clinical neuropsychology* [Technical Report]. Retrieved from https://www.asha.org/policy/TR2003-00137/

Paul, D. (2013). A quick guide to DSM-V. *The ASHA Leader, 18,* 52–54. Retrieved from https://leader.pubs.asha.org/article.aspx?articleid=1785031

U.S. Department of Justice. (2009). *A guide to disability rights laws*. Retrieved from https://www.ada.gov/cguide.htm

Reference this material as: American SpeechLanguageHearing Association. (2018). *Scope of practice in audiology* [Scope of Practice]. Retrieved from www.asha.org/policy/.

Disclaimer: The American Speech-Language-Hearing Association disclaims any liability to any party for the accuracy, completeness, or availability of these documents, or for any damages arising out of the use of the documents and any information they contain.

APPENDIX I

2020 Standards and Implementation Procedures for the Certificate of Clinical Competence in Speech-Language Pathology

Effective Date: January 1, 2020

INTRODUCTION

The Council for Clinical Certification in Audiology and Speech-Language Pathology (CFCC) is a semiautonomous credentialing body of the American Speech-Language-Hearing Association (ASHA). The charges to the CFCC are to define the standards for clinical certification; to apply those standards in granting certification to individuals; to have final authority to withdraw certification in cases where certification has been granted on the basis of inaccurate information; and to administer the certification maintenance program.

A <u>Practice and Curriculum Analysis of the Profession of Speech-Language Pathology</u> was conducted in 2017 under the auspices of the Council on Academic Accreditation in Audiology and Speech-Language Pathology (CAA) and the CFCC. The survey analysis was reviewed by the CFCC, and the following standards were developed to better fit current practice models.

The 2020 Standards and Implementation Procedures for the Certificate of Clinical Competence in Speech-Language Pathology (CCC-SLP) go into effect on January 1, 2020. View the <u>SLP Standards Crosswalk</u> [PDF] and consult <u>Changes to Speech-Language Pathology Standards</u> for more specific information on how the standards will change.

TERMINOLOGY

Clinical educator

Refers to and may be used interchangeably with supervisor, clinical instructor, and preceptor.

Individual

Denotes clients, patients, students, and other recipients of services provided by the speech-language pathologist.

CITATION

Cite as: Council for Clinical Certification in Audiology and Speech-Language Pathology of the American Speech-Language-Hearing Association. (2018). *2020 Standards for the Certificate of Clinical Competence in Speech-Language Pathology.* Retrieved from https://www.asha.org/certification/2020-SLP-Certification-Standards

The Standards for the CCC-SLP are shown in bold. The CFCC implementation procedures follow each standard.

- Standard I—Degree
- Standard II—Education Program
- Standard III—Program of Study
- Standard IV—Knowledge Outcomes
- Standard V—Skills Outcomes
- Standard VI—Assessment
- Standard VII—Speech-Language Pathology Clinical Fellowship
- Standard VIII—Maintenance of Certification

Standard I: Degree

The applicant for certification (hereafter, "applicant") must have a master's, doctoral, or other recognized postbaccalaureate degree.

Standard II: Education Program

All graduate coursework and graduate clinical experience required in speech-language pathology must have been initiated and completed in a speech-language pathology program accredited by the Council on Academic Accreditation in Audiology and Speech-Language Pathology (CAA).

Implementation: The graduate program of study must be initiated and completed in a CAA-accredited program or a program with candidacy status for CAA accreditation. The applicant's program director or official designee must complete and submit a program director verification form. Applicants must submit an official graduate transcript or a letter from the registrar that verifies the date on which the graduate degree was awarded. The official graduate transcript or letter from the registrar must be received by the ASHA National Office no later than 1 year from the date on which the application was received. Verification of the applicant's graduate degree is required before the CCC-SLP can be awarded.

Applicants educated outside the United States or its territories must submit documentation that coursework was completed in an institution of higher education that is regionally accredited or recognized by the appropriate regulatory authority for that country. In addition, applicants outside the United States or its territories must meet each of the standards that follow.

Standard III: Program of Study

The applicant must have completed a program of study (a minimum of 36 semester credit hours at the graduate level) that includes academic coursework and supervised clinical experience sufficient in depth and breadth to achieve the specified knowledge and skills outcomes stipulated in Standards IV-A through IV-G and Standards V-A through V-C.

Implementation: The minimum of 36 graduate semester credit hours must have been earned in a program that addresses the knowledge and skills pertinent to the ASHA *Scope of Practice in Speech-Language Pathology.*

Standard IV: Knowledge Outcomes

Standard IV-A

The applicant must have demonstrated knowledge of statistics as well as the biological, physical, and social/behavioral sciences.

Implementation: Coursework in statistics as well as in biological, physical, and social/behavioral sciences that is specifically related to communication sciences and disorders (CSD) may not be applied for certification purposes to this category unless the course fulfills a general the university requirement in the statistics, biology, physical science, or chemistry areas.

Acceptable courses in biological sciences should emphasize a content area related to human or animal sciences (e.g., biology, human anatomy and physiology, neuroanatomy and neurophysiology, human genetics, veterinary science). Chemistry and physics are important for the foundational understanding of the profession of speech-language pathology. For all applicants who apply beginning January 1, 2020, courses that meet the physical science requirement must be in physics or chemistry. Program directors must evaluate the course descriptions or syllabi of any courses completed prior to students entering their programs to determine if the content provides foundational knowledge in physics or chemistry. Acceptable courses in social/behavioral sciences should include psychology, sociology, anthropology, or public health. A stand-alone course in statistics is required. Coursework in research methodology in the absence of basic statistics cannot be used to fulfill this requirement.

Standard IV-B

The applicant must have demonstrated knowledge of basic human communication and swallowing processes, including the appropriate biological, neurological, acoustic, psychological, developmental, and linguistic and cultural bases. The applicant must have demonstrated the ability to integrate information pertaining to normal and abnormal human development across the life span.

Standard IV-C

The applicant must have demonstrated knowledge of communication and swallowing disorders and differences, including the appropriate etiologies, characteristics, and anatomical/physiological, acoustic, psychological, developmental, and linguistic and cultural correlates in the following areas:

- **Speech sound production, to encompass articulation, motor planning and execution, phonology, and accent modification**
- **Fluency and fluency disorders**
- **Voice and resonance, including respiration and phonation**
- **Receptive and expressive language, including phonology, morphology, syntax, semantics, pragmatics (language use and social aspects of communication), prelinguistic communication, paralinguistic communication (e.g., gestures, signs, body language), and literacy in speaking, listening, reading, and writing**
- **Hearing, including the impact on speech and language**
- **Swallowing/feeding, including (a) structure and function of orofacial myology and (b) oral, pharyngeal, laryngeal, pulmonary, esophageal, gastrointestinal, and related functions across the life span**
- **Cognitive aspects of communication, including attention, memory, sequencing, problem solving, and executive functioning**
- **Social aspects of communication, including challenging behavior, ineffective social skills, and lack of communication opportunities**
- **Augmentative and alternative communication modalities**

Implementation: It is expected that coursework addressing the professional knowledge specified in this standard will occur primarily at the graduate level.

Standard IV-D

For each of the areas specified in Standard IV-C, the applicant must have demonstrated current knowledge of the principles and methods of prevention, assessment, and intervention for persons with communication and swallowing disorders, including consideration of anatomical/physiological, psychological, developmental, and linguistic and cultural correlates.

Standard IV-E

The applicant must have demonstrated knowledge of standards of ethical conduct.

Implementation: The applicant must have demonstrated knowledge of the principles and rules of the current ASHA _Code of Ethics._

Standard IV-F

The applicant must have demonstrated knowledge of processes used in research and of the integration of research principles into evidence-based clinical practice.

Implementation: The applicant must have demonstrated knowledge of the principles of basic and applied research and research design. In addition, the applicant must have demonstrated knowledge of how to access sources of research information and must have demonstrated the ability to relate research to clinical practice.

Standard IV-G

The applicant must have demonstrated knowledge of contemporary professional issues.

Implementation: The applicant must have demonstrated knowledge of professional issues that affect speech-language pathology. Issues include trends in professional practice, academic program accreditation standards, ASHA practice policies and guidelines, educational legal requirements or policies, and reimbursement procedures.

Standard IV-H

The applicant must have demonstrated knowledge of entry level and advanced certifications, licensure, and other relevant professional credentials, as well as local, state, and national regulations and policies relevant to professional practice.

Standard V: Skills Outcomes

Standard V-A

The applicant must have demonstrated skills in oral and written or other forms of communication sufficient for entry into professional practice.

Implementation: Applicants are eligible to apply for certification once they have completed all graduate-level academic coursework and clinical practicum and have been judged by the graduate program as having acquired all of the knowledge and skills mandated by the current standards.

The applicant must have demonstrated communication skills sufficient to achieve effective clinical and professional interaction with persons receiving services and relevant others. For oral communication, the applicant must have demonstrated speech and language skills in English, which, at a minimum, are consistent with ASHA's current position statement on students and professionals who speak English with accents and

<u>nonstandard dialects</u>. In addition, the applicant must have demonstrated the ability to write and comprehend technical reports, diagnostic and treatment reports, treatment plans, and professional correspondence in English.

Standard V-B

The applicant must have completed a program of study that included experiences sufficient in breadth and depth to achieve the following skills outcomes:

1. **Evaluation**
   a. **Conduct screening and prevention procedures, including prevention activities.**
   b. **Collect case history information and integrate information from clients/patients, family, caregivers, teachers, and relevant others, including other professionals.**
   c. **Select and administer appropriate evaluation procedures, such as behavioral observations, nonstandardized and standardized tests, and instrumental procedures.**
   d. **Adapt evaluation procedures to meet the needs of individuals receiving services.**
   e. **Interpret, integrate, and synthesize all information to develop diagnoses and make appropriate recommendations for intervention.**
   f. **Complete administrative and reporting functions necessary to support evaluation.**
   g. **Refer clients/patients for appropriate services.**

2. **Intervention**
   a. **Develop setting-appropriate intervention plans with measurable and achievable goals that meet clients'/patients' needs. Collaborate with clients/patients and relevant others in the planning process.**
   b. **Implement intervention plans that involve clients/patients and relevant others in the intervention process.**
   c. **Select or develop and use appropriate materials and instrumentation for prevention and intervention.**
   d. **Measure and evaluate clients'/patients' performance and progress.**
   e. **Modify intervention plans, strategies, materials, or instrumentation as appropriate to meet the needs of clients/patients.**
   f. **Complete administrative and reporting functions necessary to support intervention.**
   g. **Identify and refer clients/patients for services, as appropriate.**

3. **Interaction and Personal Qualities**
   a. **Communicate effectively, recognizing the needs, values, preferred mode of communication, and cultural/linguistic background of the individual(s) receiving services, family, caregivers, and relevant others.**
   b. **Manage the care of individuals receiving services to ensure an interprofessional, team-based collaborative practice.**
   c. **Provide counseling regarding communication and swallowing disorders to clients/patients, family, caregivers, and relevant others.**
   d. **Adhere to the ASHA *Code of Ethics*, and behave professionally.**

Implementation: The applicant must have acquired the skills listed in this standard and must have applied them across the nine major areas listed in Standard IV-C. These skills may be developed and demonstrated through direct clinical contact with individuals receiving services in clinical experiences, academic coursework, labs, simulations, and examinations, as well as through the completion of independent projects.

The applicant must have obtained a sufficient variety of supervised clinical experiences in different work settings and with different populations so that the applicant can demonstrate skills across the ASHA *Scope of Practice in Speech-Language Pathology. Supervised clinical experience* is defined as clinical services (i.e., assessment/ diagnosis/evaluation, screening, treatment, report writing, family/client consultation, and/or counseling) related to the management of populations that fit within the <u>ASHA *Scope of Practice in Speech-Language Pathology*</u>.

These experiences allow students to:

- Interpret, integrate, and synthesize core concepts and knowledge;
- Demonstrate appropriate professional and clinical skills; and
- Incorporate critical thinking and decision-making skills while engaged in prevention, identification, evaluation, diagnosis, planning, implementation, and/or intervention.

Supervised clinical experiences should include interprofessional education and interprofessional collaborative practice, and should include experiences with related professionals that enhance the student's knowledge and skills in an interdisciplinary, team-based, comprehensive service delivery model.

Clinical simulations (CS) may include the use of standardized patients and simulation technologies (e.g., standardized patients, virtual patients, digitized mannequins, immersive reality, task trainers, computer-based interactive).These supervised experiences can be synchronous simulations (real-time) or asynchronous (not concurrent in time) simulations.

Clinical educators of clinical experiences must hold current ASHA certification in the appropriate area of practice during the time of supervision. The supervised activities must be within the ASHA *Scope of Practice in Speech-Language Pathology* in order to count toward the student's ASHA certification requirements.

Standard V-C

The applicant must complete a minimum of 400 clock hours of supervised clinical experience in the practice of speech-language pathology. Twenty-five hours must be spent in guided clinical observation, and 375 hours must be spent in direct client/patient contact.

Implementation: Guided clinical observation hours generally precede direct contact with clients/patients. Examples of guided observations may include but are not limited to the following activities: debriefing of a video recording with a clinical educator who holds the CCC-SLP, discussion of therapy or evaluation procedures that had been observed, debriefings of observations that meet course requirements, or written records of the observations. It is important to confirm that there was communication between the clinical educator and observer, rather than passive experiences where the student views sessions and/or videos. It is encouraged that the student observes live and recorded sessions across settings with individuals receiving services with a variety of disorders and completes debriefing activities as described above.

The observation and direct client/patient contact hours must be within the ASHA *Scope of Practice in Speech-Language Pathology* and must be under the supervision of a qualified professional who holds a current ASHA certification in the appropriate practice area. Guided clinical supervision may occur simultaneously during the student's observation or afterward through review and approval of the student's written reports or summaries. Students may use video recordings of client services for observation purposes.

Applicants should be assigned practicum only after they have acquired a base of knowledge sufficient to qualify for such experience. Only direct contact (e.g., the individual receiving services must be present) with the individual or the individual's family in assessment, intervention, and/or counseling can be counted toward practicum. When counting clinical practicum hours for purposes of ASHA certification, only the actual time spent in sessions can be counted, and the time spent cannot be rounded up to the nearest 15-minute interval.

Up to 20% (i.e., 75 hours) of direct contact hours may be obtained through CS methods. Only the time spent in active engagement with CS may be counted. CS may include the use of standardized patients and simulation technologies (e.g., standardized patients, virtual patients, digitized mannequins, immersive reality, task trainers, computer-based interactive). Debriefing activities may not be included as clinical clock hours.

Although several students may observe a clinical session at one time, clinical practicum hours should be assigned only to the student who provides direct services to the individual receiving services or the individual's family. Typically, only one student at a time should be working with a client in order to count the practicum hours. Several students working as a team may receive credit for the same session, depending on the specific responsibilities that each student is assigned when working directly with the individual receiving services. The applicant must maintain documentation of their time spent in supervised practicum, and this documentation must be verified by the program in accordance with Standards III and IV.

Standard V-D

At least 325 of the 400 clock hours of supervised clinical experience must be completed while the applicant is enrolled in graduate study in a program accredited in speech-language pathology by the CAA.

Implementation: A minimum of 325 clock hours of supervised clinical practicum must be completed while the student is enrolled in the graduate program. At the discretion of the graduate program, hours obtained at the undergraduate level may be used to satisfy the remainder of the requirement.

Standard V-E

Supervision of students must be provided by a clinical educator who holds ASHA certification in the appropriate profession, who has the equivalent of a minimum of 9 months of full-time clinical experience, and who has completed a minimum of 2 hours of professional development in clinical instruction/ supervision after being awarded ASHA certification.

The amount of direct supervision must be commensurate with the student's knowledge, skills, and experience; must not be less than 25% of the student's total contact with each client/patient; and must take place periodically throughout the practicum. Supervision must be sufficient to ensure the welfare of the individual receiving services.

Implementation: Effective January 1, 2020, supervisors for ASHA certification must complete 2 hours of professional development/continuing education in clinical instruction/supervision. The professional development/ continuing education must be completed after being awarded ASHA certification and prior to the supervision of a student. Direct supervision must be in real time. A clinical educator must be available and on site to consult with a student who is providing clinical services to the clinical educator's client. Supervision of clinical practicum is intended to provide guidance and feedback and to facilitate the student's acquisition of essential clinical skills.

In the case of CS, asynchronous supervision must include debriefing activities that are commensurate with a minimum of 25% of the clock hours earned for each simulated individual receiving services.

Standard V-F

Supervised practicum must include experience with individuals across the life span and from culturally/ linguistically diverse backgrounds. Practicum must include experience with individuals with various types and severities of communication and/or related disorders, differences, and disabilities.

Implementation: The applicant must demonstrate direct clinical experiences with individuals in both assessment and intervention across the life span from the range of disorders and differences named in Standard IV-C.

Standard VI: Assessment

The applicant must have passed the national examination adopted by ASHA for purposes of certification in speech-language pathology.

Implementation: Results of the Praxis® Examination in Speech-Language Pathology must be submitted directly to ASHA from the Educational Testing Service (ETS). The certification standards require that a passing exam score be earned no earlier than 5 years prior to the submission of the application and no later than 2 years following receipt of the application. If the exam is not successfully passed and reported within the 2-year application period, the applicant's certification file will be closed. If the exam is passed or reported at a later date, then the applicant will be required to reapply for certification under the standards in effect at that time.

Standard VII: Speech-Language Pathology Clinical Fellowship

The applicant must successfully complete a Speech-Language Pathology Clinical Fellowship (CF).

Implementation: The CF experience may be initiated only after completion of all graduate credit hours, academic coursework, and clinical experiences required to meet the knowledge and skills delineated in Standards IV and V. The CF experience must be initiated within 24 months of the date on which the application for certification is received. Once the CF has been initiated, it must be completed within 48 months of the initiation date. For applicants completing multiple CFs, all CF experiences related to the application must be completed within 48 months of the date on which the first CF was initiated. Applications will be closed for CFs that are not completed within the 48-month time frame or that are not submitted to ASHA within 90 days after the 48-month time frame. The Clinical Fellow will be required to reapply for certification and must meet the standards in effect at the time of reapplication. CF experiences more than 5 years old at the time of application will not be accepted.

The CF must be completed under the mentorship of a clinician who held the CCC-SLP throughout the duration of the fellowship and must meet the qualifications described in Standard VII-B. It is the Clinical Fellow's responsibility to identify a CF mentor who meets ASHA's certification standards. Should the certification status of the mentoring SLP change during the CF experience, the Clinical Fellow will be awarded credit only for that portion of time during which the mentoring SLP held certification. It is incumbent upon the Clinical Fellow to verify the mentoring SLP's status periodically throughout the CF experience. Family members or individuals related in any way to the Clinical Fellow may not serve as mentoring SLPs to that Clinical Fellow.

Standard VII-A: Clinical Fellowship Experience

The CF must consist of clinical service activities that foster the continued growth and integration of knowledge, skills, and tasks of clinical practice in speech-language pathology consistent with ASHA's current _Scope of Practice in Speech-Language Pathology_. The CF must consist of no less than 36 weeks of full-time professional experience or its part-time equivalent.

Implementation: At least 80% of the Clinical Fellow's major responsibilities during the CF experience must be in direct, in-person client/patient contact (e.g., assessment, diagnosis, evaluation, screening, treatment, clinical research activities, family/client consultations, recordkeeping, report writing, and/or counseling) related to the management process for individuals who exhibit communication and/or swallowing disabilities.

Full-time professional experience is defined as 35 hours per week, culminating in a minimum of 1,260 hours. Part-time experience should be at least 5 hours per week; anything less than that will not meet the CF requirement and may not be counted toward completion of the experience. Similarly, work in excess of 35 hours per week cannot be used to shorten the CF to less than 36 weeks.

Standard VII-B: Clinical Fellowship Mentorship

The Clinical Fellow must receive ongoing mentoring and formal evaluations by the CF mentor. Mentorship must be provided by a clinician who holds the CCC-SLP, who has the equivalent of a minimum of 9 months of full-time clinical experience, and who has completed a minimum of 2 hours of professional development/continuing education in clinical instruction/supervision after being awarded the CCC-SLP.

Implementation: Effective January 1, 2020, CF mentors for ASHA certification must complete 2 hours of professional development/continuing education in clinical instruction/supervision after being awarded the CCC-SLP and prior to mentoring the Clinical Fellow.

Direct observation must be in real time. A mentor must be available to consult with the Clinical Fellow who is providing clinical services. Direct observation of clinical practicum is intended to provide guidance and feedback and to facilitate the Clinical Fellow's independent use of essential clinical skills

Mentoring must include on-site, in-person observations and other monitoring activities, which may be executed by correspondence, review of video and/or audio recordings, evaluation of written reports, telephone conferences with the Clinical Fellow, or evaluations by professional colleagues with whom the Clinical Fellow works. The CF mentor and the Clinical Fellow must participate in regularly scheduled formal evaluations of the Clinical Fellow's progress during the CF experience. The Clinical Fellow must receive ongoing mentoring and formal evaluations by the CF mentor.

The amount of direct supervision provided by the CF mentor must be commensurate with the Clinical Fellow's knowledge, skills, and experience, and must not be less than the minimum required direct contact hours. Supervision must be sufficient to ensure the welfare of the individual(s) receiving services.

The mentoring SLP must engage in no fewer than 36 supervisory activities during the CF experience and must include 18 on-site observations of direct client contact at the Clinical Fellow's work site (1 hour = 1 on-site observation; a maximum of six on-site observations may be accrued in 1 day). At least six on-site observations must be conducted during each third of the CF experience. On-site observations must consist of the Clinical Fellow engaging in screening, evaluation, assessment, and/or habilitation/rehabilitation activities. Mentoring must include on-site, in-person observations; however, the use of real-time, interactive video and audio conferencing technology may be permitted as a form of observation, for which preapproval must be obtained.

Additionally, supervision must include 18 other monitoring activities. *Other monitoring activities* are defined as the evaluation of reports written by the Clinical Fellow, conferences between the CF mentor and the Clinical Fellow, discussions with professional colleagues of the Clinical Fellow, and so forth, and may be executed by correspondence, telephone, or reviewing of video and/or audio tapes. At least six other monitoring activities must be conducted during each third of the CF experience.

If the Clinical Fellow and their CF mentor want to use supervisory mechanisms other than those outlined above, they may submit a written request to the CFCC prior to initiating the CF. Written requests may be emailed to cfcc@asha.org or mailed to: CFCC, c/o ASHA Certification, 2200 Research Blvd. #313, Rockville, MD 20850. Requests must include the reason for the alternative supervision and a detailed description of the supervision that would be provided (i.e., type, length, frequency, etc.), and the request must be cosigned by both the Clinical Fellow and the CF mentor. On a case-by-case basis, the CFCC will review the circumstances and may or may not approve the supervisory process to be conducted in other ways. Additional information may be requested by the CFCC prior to approving any request.

Standard VII-C: Clinical Fellowship Outcomes

The Clinical Fellow must demonstrate knowledge and skills consistent with the ability to practice independently.

Implementation: At the completion of the CF experience, the applicant must have acquired and demonstrated the ability to:

- Integrate and apply theoretical knowledge;
- Evaluate their strengths and identify their limitations;
- Refine clinical skills within the *Scope of Practice in Speech-Language Pathology*; and
- Apply the ASHA *Code of Ethics* to independent professional practice.

In addition, upon completion of the CF, the applicant must demonstrate the ability to perform clinical activities accurately, consistently, and independently and to seek guidance as necessary.

The CF mentor must document and verify a Clinical Fellow's clinical skills using the *Clinical Fellowship Report and Rating Form*, which includes the *Clinical Fellowship Skills Inventory* (CFSI), as soon as the Clinical Fellow successfully completes the CF experience. This report must be signed by both the Clinical Fellow and CF mentor.

Standard VIII: Maintenance of Certification

Certificate holders must demonstrate continued professional development for maintenance of the CCC-SLP.

Implementation: Clinicians who hold the CCC-SLP must accumulate and report 30 Certification Maintenance Hours (CMHs) (or 3.0 ASHA continuing education units [CEUs]) of professional development, which <u>must include a minimum of 1 CMH (or 0.1 ASHA CEU) in ethics</u> during every <u>3-year certification maintenance interval</u> beginning with the 2020–2022 maintenance interval.

Intervals are continuous and begin January 1 of the year following the initial awarding of certification or the reinstatement of certification. <u>Random audits</u> of compliance are conducted.

Accrual of professional development hours, adherence to the ASHA *Code of Ethics*, submission of certification maintenance compliance documentation, and payment of annual membership dues and/or certification fees are <u>required for maintenance of certification</u>.

If maintenance of certification is not accomplished within the 3-year interval, then <u>certification will expire</u>. Those who wish to regain certification must submit a reinstatement application and meet the standards in effect at the time the reinstatement application is submitted.

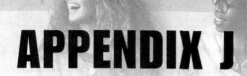

APPENDIX J

2020 Standards and Implementation Procedures for the Certificate of Clinical Competence in Audiology

Effective Date: January 1, 2020

INTRODUCTION

The Council for Clinical Certification in Audiology and Speech-Language Pathology (CFCC) is a semiautonomous credentialing body of the American Speech-Language-Hearing Association. The charges to the CFCC are: to define the standards for clinical certification; to apply those standards in granting certification to individuals; to have final authority to withdraw certification in cases where certification has been granted on the basis of inaccurate information; and to administer the certification maintenance program.

A Practice and Curriculum Analysis of the Profession of Audiology was conducted in 2016 under the auspices of the Council on Academic Accreditation in Audiology and Speech-Language Pathology (CAA) and the CFCC. The survey analysis was reviewed by the CFCC, and the following standards were developed to better fit current practice models.

The 2020 standards and implementation procedures for the Certificate of Clinical Competence in Audiology (CCC-A) go into effect on January 1, 2020. View the Audiology Standards Crosswalk [PDF] and consult Changes to Audiology Standards for more specific information on how the standards will change.

CITATION

Cite as: Council for Clinical Certification in Audiology and Speech-Language Pathology of the American Speech-Language-Hearing Association. (2018). *2020 Standards for the Certificate of Clinical Competence in Audiology.* Retrieved from www.asha.org/certification/2020-Audiology-Certification-Standards/

The Standards for the CCC-A are shown in bold. The CFCC implementation procedures follow each standard.

- Standard I—Academic Qualifications
- Standard II—Knowledge and Skills Outcomes
- Standard III—Verification of Knowledge and Skills
- Standard IV—Examination
- Standard V—Maintenance of Certification

Standard I: Academic Qualifications

Applicants for certification must hold a doctoral degree in audiology from a program accredited by the Council on Academic Accreditation in Audiology and Speech-Language Pathology (CAA) or equivalent.

Implementation: Verification of the graduate degree is accomplished by submitting (a) an official transcript showing that the degree has been awarded or (b) a letter from the university registrar verifying completion of requirements for the degree. Applicants must have graduated from a program holding CAA accreditation or candidacy status in audiology throughout the period of enrollment.

Applicants from non–CAA-accredited programs (e.g., internationally educated, PhD programs, etc.) will have their application evaluated by the Council for Clinical Certification in Audiology and Speech-Language Pathology (CFCC) to determine substantial equivalence to a clinical doctoral degree program accredited by the CAA. Individuals educated outside the United States or its territories must submit official transcripts and evaluations of their degrees and courses to verify equivalency. These evaluations must be conducted by credential evaluation services agencies recognized by the National Association of Credential Evaluation Services (NACES). Evaluations must (a) confirm that the degree earned is equivalent to a U.S. clinical doctoral degree, (b) show that the coursework is equivalent to a CAA-accredited clinical doctoral program, (c) include a translation of academic coursework into the American semester-hour system, and (d) indicate which courses were completed at the graduate level.

Standard II: Knowledge and Skills Outcomes

Applicants for certification must have acquired knowledge and developed skills in the professional areas of practice as identified in Standards II A–F, as verified in accordance with Standard III.

Implementation: The knowledge and skills identified in this standard, although separated into areas of practice, are not independent of each other. The competent practice of audiology requires that an audiologist be able to integrate across all areas of practice. Therefore, assessments used to verify knowledge and skills acquisition must require that the candidate for certification demonstrate integration of the knowledge and skills found in Standards II A–F below.

Standard II-A: Foundations of Practice

Applicant has demonstrated knowledge of:

A1. **Genetics, embryology and development of the auditory and vestibular systems, anatomy and physiology, neuroanatomy and neurophysiology, and pathophysiology of hearing and balance over the life span**

A2. **Effects of pathogens, and pharmacologic and teratogenic agents, on the auditory and vestibular systems**

A3. **Language and speech characteristics and their development for individuals with normal and impaired hearing across the life span**

A4. **Principles, methods, and applications of acoustics, psychoacoustics, and speech perception, with a focus on how each is impacted by hearing impairment throughout the life span**

A5. **Calibration and use of instrumentation according to manufacturers' specifications and accepted standards**

A6. **Standard safety precautions and cleaning/disinfection of equipment in accordance with facility-specific policies and manufacturers' instructions to control for infectious/contagious diseases**

A7. **Applications and limitations of specific audiologic assessments and interventions in the context of overall client/patient management**

A8. **Implications of cultural and linguistic differences, as well as individual preferences and needs, on clinical practice and on families, caregivers, and other interested parties**

A9. Implications of biopsychosocial factors in the experience of and adjustment to auditory disorders and other chronic health conditions

A10. Effects of hearing impairment on educational, vocational, social, and psychological function throughout the life span

A11. Manual and visual communication systems and the use of interpreters/transliterators/translators

A12. Effective interaction and communication with clients/patients, families, professionals, and other individuals through written, spoken, and nonverbal communication

A13. Principles of research and the application of evidence-based practice (i.e., scientific evidence, clinical expertise, and client/patient perspectives) for accurate and effective clinical decision making

A14. Assessment of diagnostic efficiency and treatment efficacy through the use of quantitative data (e.g., number of tests, standardized test results) and qualitative data (e.g., standardized outcome measures, client/patient-reported measures)

A15. Client-centered, behavioral, cognitive, and integrative theories and methods of counseling and their relevance in audiologic rehabilitation

A16. Principles and practices of client/patient/person/family-centered care, including the role and value of clients'/patients' narratives, clinician empathy, and shared decision making regarding treatment options and goals

A17. Importance, value, and role of interprofessional communication and practice in patient care

A18. The role, scope of practice, and responsibilities of audiologists and other related professionals

A19. Health care, private practice, and educational service delivery systems

A20. Management and business practices, including but not limited to cost analysis, budgeting, coding, billing and reimbursement, and patient management

A21. Advocacy for individual patient needs and for legislation beneficial to the profession and the individuals served

A22. Legal and ethical practices, including standards for professional conduct, patient rights, confidentiality, credentialing, and legislative and regulatory mandates

A23. Principles and practices of effective supervision/mentoring of students, other professionals, and support personnel

Standard II-B: Prevention and Screening

Applicant has demonstrated knowledge of and skills in:

B1. Educating the public and those at risk on prevention, potential causes, effects, and treatment of congenital and acquired auditory and vestibular disorders

B2. Establishing relationships with professionals and community groups to promote hearing wellness for all individuals across the life span

B3. Participating in programs designed to reduce the effects of noise exposure and agents that are toxic to the auditory and vestibular systems

B4. Utilizing instrument(s) (i.e., sound-level meter, dosimeter, etc.) to determine ambient noise levels and providing strategies for reducing noise and reverberation time in educational, occupational, and other settings

B5. Recognizing a concern on the part of medical providers, individuals, caregivers, or other professionals about hearing and/or speech-language problems and/or identifying people at risk to determine a need for hearing screening

B6. Conducting hearing screenings in accordance with established federal and state legislative and regulatory requirements

B7. Participating in occupational hearing conservation programs

B8. Performing developmentally, culturally, and linguistically appropriate hearing screening procedures across the life span

B9. Referring persons who fail the hearing screening for appropriate audiologic/medical evaluation

B10. Identifying persons at risk for speech-language and/or cognitive disorders that may interfere with communication, health, education, and/or psychosocial function

B11. Screening for comprehension and production of language, including the cognitive and social aspects of communication

B12. Screening for speech production skills (e.g., articulation, fluency, resonance, and voice characteristics)

B13. Referring persons who fail the screening for appropriate speech-language pathology consults, medical evaluation, and/or services, as appropriate

B14. Evaluating the success of screening and prevention programs through the use of performance measures (i.e., test sensitivity, specificity, and positive predictive value)

Standard II-C: Audiologic Evaluation

Applicant has demonstrated knowledge of and skills in:

C1. Gathering, reviewing, and evaluating information from referral sources to facilitate assessment, planning, and identification of potential etiologic factors

C2. Obtaining a case history and client/patient narrative

C3. Obtaining client/patient-reported and/or caregiver-reported measures to assess function

C4. Identifying, describing, and differentiating among disorders of the peripheral and central auditory systems and the vestibular system

C5. Providing assessments of tinnitus severity and its impact on patients' activities of daily living and quality of life

C6. Providing assessment of tolerance problems to determine the presence of hyperacusis

C7. Selecting, performing, and interpreting a complete immittance test battery based on patient need and other findings; tests to be considered include single probe tone tympanometry or multifrequency and multicomponent protocols, ipsilateral and contralateral acoustic reflex threshold measurements, acoustic reflex decay measurements, and Eustachian tube function

C8. Selecting, performing, and interpreting developmentally appropriate behavioral pure-tone air and bone tests, including extended frequency range when indicated

C9. Selecting, performing, and interpreting developmentally appropriate behavioral speech audiometry procedures to determine speech awareness threshold (SAT), speech recognition threshold (SRT), and word recognition scores (WRSs); obtaining a performance intensity function with standardized speech materials, when indicated

C10. Evaluating basic audiologic findings and client/patient needs to determine differential diagnosis and additional procedures to be used

C11. Selecting, performing, and interpreting physiologic and electrophysiologic test procedures, including electrocochleography, auditory brainstem response with frequency-specific air and bone conduction threshold testing, and click stimuli for neural diagnostic purposes

C12. Selecting, performing, and interpreting otoacoustic emissions testing

C13. Selecting, performing, and interpreting tests for nonorganic hearing loss

C14. Selecting, performing, and interpreting vestibular testing, including electronystagmography (ENG)/videonystagmography (VNG), ocular vestibular-evoked myogenic potential (oVEMP), and cervical vestibular-evoked myogenic potential (cVEMP)

C15. Selecting, performing, and interpreting tests to evaluate central auditory processing disorder

Applicant has demonstrated knowledge of:

C16. Electrophysiologic testing, including but not limited to auditory steady-state response, auditory middle latency response, auditory late (long latency) response, and cognitive potentials (e.g., P300 response, mismatch negativity response)

C17. Posturography

C18. Rotary chair tests

C19. Video head impulse testing (vHIT)

Standard II-D: Counseling

Applicant has demonstrated knowledge of and skills in:

D1. Identifying the counseling needs of individuals with hearing impairment based on their narratives and results of client/patient and/or caregiver responses to questionnaires and validation measures

D2. Providing individual, family, and group counseling as needed based on client/patient and clinical population needs

D3. Facilitating and enhancing clients'/patients' and their families' understanding of, acceptance of, and adjustment to auditory and vestibular disorders

D4. Enhancing clients'/patients' acceptance of and adjustment to hearing aids, hearing assistive technologies, and osseointegrated and other implantable devices

D5. Addressing the specific interpersonal, psychosocial, educational, and vocational implications of hearing impairment for the client/patient, family members, and/or caregivers to enhance their well-being and quality of life

D6. Facilitating patients' acquisition of effective communication and coping skills

D7. Promoting clients'/patients' self-efficacy beliefs and promoting self-management of communication and related adjustment problems

D8. Enhancing adherence to treatment plans and optimizing treatment outcomes

D9. Monitoring and evaluating client/patient progress and modifying counseling goals and approaches, as needed

Standard II-E: Audiologic Rehabilitation Across the Life Span

Applicant has demonstrated knowledge of and skills in:

E1. Engaging clients/patients in the identification of their specific communication and adjustment difficulties by eliciting client/patient narratives and interpreting their and/or caregiver-reported measures

E2. Identifying the need for, and providing for assessment of, concomitant cognitive/developmental concerns, sensory-perceptual and motor skills, and other health/medical conditions, as well as participating in interprofessional collaboration to provide comprehensive management and monitoring of all relevant issues

E3. Responding empathically to clients'/patients' and their families' concerns regarding communication and adjustment difficulties to establish a trusting therapeutic relationship

E4. Providing assessments of family members' perception of and reactions to communication difficulties

E5. Identifying the effects of hearing problems and subsequent communication difficulties on marital dyads, family dynamics, and other interpersonal communication functioning

E6. Engaging clients/patients (including, as appropriate, school-aged children/adolescents) and family members in shared decision making regarding treatment goals and options

E7. Developing and implementing individualized intervention plans based on clients'/patients' preferences, abilities, communication needs and problems, and related adjustment difficulties

E8. Selecting and fitting appropriate amplification devices and assistive technologies

E9. Defining appropriate electroacoustic characteristics of amplification fittings based on frequency-gain characteristics, maximum output sound-pressure level, and input–output characteristics

E10. Verifying that amplification devices meet quality control and American National Standards Institute (ANSI) standards

E11. Conducting real-ear measurements to (a) establish audibility, comfort, and tolerance of speech and sounds in the environment and (b) verify compression, directionality, and automatic noise management performance

E12. Incorporating sound field functional gain testing when fitting osseointegrated and other implantable devices

E13. Conducting individual and/or group hearing aid orientations to ensure that clients/patients can use, manage, and maintain their instruments appropriately

E14. Identifying individuals who are candidates for cochlear implantation and other implantable devices

E15. Counseling cochlear implant candidates and their families regarding the benefits and limitations of cochlear implants to (a) identify and resolve concerns and potential misconceptions and (b) facilitate decision making regarding treatment options

E16. Providing programming and fitting adjustments; providing postfitting counseling for cochlear implant clients/patients

E17. Identifying the need for—and fitting—electroacoustically appropriate hearing assistive technology systems (HATS) based on clients'/patients' communication, educational, vocational, and social needs when conventional amplification is not indicated or provides limited benefit

E18. Providing HATS for those requiring access in public and private settings or for those requiring necessary accommodation in the work setting, in accordance with federal and state regulations

E19. Ensuring compatibility of HATS when used in conjunction with hearing aids, cochlear implants, or other devices and in different use environments

E20. Providing or referring for consulting services in the installation and operation of multiuser systems in a variety of environments (e.g., theaters, churches, schools)

E21. Providing auditory, visual, and auditory–visual communication training (e.g., speechreading, auditory training, listening skills) to enhance receptive communication

E22. Counseling clients/patients regarding the audiologic significance of tinnitus and factors that cause or exacerbate tinnitus to resolve misconceptions and alleviate anxiety related to this auditory disorder

E23. Counseling clients/patients to promote the effective use of ear-level sound generators and/or the identification and use of situationally appropriate environmental sounds to minimize their perception of tinnitus in pertinent situations

E24. Counseling clients/patients to facilitate identification and adoption of effective coping strategies to reduce tinnitus-induced stress, concentration difficulties, and sleep disturbances

E25. Monitoring and assessing the use of ear-level and/or environmental sound generators and the use of adaptive coping strategies to ensure treatment benefit and successful outcome(s)

E26. Providing canalith repositioning for patients diagnosed with benign paroxysmal positional vertigo (BPPV)

E27. Providing intervention for central and peripheral vestibular deficits

E28. Ensuring treatment benefit and satisfaction by monitoring progress and assessing treatment outcome

Standard II-F: Pediatric Audiologic (Re)habilitation

Applicant has demonstrated knowledge of and skills in:

F1. Counseling parents to facilitate their acceptance of and adjustment to a child's diagnosis of hearing impairment

F2. Counseling parents to resolve their concerns and facilitate their decision making regarding early intervention, amplification, education, and related intervention options for children with hearing impairment

F3. Educating parents regarding the potential effects of hearing impairment on speech-language, cognitive, and social–emotional development and functioning

F4. Educating parents regarding optional and optimal modes of communication; educational laws and rights, including 504s, individualized education programs (IEPs), individual family service plans (IFSPs), individual health plans; and so forth

F5. Selecting age/developmentally appropriate amplification devices and HATS to minimize auditory deprivation and maximize auditory stimulation

F6. Instructing parents and/or child(ren) regarding the daily use, care, and maintenance of amplification devices and HATS

F7. Planning and implementing parent education/support programs concerning the management of hearing impairment and subsequent communication and adjustment difficulties

F8. Providing for intervention to ensure age/developmentally appropriate speech and language development

F9. Administering self-assessment, parental, and educational assessments to monitor treatment benefit and outcome

F10. Providing ongoing support for children by participating in IEP or IFSP processes

F11. Counseling the child with hearing impairment regarding peer pressure, stigma, and other issues related to psychosocial adjustment, behavioral coping strategies, and self-advocacy skills

F12. Evaluating acoustics of classroom settings and providing recommendations for modifications

F13. Providing interprofessional consultation and/or team management with speech-language pathologists, educators, and other related professionals

Standard III: Verification of Knowledge and Skills

Applicants for certification must have completed supervised clinical experiences under an ASHA-certified audiologist who has completed at least 2 hours of professional development in the area of clinical instruction/supervision. The experiences must meet CAA standards for duration and be sufficient to demonstrate the acquisition of the knowledge and skills identified in Standard II.

Implementation: The applicant's doctoral program director or designated signatory must verify that the applicant has acquired and demonstrated all of the knowledge and skills identified in Standard II.

Clinical instructors and supervisors must have:

- Current CCC-A certification,
- A minimum of 9 full-time months of experiences, and
- Completed at least 2 hours of professional development (2 certification maintenance hours [CMHs], or 0.2 ASHA continuing education units [ASHA CEUs]) in the area of clinical instruction/supervision.

Clinical instruction and supervision within a doctoral program must:

- Be conducted for a variety of clinical training experiences (i.e., different work settings and with different populations) to validate knowledge and skills across the scope of practice in audiology;
- Include oversight of clinical and administrative activities directly related to client/patient care, including direct client/patient contact, consultation, record keeping, and administrative duties relevant to audiology service delivery;
- Be appropriate to the student's level of training, education, experience, and competence;
- Include direct observation, guidance, and feedback to permit the student to (a) monitor, evaluate, and improve performance and (b) develop clinical competence; and
- Be provided on site.

Any portion of the applicant's supervised clinical experience that was not completed under an audiologist meeting the requirements above can be completed postgraduation. The applicant's postgraduation clinical instructor/supervisor must also meet the above requirements will also verify that the applicant has demonstrated and acquired the knowledge and skills for ASHA certification following completion of the required supervised clinical experience.

Applicants who apply for certification without completing a full, supervised clinical experience under a clinical instructor/supervisor who meets the requirement above within their degree program will have 24 months from their application-received date to initiate the remainder of their experience and will have 48 months from the initiation date of their postgraduation supervised clinical experience to complete the experience.

If clinical instruction and supervision are completed postgraduation, they must comply with the requirements above with the exception of on-site clinical instruction and supervision. Remote supervision or telesupervision methods may be used, provided they are permitted by the employer(s) and by local, state, and federal regulations.

The supervised clinical experience should include interprofessional education and interprofessional collaborative practice (IPE/IPP). Under the supervision of their audiologist supervisor, students'/applicants' experience should include experiences with allied health professionals who are appropriately credentialed in their area of practice to enhance the student's knowledge and skills in an interdisciplinary, team-based, comprehensive health care delivery setting.

Standard IV: Examination

The applicant must pass the national examination adopted by ASHA for purposes of certification in audiology.

Implementation: Results of the Praxis Examination in Audiology must be submitted directly to ASHA from ETS. A passing exam score must be earned no earlier than 5 years prior to the submission of the application and no later than 2 years following receipt of the application. If the applicant does not successfully pass the exam and does not report the results of the exam to ASHA within the 2-year application period, then the applicant's certification file will be closed. If the applicant passes or reports the results of the exam at a later date, then the individual will be required to reapply for certification under the standards that are in effect at that time.

Standard V: Maintenance of Certification

Individuals holding certification must demonstrate (1) continuing professional development, including 1 hour of continuing education in ethics; (2) adherence to the ASHA Code of Ethics; and (3) payment of annual dues and fees.

Implementation: Individuals who hold the CCC in Audiology (CCC-A) must accumulate and report 30 CMHs (or 3.0 ASHA CEUs) of professional development, which <u>must include 1 CMH (or 0.1 ASHA CEU) in ethics</u> during every <u>3-year certification maintenance interval</u>. Individuals will be subject to random audits of their professional development activities.

Individuals who hold the CCC-A must adhere to the ASHA *Code of Ethics* ("Code"). Any violation of the Code may result in professional discipline by the ASHA Board of Ethics and/or the CFCC.

Annual payment of certification dues and/or fees is also a requirement of certification maintenance. If <u>certification maintenance requirements</u> are not met, certification status will become <u>Not Current</u>, and then certification will expire. In order to regain certification, individuals must meet the reinstatement requirement that is in effect at the time they submit their reinstatement application.